Instrumental Clinical Phonetics

Edited by
Martin J. Ball and Chris Code

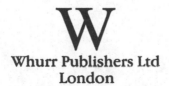

Whurr Publishers Ltd
London

© 1997 Whurr Publishers
First published 1997 by
Whurr Publishers Ltd
19B Compton Terrace, London N1 2UN, England

British Library Cataloguing in Publication Data
A catalogue record for this book is available from the
British Library.

ISBN 1 897635 18 4

Contents

Preface

It is now more than 10 years since, as editors, we brought together a group of eminent phoneticians and speech scientists to produce a volume in experimental techniques as applicable to speech pathology and therapeutics. Since that time, instrumental phonetics has, of course, developed considerably. New techniques have been adopted, approaches that in the early 1980s were in their infancy have proved themselves of worth, and procedures that were once widely used have become less important.

In this collection, therefore, we have tried to provide accounts of those instrumental techniques that are currently the most important in clinical phonetics. These techniques cover the three aspects of speech: speech production (articulatory phonetics), speech transmission (acoustic phonetics) and speech perception (auditory/perceptual phonetics), and, again, we have a group of leading authors to cover these areas. We have chapters, therefore, that deal with recording the speech signal and analysing speech acoustics through sound spectrography; others that look at aspects of speech production such as muscle inervation, airflow characteristics, laryngeal activity, and tongue palate contact patterns. We also examine the range of techniques now available for imaging the organs of speech. We also have a chapter examining two important perceptual techniques — delayed auditory feedback and dichotic listening — that have been used in speech pathology for both investigation and treatment. Finally, we look at a microcomputer-based approach to both experimentation and treatment of speech disorders.

Each chapter describes a technique in non-technical terms, outlines its role in instrumental phonetics, and details its application and impact in speech pathology and therapeutics. As such, the book should be of value to clinicians, researchers, lecturers and students in speech pathology, phonetics, linguistics and experimental psychology. It was also our intention with this collection to enlist contributors who were not simply eminent instrumental phoneticians, but who had direct experience, through research, teaching or clinical work, with the communicatively impaired.

The book presents a comprehensive coverage of major techniques. However, as with our previous collection, it was inevitable that some techniques would be left out. The criteria for inclusion were that the technique played a major role in speech pathology or was likely to develop into such a role in the near future, had a contribution to make to patient management and clinical decision making, or had contributed substantially (or was likely to) to our understanding of communication disorders.

Speech is arguably the most interesting, and certainly one of the most complex and highly skilled behaviours of which human beings are capable, and breakdown in the production or perception of speech is not only a devastating disability, but also of immense theoretical interest. It is our hope that this new collection will make both a practical and theoretical contribution to the knowledge of communication disorders, and will lead to still wider utilization of instrumental techniques by clinicians and clinical phoneticians, to the benefit of both practitioner and patient.

Finally, we would like to thank all those at Whurr Publishers who helped to bring this project to fruition. We would also like to thank our colleague Joan Rahilly who prepared the index.

Martin J. Ball
Chris Code

June 1996

Contributors

Evelyn Abberton, Department of Phonetics and Linguistics, University College London, England.

Thomas Ahrndt, Institute for Communication Engineering, Federal Armed Forces University, München, Germany.

Martin J. Ball, School of Behavioural and Communication Sciences, University of Ulster, Northern Ireland.

Chris Code, Brain Damage and Communication Research, School of Communication Disorders, Cumberland College, University of Sydney, Australia.

Alvirda Farmer, School of Education, San Jose State University, California, USA.

Adrian Fourcin, Department of Phonetics and Linguistics, University College London, England.

Michèle Gentil, INSERM, Clinique Neurologique, Centre Hospitalier Universitaire de Grenoble, France.

Fiona Gibbon, Department of Speech and Language Sciences, Queen Margaret College, Edinburgh, Scotland.

Berthold Gröne, Städt. Krankenhaus München-Bogenhausen, München, Germany.

William J. Hardcastle, Department of Speech and Language Sciences, Queen Margaret College, Edinburgh, Scotland.

Walter H. Moore (Jnr), Communicative Disorders, California State University, Long Beach, USA.

Katherine Morton, Department of Language and Linguistics, University of Essex, Colchester, England.

Mark Tatham, Department of Language and Linguistics, University of Essex, Colchester, England.

Jürgen Teiwes, Institute for Communication Engineering, Federal Armed Forces University, München, Germany.

Mathias Vogel, Entwicklungsgruppe Klinische Neuropsychologie, Städt. Krankenhaus München-Bogenhausen, München, Germany.

Campbell Yates, Professor Emeritus, Mechanical Engineering, University of Pittsburgh, Pennsylvania, USA.

David Zajac, School of Dentistry, University of North Carolina, Chapel Hill, North Carolina, USA.

Wolfram Ziegler, Entwicklungsgruppe Klinische Neuropsychologie, Städt. Krankenhaus München-Bogenhausen, München, Germany.

Chapter 1
Recording and Displaying Speech

MARK TATHAM AND KATHERINE MORTON

Introduction

The experimental investigation of speech is a very broad field. The titles of the chapters in this book show that the data we might want to examine come from a variety of sources and take a variety of forms. The soundwave itself is just the beginning, for there are several other aspects of speech that can reveal to us the nature of both normal and pathological speaking. Thus, we might want to inspect data from the neuromotor system, the aerodynamic system, the vocal tract anatomy or its configuration, as well as the final acoustic signal that results from the behaviour of these 'underlying' systems. This hierarchical approach to modelling speech production enables us to get some idea of how the final acoustic signal is derived, and, if there are errors, might help us to pinpoint their sources.

In each case, investigation of these layers in the system can involve quite different techniques and call for different approaches to the data: examining the electromyographic signals associated with muscle contraction is not the same as determining the formant structure of the acoustic signal of vowel sounds. There are, however, some principles of investigatory technique that are common to the entire field.

All the different areas of experimental work in speech involve using some instrumental technique to convert or transduce information about speech behaviour into electrical signals. Furthermore, as any scientific investigation requires careful control and interpretation of the data there can be no question that it becomes very important to have some kind of permanent record of the phenomena under investigation. This is required because it may become necessary to repeat the experiment or check the validity of any inferences that we might make.

In the laboratory study of speech we generally make two kinds of permanent record of our data:

1.   a recording of the actual or raw data, obtained as closely as possible to the original conversion of the information into electrical signals;
2.   a visual recording of the final output of any electrical or other processing of the data for inspection and measurement by the investigator.

We make a record of the raw data as close as possible in the investigatory chain to the point at which it was transduced into an electrical signal so as to minimize any distortion effects that the experimental equipment itself might introduce. This raw data recording can be rerun over and over again exactly as if the experiment itself were being run repeatedly. We need a visual record of what the researcher examines at the very end of the investigatory chain so that we can go back later and see why a particular inference was made without having to rerun the entire experiment. The raw data recording starts the chain and the visual data record ends it; in between the data has been processed and manipulated in various ways as part of the experimental procedure. The procedure itself will vary depending on the nature and source of the raw data, but the need for permanent records of the initial and final stages remains the same. Figure 1.1 illustrates the chain of events

As we shall see, the raw data record is usually a binary representation of the electrical signals transduced from the point in the speech production system under investigation. The final record is usually an image of some kind on a computer screen (soft copy) or on paper (hard copy). There are various ways in which the records at both these levels are obtained and stored, and it is important that the choices available should not be made randomly or on some basis such as cost. The wrong choice could easily result in distorted or destroyed data, or even incorrect results for the investigation.

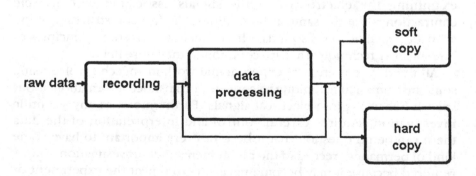

Figure 1.1. Raw data is permanently recorded before being processed and displayed — either as soft copy on a computer monitor or as hard copy on paper.

Choice among methods of recording and displaying speech signals has to be based on two major considerations:

1. the characteristics of the signal to be recorded or displayed;
2. whether or not the characteristics of the recording and displaying techniques match the signal's own characteristics without introducing distortion.

To make the necessary choices and to make the fullest use of the available equipment any researcher must have sufficient knowledge of the nature of both the data and the equipment to avoid the random or incorrect use of equipment.

Recording Speech Data Signals

Speech signals are inherently dynamic in nature and it is often the case that snapshot glimpses of speech can be very misleading. In the early days of laboratory experiments on speech, the techniques available placed severe constraints on dealing with the time-varying nature of speech. Thus, we could have a still X-ray picture of a cross-section of the vocal tract, but not a moving picture running for several seconds; or we could have a representation of a brief section of an acoustic signal from which we could measure, for example, the formant frequencies of this or that vowel sound, but not a moving image showing how in running speech formant frequencies change dynamically according to the segmental context of vowels.

As the theory of speech production has shifted in the past 20 or 30 years from a static to a dynamic focus so the focus of attention in experimental work, and therefore in the equipment used in the laboratory, has become centred on the investigation of the dynamics of speech. The two, of course, go hand-in-hand, and it would be difficult to establish whether the changes in theoretical focus have influenced the introduction of new experimental techniques or whether the availability of modern technology and the data it provides have driven the change in emphasis in the theory. What is certain, however, is that the need for permanent records at both ends of the experimental chain has become more critical and more demanding.

Analogue tape recording

The acoustic signals of speech have been recorded on tape for many years. The signal is analogue in form and the minimum of processing is needed to create a magnetic recording on tape which can be repeatedly replayed. Analogue tape recording is reliable in the sense that any distortions introduced are predictable and well understood, but it is often not appreciated that the recordings produced are not permanent. The physical and magnetic properties of the tape deteriorate with time. Magnetic deterioration is particularly troublesome in the case of the phenomenon of 'print'. This is the tendency for the magnetic image to spread into successive layers of the tape winding, producing a faint and repeated echo synchronized with the varying time occupied by each layer of tape.

For periods longer than about a year, archiving data as an analogue magnetic tape recording is not recommended. However, in the short term, analogue tape recording remains the cheapest and most easily accessible method of recording speech data. It will be several years yet before other forms of recording become as common. This is partly because of the compatibility problem: although it is easy to make a case on technical grounds for replacing analogue by digital recording there is still a vast quantity of material in analogue form that can be used for the moment only on analogue machines. Digital recording is also, for the moment, comparatively expensive.

Realistically, therefore, the first choice of a medium for recording data signals for performing experiments (rather than archiving them) must be analogue magnetic tape, and we shall devote quite a lot of space here to examining the technique and its shortcomings. Understanding the general principles of recording is important whether the medium is analogue or digital.

In analogue tape recording the medium that actually holds the data is the magnetic oxide on one side of the tape, and this tape forms part of a mechanical system at the heart of the machine. It is important for the understanding of various types of tape recorder to realize that basically the machine consists of three parts:

1.   the recording electronics;
2.   the mechanical system including the tape itself;
3.   the replay electronics.

In considering different types of analogue tape recorder we distinguish below between open-reel and cassette machines, and explain why for experimental purposes in the investigation of speech the open-reel machines are very much better. They are, however, available only as professional quality (as opposed to domestic quality) machines, and are consequently expensive. They have been almost completely displaced in the professional music recording business by digital machines which achieve higher quality and provide recordings that are much more stable in the long term. Having said that, many speech laboratories still use them, and the lower-quality cassette machines are still the norm for domestic purposes.

Direct recording

As far as we are concerned in speech research, the limiting factor in the characteristics of tape recording rests with the mechanical tape system rather than with the electronics. The characteristics of the latter are generally sufficiently sophisticated to accommodate any speech signal. The actual process of getting the signal on to the tape, and keeping it there for replaying, however, is subject to some quite severe limitations, which will have an effect on our instrumental methods.

The first parameter of tape recorders we want to consider is that of signal-to-noise ratio. This is a way of expressing the difference between the amplitudes of the highest and lowest recordable signals. As the dynamic range of speech signals of whatever kind rarely exceeds 50 dB, we might specify that our minimum requirement is for a signal-to-noise ratio of 50 dB; the decibel is a unit of intensity, related to amplitude. That is, if our highest amplitude signal is recorded just below a level that would introduce an unacceptable amount of distortion into the signal (thereby influencing any subsequent investigation of that signal), then the noise 'floor' inherent in any tape recording should be at least 50 dB below that highest level.

The second important parameter of a tape recording system is its frequency response. This refers to the machine's ability to record and replay a particular frequency range without distorting the amplitude relationships within that range. Thus, three tones of, say, 400 Hz, 1 kHz and 8 kHz of equal amplitude before recording must be reproduced after recording with their original equal amplitudes preserved. This is why frequency response specifications must be stated with reference to the recorder's ability to maintain this amplitude relationship. Generally, a typical specification might be: 45 Hz to 18 kHz plus or minus 2 dB, meaning that over the frequency range stated amplitude relationships will be held on replay within a band 2 dB greater or 2 dB less than the amplitude of a reference tone at 1 kHz. Modern tape recorders easily achieve this level of amplitude integrity provided they are well maintained.

However, it is important to note also that the ability of a tape recorder to maintain amplitude integrity depends very much on the overall amplitude of the signal being recorded. A cassette tape recorder using a good-quality tape would maintain the amplitude relationship in our example within 2 dB of the reference amplitude probably only if that reference amplitude were 20 dB lower than the maximum the machine could record at 1 kHz without more than the minimum of distortion. But raise the reference to that minimum distortion level (or 0 dB) and the same machine/tape combination might show a frequency response within 2 dB only over a range of 45 Hz to 8 or 9 kHz. This is insufficient for recording, say, the audio waveform of speech for the purpose of subsequent instrumental investigation. An open-reel tape recorder on the other hand would have no difficulty holding amplitude integrity to its maximum recording level for this given frequency range.

This illustrates a major difference between open-reel and cassette tape recorders. Their published frequency response specifications may often look identical, but usually for the cassette machine the reference level is 20 dB below the maximum level at which we will probably want to record. This means that high frequencies will play back with artificially reduced amplitude, making nonsense of any attempt to relate amplitude and frequency in a recording of the original signal. Or it means that you have to keep down the level of the recording, greatly reducing the usable signal-to-noise ratio of the recorder probably to a figure too narrow for our purposes.

With the cassette recorder, because of its miniature dimensions, the position quickly worsens as the machine ages or if it is not scrupulously maintained in a good and clean condition, so that, although it is true to say that high-frequency components of speech are generally low in amplitude anyway, an element of doubt is introduced when using a tape recorder that can achieve the required frequency response only at low amplitude settings.

Even with open-reel machines there is a general rule: better signal-to-noise ratios and better frequency response will be achieved with the widest tapes moving at the highest speeds. Consider that on a normal two-channel cassette recorder the width of each track is one-quarter (two tracks in each direction) of one-eighth of an inch (the tape width) moving at 1.875 in/s, compared with a normal two-channel open-reel machine where the tracks are one-half (two tracks in one direction only) of one-quarter of an inch (the tape width) moving at 7.5 in/s (usually), or better at 15 in/s. The area of tape passing across the recording and replay heads in a given time is critical: the more the better. Less than one thirty-second of the area of tape passes under a recording head per track on a cassette machine in a given time than on an open-reel machine running at 15 in/s. There are a few cassette recorders available that run at a speed of 3.75 in/s, which might just make acceptable recordings for instrumental analysis, but these are rare and problems of compatibility with other recorders arise.

Distortion in tape recording is another parameter that must be taken into consideration. In general, the most disturbing form of distortion occurs when the oxide on the tape becomes magnetically saturated. This happens if we attempt to record a signal of too great an amplitude (see below). Most tape recorders are satisfactory from this point of view provided no attempt is made to record a signal above the 0 dB reference point indicated on the machine's recording meters. Such a level should give a distortion level of less than 1% which should not bother us unduly in subsequent analysis of the replayed signal.

FM recording

The above description of the characteristics of analogue tape recorders refers to ordinary or direct recording machines. They are referred to as direct recording machines because the raw signal does not undergo any special transformation as part of the recording or replaying process.

The usual lowest frequency that can normally be recorded accurately is seldom below about 35 Hz. Many of the signals that we need to record for instrumental analysis, however, contain components below this frequency, and indeed may contain frequencies as low as 0 Hz; that is, the analysis may contain periods where there is no change in signal. Such steady state signals are rather like the signal you would get by connecting two wires to a battery: a constant (not changing) amplitude of about 1.5 volts. Speech signals that come into this category include the aerodynamic signals of air pressure and airflow (see Chapter 4), glottograph signals (Chapter 5), and some components of electromyography signals (Chapter 3).

Clearly, an ordinary tape recorder is going to be unsuitable for recording signals of this kind: it will simply fail to record the low frequency components of the signal or will hopelessly distort them. This is an area of data recording where digital techniques have, in speech research, already completely displaced the older analogue techniques. A few laboratories still use an analogue technique known as FM (frequency modulation) recording when the signal has a predominance of low-frequency components. The technique was described fully in the first edition of this book (Code and Ball, 1984). All we need take note of here is that there are many data signals derived from speech production, other than the acoustic ones, which cannot be successfully recorded on to analogue tape. Under these conditions a move must be made to digital techniques.

Noise reduction

Many analogue tape recorders, especially cassette machines, incorporate a noise reduction system. All of these alter amplitude relationships in the incoming signal in order to compress a signal's dynamic range to make it easier for the tape to accommodate it. They are primarily designed for music recording where the dynamic range of the signal may well exceed 90 dB (much wider than the dynamic range of speech). On replay, the compression is reversed to expand the recorded signal back to its original dynamic range. Provided that the expansion is a perfect mirror image of the compression, then in theory what comes out of the machine will be identical to what went in.

In practice, such an ideal situation is never achieved, and, depending on which noise reduction system is being used, amplitude/frequency integrity is more or less disturbed and several intrusive forms of distortion are introduced. For instrumental analysis of any speech signal (as opposed to just listening to a recording) the only advice possible is: do not use any noise reduction system. If your tape recorder cannot achieve a better signal-to-noise ratio than, say, 50 dB (and many cassette machines, especially the portable ones, cannot) without the help of noise reduction then the machine is unsuitable for any of the research techniques described in this book.

Digital recording

Digital recorders work by converting the analogue signal of the speech waveform into a binary representation. It is this binary representation that is recorded on to the recorder's magnetic tape. On playback the binary representation is read from the tape and converted back into analogue form before being amplified and sent to loudspeakers or earphones. Alternatively, the binary representation can be transferred directly to a computer.

Analogue to digital conversion

All signals connected with speech (with the exception of some components that originate from neural signals) are analogue in form. That is, amplitude variations in the signals exhibit transitions that are smooth and continuous in nature. Digital tape recorders, by contrast, expect to record signals by sampling the signal's amplitude level at particular discrete moments in time. For each time interval a number is recorded that is a rounded measurement of the average amplitude during the time interval sampled. The analogue signal's smooth (or continuous) amplitude changes in time are therefore converted into discrete (or discontinuous) amplitude measurements.

Figure 1.2 shows the relationship between an original analogue waveform (in this case a simple sine wave) and the quantized version resulting from sampling amplitude levels during discrete periods or slices of time. Notice the loss of the smoothness that is characteristic of analogue signals, and how the digital signal exhibits jagged discontinuities of amplitude. The process of changing from smooth to discontinuous representation of amplitude is called analogue to digital conversion, and we speak of digitizing or sampling the original analogue signal. There are two parameters to the analogue to digital conversion process: frequency response and dynamic range. Frequency response is determined by the sampling rate and dynamic range (the range of amplitudes that can be faithfully represented) is determined by the number of different discrete levels of amplitude to which the converter is sensitive.

Analogue to digital converters enable us to sample signals at different

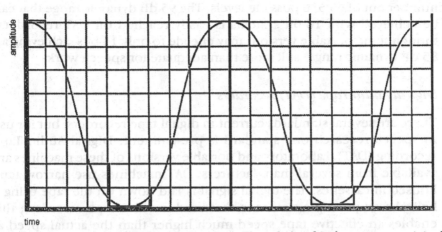

Figure 1.2. Analogue to digital conversion. The relationship between an original analogue waveform (a simple sine wave) and its quantized version.

rates, but clearly the more often the incoming signal is sampled the less obtrusive will be any discontinuities. In fact, it is possible to imagine sampling, which occurs so frequently that the original smoothness of the analogue representation is almost completely preserved; indeed, it would be preserved completely in theory at an infinitely high sampling rate. It helps to understand sampling theory if we imagine analogue representation to be simply a special case of a digitized representation: one where the sampling rate has been infinite.

In general, to capture a given frequency range a digital device needs to sample the input signal at a rate somewhat more than twice as often as the highest frequency in the incoming analogue signal; this is known as the Nyqvist rate. So, if we expect speech to have its highest frequency component around 12 kHz, then it must be sampled at least 25 000 times per second. Fortunately, no digital tape recorder's analogue to digital converter samples this slowly. They all accommodate input frequencies up to 20 kHz because all are basically designed to cover the entire range of human hearing (20 Hz to 20 kHz) and music signals. So, at least with digital tape recorders, we need not worry about frequency response. There are some established standards of sampling rate for digital audio. Thus, for example, for a CD (compact disc) the sampling rate is 44.100 times per second — or 44.1 kHz — enabling an audio signal up to about 22 kHz to be represented. Digital Audio Tape (DAT) recorders (see below) sample at rates of 48, 44.1 and 32 kHz, enabling signals up to about 24, 22 and 16 kHz respectively to be represented.

The dynamic range available in the analogue to digital conversion process is expressed in terms of bits (binary digits). CD audio has a 16-bit dynamic range covering 65 536 possible discrete levels, meaning that for the CD standard the audio signal is sampled 44 100 times each second and its amplitude in any one sample is expressed as a rounded number out of 65 536 possible levels. The 95 dB dynamic range that can be achieved with 16-bit systems is easily reached on DAT recorders, though some portable versions may encode to only 14 bits, achieving an 85 dB dynamic range: still more than adequate for speech work.

Digital Audio Tape (DAT) recorders

There are several standards current in digital tape recorders, but for use in speech research one standard is pre-eminent: Digital Audio Tape recording (DAT). Laboratory and portable versions of these machines are available from several manufacturers. DAT machines use narrow tape housed in cassettes. The digital signal is laid down on the tape using a helical scan principle similar to that used in video tape recorders; this enables an effective tape speed much higher than the actual speed at which the tape is pulled through the mechanism. Many DAT machines have a so-called long-play mode which reduces the tape speed to achieve longer recording times. In this mode the sampling rate is reduced from a standard 44.1 kHz to 32 kHz with a consequent drop in upper frequency response to about 15 kHz. Long-play mode should generally be avoided, not because of the restricted frequency response, but because it cannot be regarded as a true standard and interchangeability of cassettes between machines is made more difficult.

A DAT recorder can be regarded as a multi-stage system. The various stages, following the progress of a signal through the system, are:

1. analogue to digital conversion;
2. signal conditioning, the digital signal suitable for recording on the tape;
3. the actual recording;
4. replaying the recording;
5. digital to analogue conversion.

It is at stage 5 that the digital signals being replayed from the tape are converted back into analogue signals. Thus, a DAT recorder accepts analogue signals as input and outputs analogue signals. This is entirely suitable for music purposes, particularly in a domestic environment, but there are problems in using DAT in a speech laboratory.

Sometimes we may want simply to copy a recording. In this case we would not wish to take an original digital recording, convert it to analogue, and then reconvert it to digital form before making the copy. Check to make sure that you can directly input and output a digital signal; if you can then use this direct digital connection. This facility is useful for more than copying between recorders. We can record a signal that is already in digital format (say, straight from a computer) or take a digital signal directly from a DAT recording into a computer. Playing the

DAT recording directly into a computer is the normal situation in a speech laboratory; it is the commonest route to processing and subsequently displaying recorded speech data. Remember: when setting up such a system it is crucial to ensure that the sampling rates and bit levels are matched for the sending and receiving equipment; failure to do so will result in pitch and amplitude anomalies.

From the point of view of actual operation the digital machine is the same as an analogue machine, with one exception: when recording it is extremely important not to try to record a signal of too high an amplitude — overload distortion on a digital tape recorder is far, far worse than on an analogue machine. However, as the dynamic range of digital machines is greater than that for analogue machines, the recording levels can be kept down to make sure that this does not happen.

One thing it is necessary to be aware of with DAT recorders is that editing (see below) on digital machines is quite different from editing on analogue machines. Physical editing in the form of tape splicing is not possible at all because of the helical scanning system adopted for digital recording. Electronic editing during copying from one DAT recorder to another, while possible and extremely accurate, is difficult and requires expensive special equipment. Therefore, editing is best done once the signal has been passed to a computer for processing and subsequent display.

Direct to disk recording

As virtually all processing and experimental work with speech signals, whether audio or of some other type, is now carried out by computers, it may sometimes be useful to set up a system where signals from transducers such as microphones, electro-glottographs, etc., are taken directly to the computer without recording on to tape. Although it is good practice to record the data, it is now possible to bypass tape and make recordings directly to the computer's hard disk. For lengthy quantities of data, though, a tape recorder is needed because, although hard disk drives of capacities of one or more gigabytes are commonplace, it is very easy to fill up the available space. Data exchange with other laboratories is still easier using a format such as DAT, although for this purpose CD-ROM (compact disk — read only memory) should also be considered (see below).

Direct to disk recording requires a sound card to be installed in the host computer. For our purposes the term 'sound card' here is somewhat of a misnomer because we can use the card to enable us to input and output speech signals other than the audio. All of the signals used for the experimental work described in this book can be accepted by these cards.

There are many sound cards available and there is a variety of different standards in use, but we recommend cards with variable sample rates for the analogue-to-digital and digital-to-analogue converters, and an amplitude resolution of 16 bits. Many such cards also provide an interface for a CD-ROM drive, at least one of which should be available in speech laboratories as many databases are being made available to the speech research community in this format. Sound cards have on-board means of accepting analogue signals direct from audio sources and other forms of data sources in speech investigation. Their function is to condition the signal to make it suitable for storage as data files on the machine's hard disk. They perform the additional function of enabling hard disk files to be read and converted back to analogue form for listening or other purposes. Cards are available with both analogue and digital input and output channels.

Sound cards often have on board a digital signal processing (dsp) chip. This is a processor that has been optimized for the kind of processing needed for manipulating audio (and similar) signals at high speed. Much of the commercially available software for laboratory computers uses dsp facilities for transforming signals for display, for example, as spectrograms, which require high-speed and powerful processing if they are to be made available in real time; that is, while the utterance is actually being made.

CD-ROM recordings

CD-ROMs store audio and textual data on compact disks. If the speech data is accompanied by a video signal this can also be stored on CD-ROM, although in this case a video card with sound will be needed for processing. Making your own CD-ROMs from data on your hard disk is a possibility, although the drives necessary for this are still comparatively expensive. Most speech laboratories currently have read-only CD-ROM drives, and rely on obtaining from elsewhere the material already recorded on CDs. Make sure your CD-ROM drives have software enabling the material to be transferred to hard disks and at the same time converted if necessary from one standard to another. For example, it might be necessary to change the sampling rate so that the material can be further processed by additional software. The standard capacity of a CD-ROM is around 640 Mbytes, although increased capacities are available.

A word of caution if you feel you would like to use the soundtrack of a video available on CD as data in an experiment. The audio that accompanies these videos is compressed so that it takes up less space on the CD. There are standards for video compression, which include a specification of how the audio also is to be compressed by as much as 11:1; that is, such that it occupies less than 10% of the CD's capacity than it would occupy if uncompressed. The protocols for compression and subsequent expansion are called MPEG-1 and MPEG-2 (after the Motion Picture Experts Group, which worked them out) and these protocols are incorporated in the processing carried out by the video card installed in the computer or video player.

The problem from the point of view of the researcher is that the three levels of audio compression specified by the protocols all rely on a coding scheme which is described as 'perceptual', and this term is not well defined. The audio signal is transformed from the time domain (where it looks like waveforms on a screen) to the frequency domain (where if displayed it looks like spectrograms). It is then manipulated to remove what MPEG consider to be perceptually redundant components of the signal. At this point, it is converted back to a time domain representation, recoded and recorded. On playback the final analogue signal fed to the loudspeakers is said to be perceptually satisfactory. However, no one really knows exactly which elements of a speech signal are or are not perceptually redundant. In any case, compression of such a severe nature where a considerable portion of the signal is irrecoverably removed (whether perceptually relevant or not) renders such signals completely useless for serious speech research. It is worth noting that some analogue broadcast TV and radio signals, especially those from satellites, and all digital broadcast TV and radio signals are similarly compressed and thus present similar problems.

Many speech laboratories can now access the Internet system for linking computers worldwide and exchanging data. Most of the data available on the Internet is text and for that reason the capacity of the system for transmitting data is strictly limited. But as users increasingly want to transmit data that is not text — including binary coded audio data — standards are being set up to enable the compression of these wider bit rate data types so that they can be sent around the Internet as easily as text. The same warning holds here as in the case of video CDs. The compression systems for audio on the Internet will often follow the MPEG standards, with similar distortion of the signal. If you intend to exchange audio data with other researchers on the Internet you should make sure that you understand how the various compression systems alter your data.

The audio recording session

In this section, we discuss some of the essential techniques and equipment for making audio recordings. In most cases, simple precautions will make the difference between a recording that is unusable for instrumental analysis purposes and one which is entirely suitable for detailed analysis. You should treat data as a valuable re-usable resource: it makes sense to have your recordings of the highest possible quality and made with care.

Making the recording

The majority of recordings that the speech pathologist will make during the course of his or her duties or research will be of the audio waveform of patients and of normal speech for comparison purposes. There are good ways and bad ways of making a recording, especially when the material is to be analysed instrumentally. Listening to a recording will not normally provide a good judgement as to its quality; this is part of the problem we noted earlier with digital perceptual coding compression techniques. The reason for this is quite simple: a subjective impression will tend to overlook the imperfections in any recording, unless they are very gross, but these imperfections will show up in any instrumental analysis that might follow. This may lead to difficulties and inaccuracies in measurements. The only way to ensure a good recording is to know what factors influence the quality of recordings, and try to make sure you have obtained the best conditions possible.

Location

Echo is one of the biggest problems likely to be encountered. Ideally, recording should be made in a studio especially designed for audio. Unfortunately this is going to be available to very few clinicians. The next best thing is to select the quietest, most heavily furnished room possible, and preferably one certainly no larger than the average-sized living room. The idea is that heavy furnishings (particularly soft chairs, carpets and curtains) absorb unwanted reflections that bare walls, floor, windows and ceiling would normally produce, and in addition provide some kind of insulation against noises coming into the room from outside. Listen carefully for such unwanted noises. Normally we tend not to notice them ourselves, but the microphone will mercilessly pick them up. Listen out especially for the noise of people walking along corridors, aircraft and traffic noise, and particularly for the drone of air - conditioning systems. These have become so much a part of our lives that, on hearing a recording of 'silence' made in a normal room, the amount of background noise is striking.

Microphones

Having chosen the quietest, least reverberant (or deadest) room you can find, further echoes and outside noises can be minimized by carefully selecting microphones and using them properly. Omni-directional microphones (which pick up sound from all around them) are usually not suitable. After all, the signal is usually coming from just one direction: from the lips of the subject. Choose a directional microphone and make sure it is pointing roughly at the subject, although not in such a way that it gets blown on to directly; the subject should be talking across the microphone. There is no need to go into the vast array of types of microphone available; most these days, except the very cheapest, are good enough.

Select a microphone that has a reasonably flat frequency response over the speech range (say, 75 Hz to 12 kHz, ±3 dB). There is one kind of reliable and excellent microphone that satisfies almost all the conditions for our recordings; this is the battery-powered electret microphone mounted with a lapel clip or slung on a cord around the neck. Choose the directional type. Such a microphone has the additional advantage that almost automatically you are likely to mount it in precisely the right place, about 40 cm from the subject's mouth, not immediately in front of him or her (to avoid breath noises), and not on some reverberant surface like a table. In fact the only disadvantage with this kind of microphone is the possible pickup of the rustle of clothes, so check on this.

One further point on microphones: it is often necessary to record a conversation between two or more people, say between the clinician and patient. In this case, you must use two microphones connected preferably to the two separate channels of a stereo recorder. In this way you will find that on playback it is very easy to keep the two signals almost separate with just enough 'breakthrough' for you to hear what is going on by listening to just one channel. If more than two people are to be recorded, then the best practice is to have a microphone for each, with the signals mixed electronically using a microphone mixer before recording on one or two channels. We do not recommend placing a single omni-directional microphone on a table in the middle of a group of subjects. The mix of signals is difficult to decode because directionality is missing and this will become apparent when you come to analyse the recording. Good microphone technique cannot be overemphasized. Try making several recordings with different microphone positions; analyse them, say by making spectrograms, and see how different the signals are.

Stereo recorders are readily available these days to provide two-track recording as described above in either the analogue cassette format or in the higher-quality DAT format. If you are going to do a great deal of recording and your experiments are particularly important it is well worth investing in a DAT recorder.

One word of warning: compatibility between recorders is not guaranteed, and you should be careful to ensure you can play back recordings either on the machine used for making them or on another machine you have previously tested for compatibility. Do not rely on specification sheets to indicate the compatibility of two apparently identical tape recorders, particularly the cassette type. There can be a slightly different alignment of the record and playback heads, which will make tapes recorded on the one machine reproduce badly on the other. A good diagnostic with an analogue machine, which you should listen out for, is loss of high frequencies on playback on the second machine when the tape played back perfectly satisfactorily on the original machine.

Using the gain control

Avoid using automatic gain controls for recording. These come labelled in several different ways, so if in doubt consult a competent engineer to ask whether automatic gain control (often cued AGC) is used on the machine, and if so then how to switch it off. The trouble with automatic gain control is that, although such a system takes much of the work out of making a recording, it will considerably distort the amplitude relationships of the recordings you make and will faithfully record the background noise you have gone to such pains to remove. The reason for this is that when there is no intended speech signal the AGC increases sensitivity in an attempt to find one — the system is not intelligent enough to distinguish between wanted and unwanted sounds. AGC systems are commonest on portable recorders, even DAT machines.

Having decided never to use AGC, you are now faced with using the manual gain control for recording. Imagine that a tape recorder looks at the amplitude of sound through a window. That window has a top and a bottom. The top and bottom are represented on the meter used in conjunction with the gain control. The window top is marked 0 dB and corresponds to the point where the meter scale usually changes to red (this applies both to meters like dials with pointers and to luminous displays). The bottom of the window is the far left of the meter (or bottom if it is mounted vertically). If you have the gain control too low the signal will be at the bottom of the window and insufficiently 'seen' by the recorder. On the other hand, if you have the gain control too high then the signal will overshoot the window resulting in considerable unwanted distortion, and giving an unusable recording. The control must be manipulated to get the signal within the window.

How do you do this? Consider what speech sound is again for a moment. It has a certain amplitude range, and we already know that most tape recorders can cope with that range. Some sounds have more amplitude than others, so tape recorders need to be set so that the loudest sounds just kick the display to the 0 dB mark and leave the rest to get on with it. So how do we know what the loudest sound is going to be before it has happened? Research shows that the speech sound usually with the highest intrinsic amplitude is the [a] sound in a word like cart. If possible, get the subject to say this sound, or a word containing this sound, several times into the microphone before you begin the recording session proper. Adjust the gain control carefully so that the meter just registers 0 dB, and no more. Make sure the subject is talking in what you expect to be a normal voice. Let the subject practise using a microphone beforehand to make the voice as normal as possible.

Once you have set the gain control before the actual session begins do not touch it again, unless you can see during the session that you had obviously set it wrongly. The point here is that the gain control improves or worsens the recorder's sensitivity to signals. If you change the setting during the recording, you will not be able to compare the amplitudes of anything recorded before the change with those of anything recorded after the change and you may want to do this. If it is absolutely necessary to make a change and the session cannot be restarted then do so deliberately and quickly, making a note of what you did and when you did it. But preferably start the session over again.

Listening to a recording

No tape recorder with built-in loudspeakers is good enough for listening purposes, except for the crudest monitoring. To listen seriously to any recording you need the highest fidelity playback system available or affordable. Only the best systems will accurately preserve the amplitude and frequency relationships that make up the speech to which you are trying to listen. Failing a good loudspeaker system, use headphones. The fidelity of headphones can often be deceptive; they sound better than they really are objectively. But many people prefer them for auditory analysis purposes because, by putting you closer to the signal being replayed, some find that concentration on listening is much better and that it is easier to be more objective in making judgements of what is being listened to. It is really up to you which you prefer, but try to ensure the best fidelity possible. Once again, it is a question of looking for the flattest adequate frequency response curves.

Tape editing

The need for editing arises when portions of a recording need to be removed, or sections from several different recordings need to be put together on to a single tape. There are two ways of doing this: one is by physically cutting the tape and splicing it together again in the required sequence, and the other is to accomplish the same thing by electronic means. Cutting and splicing tape is a very time-consuming business and can really only be done successfully if the original recording is made in the open-reel format at as high a tape speed as possible (to give the most room for locating the edit point on the tape). If you do go in for physically editing the tape in this way, make sure you get plenty of practice beforehand and never edit your original recording (you may make a mistake and destroy it). Always work on a copy of the tape. That way if you mess things up, you just make another copy and begin again.

Remember, though, that copying tape results in degradation of the signal, so you must have an exceptionally clean recording to begin with.

Furthermore, if your final spliced tape contains many joins or is to be kept for more than a few weeks, you cannot guarantee that your splices will hold and a copy of the edited tape must be made. You will then work from this final copy. This final tape is a copy of a copy, with attendant multiplied degradation. Having made these warnings, though, it is not likely that you will be using an open-reel recorder. It is more likely that you will have to deal with a cassette machine or a DAT recorder.

Electronic editing is better than physically splicing tape and is all that you can do with cassette and DAT. Electronic editing is done by connecting two tape recorders together, taking the signal out from the machine holding the original tape and putting it into the second machine. The sections of the original recording to be edited must be found by careful listening, and then copied on to the new tape on the second recorder with its controls set to record. It is worth noting that, unlike the situation with analogue recording, copying digital recordings should not result in any degradation in quality. Provided the binary representation can be read satisfactorily, a perfect copy can be made with no introduction of noise or distortion.

Displaying speech data signals

The output of instruments used for analysis in the laboratory is often presented in some visual form. This requires connecting the instruments or tape recorders to a computer via the sockets on the installed sound card, using analogue inputs for analogue material and digital inputs for digital material. It is important to make sure in advance that the signals being presented to the card are the type that it is expecting. In particular, it is important to distinguish between analogue and digital signals, and in the case of analogue signals to make certain that the voltage levels are correct.

The computer will need to be running a software package controlling the sound card drivers and checking that the signal is brought into the computer without introducing distortion. Often at this point there will be the option of making a copy of the original recording directly on to the hard disk for displaying and analysing later, or displaying now and saving to the hard disk later. Choosing which will depend on the purpose of the experiment. You may want to keep long unedited portions of the material on the hard disk; in which case you may want to make the disk copy now. Check to see there is enough file space. But you may want to inspect and edit the data before committing it to disk; in this case you will want to display now, inspect and then decide whether to commit to disk.

Temporary display

Software packages for inputting data, editing it and analysing it all have a means of displaying the data on the computer screen. The software provides for displaying both raw and processed data in separate windows. Often, data in various stages of processing or analysis can be displayed alongside one another; there are many possibilities. For complex and detailed data it pays to have large, high-quality display monitors. This is the only part of the computer you actually look at, and it is worth spending a large proportion of the budget on it. It is not uncommon, especially with PCs, to spend more money on the display than on the computer itself in the laboratory environment. There is a great deal of difference between the requirements of office usage of PCs and their use in speech laboratories.

Software for displaying and analysing speech varies considerably, not just in terms of its functionality, but in terms of its ergonomics, or ease of use. You will sometimes get the impression that the software designer was unfamiliar with its actual usage in a speech laboratory. But having said that, there are many excellent general-purpose packages available. These are too numerous to discuss here, but they range from simple programs that simply control the sound card for inputting and outputting soundwaves, through waveform display and editing, to complex signal processing and displays. You will have to see what is available at the time of your experiment and choose accordingly.

In general, it is probably better to adopt programs that use standard computer configurations and also standard sound cards to ensure compatibility with other laboratories. Make sure that the software saves files in standard formats also; once again, this is to ensure compatibility with files produced by other researchers. You might want, for example, to exchange recordings in binary representation on floppy disks rather than as tape recordings.

For specialist work that goes beyond the simple editing of audio signals and perhaps spectrographic displays, you should look to software prepared by researchers in the field, and often marketed by themselves or made available free. There are many speech software packages available on the World Wide Web for free downloading and a systematic and regular search of the Internet is well worthwhile. You will soon get the hang of where to look and which WWW servers to visit regularly for the latest in software. But check on compatibility and how the data has been pre-processed, for example compression as mentioned above.

Permanent display

The computer screen is useful as a temporary display for viewing your sound files and is essential for editing sessions, but you will want to save many of the displays you generate as permanent records on paper. Although there are still a few around, the days of strip chart recorders have gone. These machines were very useful indeed; the paper format was ideal, matching the fact that speech unfolds in time, and the only limit to the length of time displayed was the length of paper on the roll. Today, however, page printers are almost universal.

A page printer is one that, as its name suggests, prints single pages, usually in A4 format with either portrait or landscape orientation. The commonest of these are the laser printer and the ink-jet printer. Laser printers compose an entire page prior to printing, whereas ink-jet printers generally print the page while data is being received (meaning you can actually see the page being continuously printed). Strictly speaking, the term 'page printer' should not be applied to an ink-jet printer for this reason. The print quality obtainable from a laser printer is superior to that from an ink-jet printer in both black-and-white and colour.

Most signal processing software will enable you to dump what is on the screen to a printer with automatic adjustments to format and aspect ratio to make sure that what is on the screen looks right when printed on paper. In the case of colour laser or ink-jet printers it is often possible to produce a printed image with different colours from those appearing on the screen. It may well be the case, for example, that colours appropriate for a screen are not suitable for a display on paper. The software will make adjustments automatically for printing the data at the appropriate printer resolution (the number of dots per inch). In general, the quality of print obtained by printing the file directly from disk is better than simply dumping a screen print to paper.

One additional piece of software that is very useful is a screen capture program. These enable you to 'grab' part of all or the screen display and send it to a printer or save it to a file in a standard graphical format. There are two reasons why you may want to do this:

1. To enable a quick printout of what is displayed in the screen or in a window on the screen — sometimes more useful than having the analysis software print the file from disk.
2. To produce an illustration in, say, a text article being produced in a word processor or desktop publishing program. The text processor simply loads and sometimes resizes and rescales the picture for placing at the desired location in the text.

Similarly, material on paper may be transformed into a graphics file for illustration purposes by using a scanner. These devices are able to accept paper illustrations in either colour or black-and-white for creating a standard format graphics file on your hard disk. Scanners operate at resolutions varying from 150 to 1200 dots per inch, but, of course, cannot improve on the resolution of the original picture.

Do not expect that a screen image will be more detailed on paper than it is on the screen. Screens have an aspect ratio of 4:3 and resolutions of 640×480, 800×600, 1024×786, 1280×1024, or 1600×1200 pixels, whereas printers have resolutions of 300, 400 or 600 dots per inch: the screen has comparatively low resolution, therefore, compared with what is possible on paper. In addition, the window in which your data is displayed on the screen will have fewer pixels available than the entire screen. This means that some of the details in the signal will not show on the screen.

Conclusion

These are the main points we have been making in this chapter covering the means of recording and displaying speech signals:

1. Be sure you are fully aware of the characteristics of the speech signals you wish to record and display.
2. Choose the right machine for the recording job in hand, making sure in particular that you understand the limitations of cassette recorders.
3. If possible now, and certainly in the future, use a digital recorder. You will never have any worries about quality if you do, although editing may be difficult. Failing a digital recorder, open-reel analogue is better than standard cassette analogue (although the former is now comparatively rare).
4. Check the frequency range of your data signal. If there are components lower than about 35 Hz you will need a frequency modulation tape recorder or digital machine designed for the purpose. Such signals can often be recorded in a direct-to-disk session using the sound card of a computer.
5. Make sure you have the highest-quality display you can afford on your computer. You cannot expect to make accurate observations of the data if the display is unable to show the signals without distortion.
6. For the highest-quality permanent records choose a laser printer rather than an ink-jet recorder.

Reference

Code C, Ball MJ. (Eds), Experimental Clinical Phonetics. London: Croom Helm, 1984.

Chapter 2
Spectrography

ALVIRDA FARMER

Introduction

The purpose of this chapter is to provide a brief description of spectrography with a review of some of the research that has used this technique to study the speech of individuals with various speech and/or language disorders. We aim for a discussion that will provide advanced undergraduate or graduate students with information from which they could launch their own research. Students at these levels should be familiar with linear source-filter theory, digital signal processing, and the acoustic structure of the speech signal. Four of many sources for this information are Kent (1993), Kent and Read (1992), Ohde and Sharf (1992) and Lass (1996). The reader who has not had the opportunity to use a spectrograph may also find the laboratory exercises in Orlikoff and Baken (1993) a valuable introduction to acoustic analyses.

Since its development in the late 1940s, the sound spectrograph or sonograph analyser has been the single most useful device for the quantitative analysis of speech. While early applications of the spectrograph focused on the parameters of normal speaking patterns (Lehiste, 1967; Potter *et al*, 1966), this instrument has more recently been used to study just about every speech and language disorder. Until the mid-1980s most of this research used the electro-mechanical sound spectrograph (Baken, 1987; Farmer, 1984; Kent and Read, 1992). Research using this instrumentation was time-consuming and somewhat tedious as measures were produced relatively slowly and analysed by hand. Further, the sound spectrograph was limited in the number of analysis techniques as compared with those provided by newer instrumentation.

The development of digital signal processing or the ability to convert analogue to digital (A/D) signals for analysis has produced a radical change in spectrography. Microcomputers coupled with A/D converters permit the automatic analysis of digitized sound signals. Various programs are available that not only can display acoustic signals as wide-

or narrow-band spectrograms but also allow creation and analyses of several frequency, spectral and amplitude windows, which are summarized in Table 2.1.

There are several programs for IBM compatible and Macintosh computers that were compared and evaluated by Read, Buder and Kent (1990, 1992). Their observations are informative for prospective consumers, and they suggested improvements that programmers will probably incorporate in newer versions of these software packages. A screen from one of these systems (the Kay CSL") is shown in Figure 2.1.

Acoustic Measurements

Various segment durations, formant frequencies and vocal quality parameters have been analysed in speech and/or language disorders. Increased use of transitional patterns as well as vocal quality parameters (e.g, jitter, shimmer) has emerged in more recent literature. The type of acoustic measure will indicate which analytic technique should be used.

Table 2.1. Summary of analysis techniques for acoustic measures.

Technique	Description
Waveform	Graphic display of amplitude versus time function for a continuous signal
Envelope	Display of total distribution of frequencies contained in a sound signal
Wide-band spectrogram	Display of acoustic signal through a wide-band pass filter (around 200–300 Hz) which provides good time but poor frequency resolution
Narrow-band spectrogram	Display of acoustic signal through a narrow filter (around 29 Hz) which provides good frequency but poor time resolution
FFT spectrum	Fast Fourier Transform is a power spectrum from a specified location of the waveform displaying frequency on the abscissa and intensity on the ordinate
LPC spectrum	Linear Predictive Coding displays a spectral envelope based on a weighted linear sampled sum to predict following values
Cepstrum	Displays an inverse spectrum of an FFT in which the horizontal axis is called 'quefrequency'
Waterfall	Shows a plot of spectra over time (actually has the appearance of a number of 2-dimensional mountain ranges rather than a waterfall)

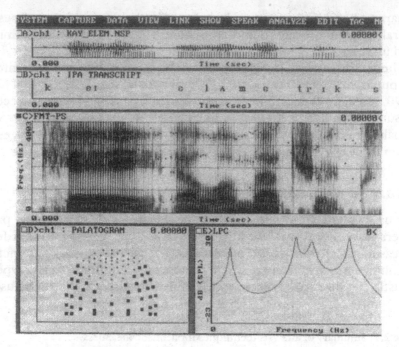

Figure 2.1. A sample screen from the Computerized Speech Lab (Kay's CSL™).

Voice onset time and other segment durational analyses

The most frequently used segmental analysis has been voice onset time (VOT). After Lisker and Abramson's (1964) classic study using VOT to delineate voicing contrasts across languages, VOT has been used to study a variety of speech and language disorders. VOT is defined by Lisker and Abramson as the difference in time between the release of complete articulatory constriction and the onset of quasi-periodic vocal fold vibration. Generally, VOT is used to measure to stop consonants, and Figure 2.2 shows a spectrogram of the words 'tot — dot', where the VOT differences are clear. However, the voicing contrast of fricatives has also been compared (Code and Ball, 1982). VOT has been used frequently because it has implications for both linguistic (categorical contrast) and motor (timing difference) components. Once measured with a ruler and conversion table, VOT can now be marked by cursors to obtain an automatic digital notation in milliseconds. VOT usually measured from a wide-band spectrogram can be analysed from waveform, envelope or waterfall displays (Kent, 1993).

A number of studies have used segment duration to analyse speech disorders. Segments have ranged from individual sounds to extended sentences and can be measured by placing cursors at the beginnng and end of the segment being studied. Segment durations generally follow known patterns in a language. For example, a frequently studied

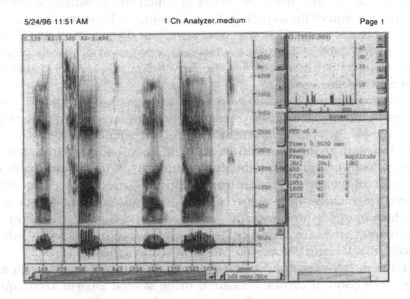

Figure 2.2. A sample screen from Soundscope 1.27 depicting an analysis of 'a tot a dot'. VOT for /t/ in 'tot' is shown in the upper left hand corner. The FFT is displayed in the upper right hand window.

segment, vowel duration (VD), is affected by several intrinsic and extrinsic factors. These factors include degree of vocalic laxness/tenseness with tense vowels being greater in duration; degree of openness with constricted vowels being longer in duration; degree of diphthongization; and influences exerted by releasing and arresting consonants due to their segmental features of voicing, place of production, manner of production, and position of words in sentences (Delattre, 1962; House and Fairbanks, 1953; Lehiste, 1976; Umeda, 1975; Zimmerman and Sapon, 1958). Segment durations can be analysed using wide-band spectrograms, waveforms, envelopes and waterfall techniques (Kent, 1993).

Formant frequency

The speaking voice is heard as the Fo and its harmonics which are multiples of the Fo. Some of the harmonics are emphasized because of the resonant characteristics of the vocal tract. These high-energy harmonics are called formants. While most voices have several formants, clinical research has generally been concerned with F1 and F2. F1 is related more to tongue height, and F2 is related more to anterioposterior position of the tongue. The frequencies of formants are influenced by three factors: the degree of constriction created by the height of the tongue; the distance from the larynx at which this constriction occurs; and the amount of lip-rounding, lip-protrusion or lip-spreading present (Stevens and House, 1955). The relationship or distance between F1 and F2 has been used to describe the normal production of vowels (Eguchi and Hirsh, 1969; Peterson and Barney, 1952). Figure 2.3 shows the formants of some vowels.

Anti-resonance may result from extra leakage of the vocal tract, such as nasalization, which causes a major reduction in the magnitude of the envelope of the speech spectrum (Shoup and Pfeifer, 1976). Schwartz (1971) lists four of the main features of vowel spectra in nasalized speech. They include: (1) reduction in intensity of the first formant; (2) presence of one or more antiresonances in the spectrum; (3) presence of extra resonances or presence of reinforced harmonics at frequencies at which energy is not normally expected; (4) a change of shift in the centre frequencies of formants. These can be seen in Figure 2.4, where nasalized and normal versions of the vowel ɑː are shown.

Formant frequency as well as formant amplitude, bandwidth and frequency contour can be measured using several analytic techniques. FFT is preferred for formant frequency, amplitude and bandwidth; waveform, narrow-band spectrograms, cepstrum and waterfall techniques can be used to plot Fo contour; narrow-band spectrograms, FFT and waterfall techniques all measure harmonic spectra (Kent, 1993). These measures are automatically performed by the computer and are menu driven.

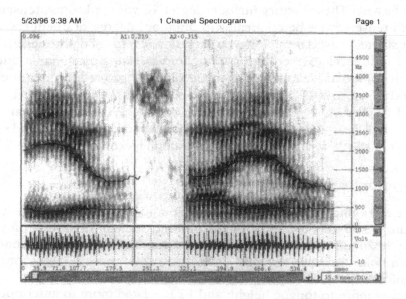

Figure 2.3. A 1 channel spectrogram screen from Soundscope 1.27 showing first and second formants of the speech sample /ios aio/.

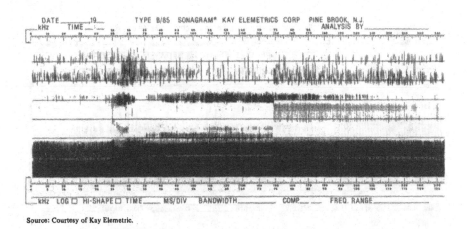

Source: Courtesy of Kay Elemetric.

Figure 2.4. Spectrogram of the vowel \ɑ:\ spoken with normal (at the right) and nasal (at the left) voice quality.

Vocal quality

Vocal abnormalities are visually apparent on the spectrogram and may include lack of vocalization, extraneous vocalization, intermittent vocalization, sudden pitch breaks, loss of harmonic components and added noise components. Figure 2.5 shows a spectrographic analysis of hoarse voice. Newer techniques provide methods for measuring specific components in voicing. Waveform, wide- and narrow-band spectrograms, FFT, LPC, cepstrum and waterfall techniques measure voicing energy and noise in the voiced signal; amplitude rise time can be analysed using waveform, envelope and waterfall techniques; jitter and shimmer can be calculated with the waveform technique. Waveform, FFT and LPC techniques are preferred measures for signal/noise ratio (Kent, 1993). These measures are also performed automatically. In addition, Computer Speech Lab (CSL) offers an optional program, Multi-Dimensional Voice Program (MDVP), which graphically displays 22 extracted voice parameters against a normative database and the Voice Range Profile, which plots 'voice maps' or a phonetograph. Visi-Pitch, a dedicated clinical instrument, will calculate Fo, perturbation, intensity and voicing percentage.

It should be noted that there is one caveat for those using commercial programs to ascertain perturbation measures, especially for voice disordered subjects. As available computer programs use varying algorithms and Fo markings to compute perturbation, values for many analyses will differ from system to system and may be invalid. For a discusssion of this problem see Bielamowicz, Kreiman, Gerratt, Dauer and Berke (1996).

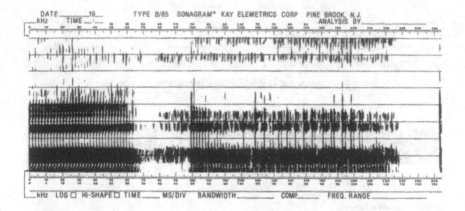

Figure 2.5. Spectrogram of vocal abnormalities in hoarseness with the vowel \ɑ: \. Note intermittent vocalization, loss of harmonic components and antiresonance.

Applications in Speech Pathology

As mentioned earlier, almost every speech and language disorder has been studied via the spectrograph. Studies for six categories of speech-language disorders are summarized in this section to demonstrate the various uses of spectrography. These studies are listed in chronological order to demonstrate the development of interest in acoustic parameters in various disorders.

It should be noted that, while exhausting, these tables are not exhaustive. However, the selected studies are intended to provide the reader with an overview of acoustic research and titillate her or his interest in conducting further studies in these areas.

Stuttering

During the 1970s a considerable area of interest in stuttering research focused on speech motor timing using acoustic measures to compare stutterers' fluent speech with that of control subjects or to compare pre- and post-treatment speaking parameters within stuttering groups. While segment duration measures are still being used in stuttering research, more recent studies have looked at vowel centralization, transitional durations, speaking rates and vocal characteristics. The summary of research in Table 2.2 demonstrates the development of interest in acoustic parameters in stuttering speakers over the past 20 years. Numbers of child and adult subjects are designated to give the reader a sense of the stuttering population that has been studied.

Table 2.2. Summary of selected studies examining acoustic parameters of stuttering speakers' speech.

Study	Findings
Agnello, Wingate and Wendell (1974)	VOT and voice termination time (VTT) were compared among 12 child SSs, 12 child NSs, 12 adult SSs and 12 adult NSs. VOT and VTT differed between adults and children; child SSs used longer VOTs than child NSs; adult SSs lagged in VOT time and had slower VTTs than adult NSs.
Di Simoni (1974)	VDs and fricative durations were analysed for 6 adult SSs and NSs. SSs' VDs were longer than those of NSs in published norms. Fricative durations were significantly longer for SSs than NSs. VD-consonant relationships were maintained by the SSs.
Hillman and Gilbert (1977)	VOT for voiceless consonants was compared among 10 presumably adult SSs and NSs. SSs used longer VOTs than NSs.
Brayton and Conture (1978)	Seven of 9 adult SSs had significantly longer VDs in noise and rhythmic stimulation conditions as opposed to a natural reading condition. An inverse relationship was found between number of disfluencies and VD.
Metz, Conture and Caruso (1979)	Five adult SSs VOTs for one-third of the sound/sound clusters were significantly different from those of NSs. With the exception of /tw/, aspiration duration and frication of SSs were not different from NSs.
Farmer and Brayton (1979)	VDs were compared among 6 disfluent and 7 fluent individuals with Down's syndrome. Disfluent speakers had significantly shorter and less variable VDs.
Colcord and Adams (1979)	Voicing duration and vocal SPL were compared among 8 adult SSs and NSs during reading and singing. Both groups significantly increased voicing during singing; NSs, but not SSs, increased SPL during singing.
Starkweather and Meyers (1979)	Seven subsegments of intervocalic intervals were compared for 16 child and adult SSs and NSs. SSs were slower than NSs in transitional subsegments corresponding to tongue and laryngeal movements but not in steady-state subsegments.
Healey and Adams (1981)	Ten child SSs and NSs were not significantly different for consonant duration, VD, pause duration and utterance duration in two rate conditions.
Watson and Alfonso (1982)	Laryngeal reaction time and VOT were compared among 8 adult SSs and 8 adult NSs. No significant group differences were found.
Klich and May (1982)	Vowels for 7 adult SSs were more centralized than those for NSs, especially in the reading condition.

Ramig (1984)	Post-therapy, 9 adult SSs reduced rate of words in sentences with the exception of the word at the end of the sentence.
Healey and Gutkin (1984)	VOTs, Fo at vowel onset, average vowel Fo, speech and change of Fo were compared among 10 adult SSs and NSs. VOTs for voiced stops and range of Fo change for voiceless stops were significantly longer for SSs than NSs.
Falck, Lawler and Yonovitz (1985)	Fo, variation around the mean Fo and number of voiced data points contained within each temporal segment in identical samples of speech prior to fluent and disfluent moments were significantly different for 7 adult SSs.
Mallard and Westbrook (1985)	Nine SSs demonstrated extended VDs after Precision Fluency Shaping therapy.
Robb, Lybolt and Price (1985)	Fo and VOT did not significantly change from pre-therapy to 2-month follow-up in 12 SSs. Voicing time increased 12%.
Zebrowski, Conture and Cudahy (1985)	Vowel consonant (VC) transition duration, rate of VC transition, stop-gap, frication and aspiration durations, VOT, consonant-vowel (CV) transition duration, rate of CV transition and VD were compared among 11 child SSs and NSs. None of the temporal measures was significantly different.
Pindzola (1986)	Movement rates of formant frequencies and extent of articulatory change were not significantly different for 10 adult SSs and NSs.
Winkler and Ramig (1986)	Nine child SSs and NSs were not significantly different for frequency of interword silent intervals, interword pause duration, VD, consonant duration of voiceless fricatives and total utterance duration during sentence production. SSs had significantly longer and more frequent pauses than NSs during narrative production.
Healey and Ramig (1986)	Twenty-two adult SSs had longer and more variable VOTs, VDs, consonant and phrase durations than NSs. Greater differences were found in the isolated phrase condition than in the extracted reading passage phrase condition.
Howell and Vause (1986)	F1, F2, F3, VD and intensity were compared for fluent and preceding disfluent vowels in syllables in 8 adult SSs' speech. Stuttered vowels which sounded like schwas had similar spectral properties but were shorter in duration and lower in amplitude than non-stuttered vowels. When amplitude and duration of stuttered vowels were increased, they were perceived as the target fluent vowels.

McKnight and Cullinan (1987)	VOTs, VDs, fricative durations and sentence durations were significantly longer and more variable in 17 child SSs with other speech or language disorders than for SSs only and NSs.
Sacco and Metz (1987)	Fo declination during the first 50 msec in vowels following voiced-stop productions did not significantly change after an intensive therapy program for 53 child and adult SSs.
Prosek, Montgomery, Walden and Hawkins (1987)	F1 and F2 measures did not indicate that 15 adult SSs used vowel centralization more than NSs nor within SSs' group for fluent and disfluent vowels.
Adams (1987)	VOTs, VDs and initial consonant durations were significantly longer for 5 child SSs than NSs.
Borden, Kim and Spiegler (1987)	Stop-gap, VOT and VDs were measured. Stop-gap and VD durations were significantly longer for 8 severe adult SSs than NSs.
Healey and Ramig (1989)	VOT, VD, consonant and phrase durations were compared for 17 adult SSs divided into short-term and long-term treatment groups. No significant differences for temporal measures were found, and results did not differ by treatment group or severity of SSs.
Viswanath (1989)	Total articulation time (TAT) and total pause time (TPT) were analysed for 4 SSs and 4 NSs. TAT and TPT decreased as stuttering events were reduced.
Metz, Schiavetti and Sacco (1990)	VOT and sentence duration were found to be the acoustic parameters most highly correlated with speech naturalness in 20 child and adult treated SSs and 20 NSs.
DeNil and Brutten (1991)	VOTs were compared under a normal and time and linguistic pressure condition for 10 child SSs and 10 NSs. No differences were found between groups, but SSs' VOTs were significantly more variable than those of NSs.
Zebrowski (1991)	Ten child SSs did not differ from NSs for duration of sound/syllable repetitions, sound prolongations, and number of repeated units per repetition for sound/syllables or whole words.
Onslow, van Doorn and Newman (1992)	Interphonatory interval, VD, VOT and articulation rate were not significantly different for pre- and post-treatment measures in 10 child SSs. However, VD and articulation rate were less variable post-treatment.
Hall and Yairi (1992)	Fo, jitter and shimmer were compared for 10 child SSs and NSs. SSs differed from NSs on shimmer.

Howell and Williams (1992)	Syllable repetitions in 24 child and 8 teenage SSs were compared with the following fluent vowel. F1 and F2 did not differ in either group. Fluent vowel intensity was greater than nonfluent vowels for teenagers. Excitation spectra fell off more rapidly with frequency than in disfluent vowels. Fo of children's speech was higher for disfluent vowels.
Yaruss and Conture (1993)	F2 of sound/syllable repetitions in 13 child SSs were nonmeasurable, missing or different in direction from fluent transitions. F2 transitions did not predict chronicity of stuttering.
Zebrowski (1994)	Duration of sound/syllable repetitions and prolongations were approximately three-quarters of a second in 14 child SSs.
Jancke (1994)	VOT and duration of phonation did not differ between 18 adult SSs and NSs. SSs had more variable VOT and phonation duration.
Throneburg and Yairi (1994)	Durations of spoken units and silent intervals were compared in the speech of 20 child SSs and 20 child NSs. Duration of spoken units were similar between groups, but SSs' silent intervals were significantly shorter than those of NSs.
Viswanath and Neel (1995)	Gap duration, VOT, VD and vowel spectra were analysed for 6 adult male SSs' stuttering events. VOTs for consonants without vowels were longer than for consonants with vowels. F1 was lower in shorter vowel fragments than in resolved vowels.

SSs = stutterers; NSs = non-stutterers

To paraphrase a well-known physical law: for every result in stuttering research there is an opposite and often equal result. This law is well illustrated in acoustic studies. One of the best examples is VOT, which was found to be longer in stutterers (Adams, 1987; Agnello *et al*, 1974; Healey and Gutkin, 1984; Healey and Ramig, 1986; Hillman and Gilbert, 1977) and not significantly different between stutterers and non-stutterers (Borden *et al*, 1987; Jancke, 1994; Zebrowski *et al*, 1985). Mixed results were found by Metz *et al* (1979) with fewer VOT differences than similarities. McKnight and Cullinan (1987) found VOT differences when comparing stutterers only with stutterers who had other speech or language disorders which suggests that carefully subtyping disfluent subjects might resolve some of the conflicts found in the research. Pre- and post-treatment comparisons have shown no change in VOT (Healey and Ramig, 1989; Onslow *et al*, 1992; Robb *et al*, 1985). Even where no significant differences in duration may be found, VOT is generally more variable for stutterers than non-stutterers (De Nil and Brutten, 1991; Jancke, 1994) which reflects the inconsistency in stutterers' 'fluent' speech.

The second most frequently studied segment in stutterers' speech has been VD. Longer and more variable VDs have been observed in child and adult stutterers' speech (Adams, 1987; Borden *et al*, 1987; Di Simoni, 1974; Healey and Ramig, 1986), but no difference in VD was found for child stutterers and non-stutterers by Healey and Adams (1981) or Zebrowski *et al* (1985). Brayton and Conture (1978) found an inverse relationship between number of disfluencies and VD and an increase of VD when stutterers spoke in noise or to rhythmic stimulation. Farmer and Brayton (1979) found that disfluent Down's syndrome speakers had significantly shorter and less variable VDs than fluent Down's syndrome speakers, and McKnight and Cullinan (1987) found that VDs were longer and more variable in child stutterers who had additional language and speech problems than in children who were stutterers only. Two pre- and post-treatment comparisons (Healey and Ramig, 1989; Onslow *et al*, 1992) found no difference in VD, although Onslow *et al* observed less variance in VD post-treatment. In contrast, Mallard and Westbrook (1985) observed an increase in VD after Precision Fluency Shaping treatment.

Other measures of duration have been compared between stutterers and non-stutterers. Significant differences have been found (Di Simoni, 1974) and no significant difference has been found (Metz *et al*, 1979; Winkler and Ramig, 1986; Zebrowski *et al*, 1985) for frication. McKnight and Cullinan (1987) found a difference in frication between their stuttering group with other speech and language problems and stuttering-only children. Stopgap, vowel-consonant transition, consonant-vowel transition, rates of both these transitions, and aspiration were not found to be significantly different between stutterers and non-stutterers (Zebrowski *et al*, 1985). Consonant and phrase durations were significantly longer and more variable for stutterers than non-stutterers (Healey and Ramig, 1986). Sound prolongations and sound/syllable repetitions between child stutterers and non-stutterers were not observed to be different (Zebrowski, 1991), and were observed to be about 0.75 s in duration in child stutterers (Zebrowski, 1994). Throneburg and Yairi (1994) measured spoken repetition units in preschool stutterers and non-stutterers, also finding unremarkable differences between spoken units. However, they consistently found that the silent interval between repeated units was significantly shorter in stutterers. In an analysis of repetition fragments in adult stutterers, Viswanath and Neel (1995) found shorter VOTs for stops occurring without vowels than for stops occurring with vowels. Post-treatment word rate has been found to be reduced (Ramig, 1984), but no difference has been found between pre- and post-treatment interphonatory and articulatory rates (Onslow *et al*, 1992).

Formant research has addressed vowel centralization, which was reported by Klich and May (1982). Howell and Vause (1986) compared fluent and preceding disfluent vowels, finding no difference between spectra but noting that disfluent schwa-like sounding vowels had shorter VD and less amplitude. Howell and Williams (1992) reported similar findings for teenage and child stutterers. Viswanath and Neel (1995) noted two types of vowels in the repetitions they studied. Vowels longer than the resolution vowel did not differ in spectral shape, but vowels shorter than resolution vowels had lower F1s. Yaruss and Conture (1993) analysed F2 in sound/syllable repetitions and found that they were non-measurable, missing or different in direction from fluent transitions.

Fo has been the most frequently studied vocal characteristic in stutterers. Range of Fo change for voiceless stops has found to be larger for stutterers (Healey and Gutkin, 1984); Fo between fluent and disfluent segments was different (Falck *et al*, 1985); Fo in child stutterers was higher for disfluent than fluent vowels (Howell and Williams, 1992). However, Hall and Yairi (1992) found no significant difference in Fo for child stutterers and non-stutterers. Neither Robb *et al* (1985) nor Sacco and Metz (1987) found Fo differences post-treatment. More recently, Hall and Yairi (1992) compared jitter and shimmer between child stutterers and non-stutterers and found a significant difference only for shimmer.

There are many possible reasons for the differences found in acoustic research in stuttering. Subject selection alone presents a number of problems including age, treatment history, severity, type of stutterer, and presence of other types of speech and language disorders. Many of the cited studies used a small number of subjects and did not clearly delineate subject characteristics. Type and length of stimuli, as well as choice of procedures, may all affect acoustic results. A recent article by Armson and Kalinowski (1994) challenged the basic premise on which much of this research was based. They delineated problems with variables that must be considered in designing stuttering research and offered alternative suggestions for future research. Instead of being intimidated by this state of affairs, students considering acoustic research in stuttering should be challenged by the number of unresolved questions.

Dysarthrias

It has been 30 years since Lehiste (1965) published her classic monograph on acoustic analysis of dysarthric speech. Although she used articulatory features as opposed to acoustic terms to describe aberrant speech patterns, her findings may be of interest to the student wishing to pursue similar research with dysarthric speakers. More recent research in dysarthrias focuses on acoustic features.

Unlike stuttering research, acoustic measures of dysarthric speech are generally consistent. This is expected as lesions at different levels of the nervous system affect the speech mechanism in predictable ways resulting in fairly consistent speech patterns. To date, most of the acoustic research has been descriptive either of a speech parameter or speech pattern in one type of dysarthria or a comparison of parameters and patterns among several types of dysarthria. Three studies (Mulligan *et al*, 1994; Ramig *et al*, 1990; Seikel *et al*, 1991, 1992) have compared repeated measures over time to document degeneration or stability in dysarthric conditions, and three studies (Adams, 1994; Farmer and Green, 1978; Turner and Weismer, 1993) have compared repeated measures under speech rate, white noise and delayed auditory feedback conditions, respectively.

Although reductionism was touted during the 1970s and 1980s as the preferable way to study the nervous system and its disorders, theoretically the premise for acoustic research in dysarthria as well as other speech disorders is alive and well (Weismer and Liss, 1991a). The reductionist point of view argued against using acoustic analysis alone to study movement disorders. All students, especially those interested in acoustic research, should read Weismer and Liss's epitaph on reductionism in speech research. The considerable interest in using acoustic analysis to study speech parameters in dsyarthria is illustrated in Table 2.3.

A number of duration measures have been made of dysarthric speech. In cerebral palsied speakers VOT was found to be longer and more variable for athetotic subjects (Farmer, 1980), shorter and less variable for spastic than ataxic and flaccid subjects (Morris, 1989), but was not a major contributor to intelligibility differences in mixed subjects (Ansel and Kent, 1992). Measures of VOT, VD, frication and segment durations in ataxic speakers showed prolongations and a tendency towards equalized syllable durations (Kent *et al*, 1979). VOT, VD and stop-gap durations were all found to be longer and more variable in ALS speakers (Caruso and Burton, 1987; Turner *et al*, 1995). Rate and duration differences were observed between Parkinson's and Shy-Drager syndrome subjects with the former using shorter segments and more rapid speech, while the latter used normal segmental lengths but slower speech (Ludlow and Bassich, 1983). Lieberman *et al*. (1992) found a relationship between VOT overlap, higher syntax, cognitive and response time tasks between mild and moderate Parkinsonism subjects. LaPointe *et al*, (1994) found that subjects with spasmodic torticollis generally had slower rates, shorter fricative and longer vowel durations than a control group. Syllable duration and within-utterance pause time have also been found to be longer in some traumatic brain-injured patients than in normal speakers (Campbell and Dollaghan, 1995). Increased segmental durations have also been documented in the speech of some subjects with multiple sclerosis (Harteluis *et al*, 1995).

Formant relationship, transition and slope analyses have yielded important information particularly regarding intelligibility in several

Table 2.3. Summary of selected studies examining acoustic parameters in the speech of dysarthric subjects.

Author(s) (Year)	Findings
Lehiste (1965)	Described 22 articulatory features found in 10 dysarthric speakers.
Farmer and Lencione (1977)	Durations of a prevocalization were analysed in 8 predominately athetoid and 2 predominately spastic cerebral palsied speakers. Prevocalizations occurred more frequently in athetoid Ss, before voicing than place errors and before voiced than voiceless stops.
Farmer (1977)	VOTs and prevocalizations were measured in three athetotic cerebral palsied Ss. All Ss demonstrated distinctive categorical voicing with wide intersubject variation for voiceless stops. Prevocalizations occurred more frequently and were generally longer before voiced stops.
Farmer and Green (1978)	Word, interword and total utterance durations were compared for 1 spastic and 2 athetotic cerebral palsied speakers in two control and one white noise masking conditions. Individual differences were observed among Ss with the spastic speaker generally decreasing duration and the athetotic speakers increasing duration in the noise condition.
Kent, Netsell and Abbs (1979)	F1, F2, VOT, VD, frication and segment durations were analysed for 5 ataxic dysarthric Ss. Prolongations and a tendency toward equalized syllable durations were found. Vowel formant structure was essentially normal except for transitional segments. Intonation patterns were abnormal.
Farmer (1980)	VOTs were compared between 5 spastic and 5 athetotic cerebral palsied speakers. VOTs for /p, t, g/ were longer and more variable for the athetotic Ss.
Kent and Rosenbek (1982)	Wide- and narrow-band spectrographs were used to illustrate prosodic disturbances in 5 ataxic dysarthric, 7 apraxic, 20 Parkinsonian dysarthric and 3 right hemisphere damaged Ss. Prosodic patterns resembled descriptive terms generally used to describe the speech of Ss with these disorders.
DeFeo and Schaefer (1983)	F2 transitions and frequencies of burst noise in stops were analysed in the speech of 1 Moebius syndrome child to verify lingua-interdental compensation for bilabial valving.
Ludlow and Bassich (1983)	A number of Fo, rate, duration and quality measures were compared between 7 Shy-Drager, 7 Parkinson's dysarthric speakers and 7 Cs. Differences were found in rate, Fo and vocal quality measures among the groups.

Weismer (1984)	Tutorial article in which author describes with spectrograms characteristics of a speaker with Parkinson's disease and a speaker with spastic dysarthria.
Caruso and Burton (1987)	VOTs, VDs and stop-gap durations were compared for 8 dysarthric speakers with amyotrophic lateral sclerosis and 8 Cs. All measures were longer and more variable for the experimental group.
Kent, Kent, Weismer, Sufit, Brooks and Rosenbek (1989)	F2 slope was analysed in 35 SSs with ALS and found to be correlated with intelligibility. Less intelligible ALS speakers had longer and flatter slopes than C SSs.
Morris(1989)	VOT was compared among 5 spastic, 5 flaccid, 5 ataxic and 5 hypokinetic dysarthric Ss. All Ss exhibited overlap in their productions. Spastics used the shortest VOTs. Ataxic and flaccid groups used the most variable VOTs.
Ramig, Scherer, Klasner, Horii and Titze (1990)	Acoustic measures of phonatory instability, phonatory limits and nasal-oral amplitude ratio were measured 5 times over 6 months in 1 S with ALS. Acoustic measures reflected the progression of ALS over time.
Seikel, Wilcox and Davis (1991, 1992)	VOT, VD and duration of articulatory closure were analysed for three dysarthrics with motor neuron disease over four recording sessions. Little change was observed.
Ansel and Kent (1992)	VOTs, VDs, nasalization, noise durations rise times, F1-F2 difference and F1 frequency location were analysed for 16 adult males with mixed cerebral palsy. Multiple regression analysis indicated that fricative-affricative and three vowel contrasts contributed most to variability in intelligibility estimates.
Kent, Kent, Rosenbek, Weismer, Sufit and Brooks (1992)	F1 and F2 transition duration, frequency extents of trajectories, Fo, jitter, shimmer and S/N ratios were studied in 10 women with amyotrophic lateral sclerosis. Results showed that the mean slope of F2 was reduced as compared with Cs; Fo, jitter, shimmer and S/N ratios were abnormal in the experimental group.
Lieberman, Kako, Friedman, Tajchman, Feldman and Jiminez (1992)	VOTs were compared between 20 mild and 20 moderate Ss with Parkinson's disease. Two mild and 7 moderate Ss exhibited overlap. VOT errors were correlated with higher syntax errors, longer response times and increased errors on cognitive tasks.
Weismer, Martin, Kent and Kent (1992)	Formant trajectories were compared between 25 males with ALS and 15 C Ss. ALS speakers had shallower slope transitions, exaggerated formant trajectories at onset of vocalic nuclei and more interspeaker variability of formant transitions than did Cs.
Turner and Weismer (1993)	Three speaking rates were analysed between 9 Ss with ALS and 9 C Ss. ALS Ss used pause duration and frequency as opposed to articulation change in varying

	rate. Phrase duration to phrase length in syllables was related in both groups but less so in ALS Ss.
Adams (1994)	The speech of 1 S with hypokinetic dysarthria was compared for normal and DAF conditions. Spectrographic analysis indicated that increased duration under the DAF condition contributed to improved intelligibility.
Hakel, Healey and Sullivan (1994)	Fo measures were compared using 5 different speech analysis systems for 6 hypokinetic and 5 mixed types of dysarthric Ss as well as 6 Ss with hyperfunctional voice disorders. Differences among means and standard deviations are reported for disorder and severity.
Mulligan, Carpenter, Riddel, Delaney, Badger, Krusinski and Tandan (1994)	F2 formant trajectories were compared for 7 dysarthric and 7 nondysarthric ALS Ss over a 6-month period. F2 transition rates of less than 4Hz/msec were seen only in dysarthric Ss.
LaPointe, Case and Duane (1994)	Rate, duration and Fo measures were analysed for 75 Ss with spasmodic torticollis (ST) and 20 Cs. Generally, ST Ss had slower speech movements and rates, shorter durations for /s,z/ and /a/ prolongation. Female ST Ss tended to have lower Fos and a lower Fo ceiling than C female Ss.
Harteluis, Nord and Buder (1995)	Rate, relative timing and formant meaures were analysed in 3 male and 2 female adult MS speakers and 1 male and 1 female normal speakers. Relative timing and formant analyses differentiated among MS subgroups.
Turner, Tjaden and Weismer (1995)	F1, F2 and VD were compared between 9 ALS Ss and 9 normal speakers for 3 speaking rates. ALS speakers showed restricted vowel space and less variability with rate changes than normal speakers as well as longer VDs across rate conditions. Vowel space was reported to account for 45% of variance in speech intelligibility.
Dromey, Ramig and Johnson (1995)	A number of measures including VD and F2 trajectories were compared from the speech of one Parkinsonian subject whose treatment emphasized increased vocal intensity. Along with increase in vocal intensity, VD increased and F2 showed more normal patterns.
Campbell and Dollaghan (1995)	Syllable duration and within-utterance pause time were found to be longer in some TBI Ss as compared with normal Ss.

NAs = non-fluent aphasics; FAs = fluent aphasics; C = control subjects; ALS = amyotrophic lateral sclerosis; MS = multiple sclerosis dysarthric populations. Vowel contrast has been found to be a major contributor to intelligibility in speakers with mixed cerebral palsy (Ansel and Kent, 1992). Longer transition durations have been observed in the speech of ataxics (Kent *et al*, 1979). Longer and flatter F2 slopes were found to be correlated with poorer intelligibility of ALS speakers (Kent *et al*, 1992; Kent *et al*, 1989; Weismer *et al*, 1992). Mulligan *et al* (1994) found flatter F2s in dysarthric ALS subjects. Prosodic patterns from narrow-band spectrograms were found to resemble the descriptive terms traditionally applied to ataxic, apraxic and right hemisphere-damaged speakers (Kent and Rosenbek, 1982).

Measures related to vocal characteristics have been used to differentiate Parkinsonian and Shy-Drager speakers (Ludlow and Bassich, 1983), track degeneration in the speech of ALS subjects (Ramig *et al*, 1990) and describe speech in mixed cerebral palsied speakers (Ansel and Kent, 1992), ALS subjects (Kent *et al*, 1992), hypokinetic and mixed dysarthrias (Hakel *et al*, 1994) and spasmodic torticollis (LaPointe *et al*, 1994). While Fo, shimmer, jitter and H/N (harmonic-to-noise) ratio have verified perceptually apparent voice disorders in these subjects as well as shown a relationship with severity, Ludlow and Bassich (1983) noted that acoustic analyses may highlight problems not necessarily detected in perceptual analyses.

Acoustic research of the dysarthrias has evolved with instrumental technology to a level where multiple measures (e.g. Ansel and Kent, 1992) can identify critical parameters affecting intelligibility in various types of dysarthric speakers. For example, the relationship between F2 slope and intelligibility in ALS, which has been studied by the Kents and colleagues, alone suggests a number of research pursuits. As can be seen in Table 2.3, a number of acoustic measures have not been applied to the study of a variety of dysarthrias, and students should generate a plethora of questions in this area.

Acoustic measures were used by Dromey, Ramig and Johnson (1995) to document speech behaviour changes in a Parkinsonian subject whose treatment focused on increasing vocal intensity. As expected, VD increased and F2 patterns became more normal in conjunction with increased vocal intensity.

Apraxia and aphasia

The dysarthric research was based on the fact that motor control of speech was disordered at some level in the nervous system which ultimately affected muscle groups required to produce speech. Acquired apraxia of speech is considered to be a neurogenic phonological disorder that impairs the ability to select, programme and/or execute the musculature to produce coordinated and properly sequenced speech using normal prosody. Although apraxia can occur alone, it usually appears in conjunction with non-fluent aphasias (NAs). The language disorder of aphasia includes several fluent aphasias (FAs) in which sound production may be disordered. The postulate was that apraxic errors are more phonetic in nature, and sound production errors (also known as literal paraphasias) occurring in fluent aphasics are more phonemic in nature. VOT has been used as the acoustic bellwether for testing this premise. It was thought that phonemic errors (voicing substitutions) would occur in FAs, and overlay or VOTs falling between the upper limit for voiced stops and below the lower limit for voiceless stops would be produced by apraxic and/or NAs. Although the research has not found a pure theoretical division of VOT errors, it has raised a number of interesting questions concerning the nature of sound production in the aphasias. While VOT was of prime interest in early acoustic research in acquired apraxia of speech and aphasia, other measures have provided valuable knowledge concerning these disorders as shown in Table 2.4.

Instead of finding a phonemic-phonetic contrast, studies (Baum *et al*, 1990; Baum and Ryan, 1993; Blumstein *et al*, 1980; Freeman *et al*, 1978; Itoh and Sasanuma, 1984; Shewan *et al*, 1984) have found that most frequently NAs, less frequently FAs and very rarely control subjects produce overlapping VOTs. Both NAs and FAs exhibit voiced-voiceless substitutions. Similar findings were reported by Gandour *et al* (1992a) who analysed VOT in Thai speakers who have three bilabial and alveolar and two velar word initial stops. In an attempt to resolve the VOT issue, Baum *et al* (1990) correlated CT scan findings with VOT production and found that subjects with considerable overlap shared common lesion sites including Broca's area, the anterior limb of the internal capsule and the lowest motor cortex areas for the tongue and larynx leading them to conclude that these areas probably play an important role in integrating articulatory movements. The fact that subjects with posterior lesions show infrequent VOT overlap continues to be an interesting but unexplained issue.

VDs have been found to be generally longer and more variable in apraxic and NA speakers than in control or FA subjects (Baum, 1992, 1993; Collins *et al*, 1983; Duffy and Gawle, 1984; Gandour *et al*, 1992b; Kent and Rosenbek, 1983). Collins *et al* (1983) reported that apraxics decreased VD as words increased in length, and Baum (1992) noted a decrease in two- but not three-syllable words for NAs. Baum (1993) also observed that NAs did not reduce VD in a fast-rate speaking condition. Fricative analysis has indicated that NA and FA subjects maintain the same intrinsic duration and consonant-vowel ratio relationships among fricatives as do control subjects (Baum *et al*, 1990). Two studies found that NAs delayed voicing onset or had inconsistent periodicity for voiced fricatives (Baum *et al*, 1990; Code and Ball, 1982).

Although Ryalls (1982) found restricted intonation ranges in NAs,

Table 2.4. Summary of selected studies of acoustic parameters in the speech of subjects with acquired apraxia of speech and aphasia.

Author(s) (Year)	Findings
Freeman, Sands and Harris (1978)	One apraxic subject produced VOTs with voicing lags although small differences were found between voiced and voiceless stops.
Blumstein, Cooper, Goodglass, Statlender and Gottlieb (1980)	Four Cs, 9 FAs and 1 dysarthric maintained voiced-voiceless contrasts while 4 NAs showed marked overlay of VOTs.
Code and Ball (1982)	Duration of voiced and voiceless frication was longer for 1 NA than for 1 C. Vocal fold vibration was absent from some voiced fricatives in NA.
Ryalls (1982)	Eight NAs demonstrated significantly restricted ranges of intonation as measured from the fifth harmonic of narrow band spectrograms when compared with 11 Cs.
Collins, Rosenbek and Wertz (1983)	Eleven apraxic and 11 Cs decreased VD as word length increased. VD and word length were significantly longer in apraxic than C Ss.
Kent and Rosenbek (1983)	Seven apraxic Ss demonstrated prolonged vowels, stressing of normally unstressed vowels, inappropriate pause insertion and prolongation of transitions.
Ryalls (1984)	Five NAs used significantly higher Fos than Cs, and both 7 FAs and NAs had significantly greater inter- and intra-speaker Fo variability than Cs.
Itoh and Sasanuma (1984)	VOT was compared among 4 apraxic, 6 FA and 5 C Ss. Apraxic Ss had considerable overlay; FAs and Cs had little overlay.
Duffy and Gawle (1984)	VD was compared among 5 apraxic (1 predominately fluent), 4 aphasic (2 FA, 2 NA) and 5 C Ss. The apraxic group had the longest VD before both voiced and voice-less final consonants. The aphasic groups, VDs were longer than those of the C Ss in both final consonant conditions.
Shewan, Leeper and Booth (1984)	VOT was compared among 9 Broca's aphasics, 6 conduction aphasics and 9 C Ss. All groups produced categorical VOTs with both aphasic groups producing more voiced for voiceless substitutions and more overlay VOTs than the C group.
Ziegler and von Cramon (1986)	One apraxic subject showed a deficit in coarticulation as measured by formant frequencies and reflection coefficients when compared with Cs.

Ryalls (1986)	Midpoints of F1 and F2, VD and Fo were measured. No significant difference in formant frequencies was found for 5 NAs, 7 FAs and 7 Cs. NAs and FAs were significantly more variable in vowel production.
Tuller and Story (1988)	Anticipatory coarticulation of vowels in fricatives was compared among 5 NAs, 5 FAs and 5 Cs. NAs and FAs differed from Cs in extent but not pattern. NAs showed later anticipatory coarticulation than did FAs, but FAs showed a lack of carry-over coarticulation.
Gandour, Petty and Dardarananda (1989)	Syllable, phrase and sentence timing, intensity dB variation and Fo contours were analysed in 1 NA Thai speaker. Timing and intensity were differentially impaired, but tonal contours were normal.
McNeil, Liss, Tseng and Kent (1990)	VDs, consonant, stop gap, other segment durations and F2 trajectories were compared among 3 apraxic,2 conduction aphasic and 3 C speakers in different rate conditions for on-target productions. Apraxics and aphasics were less efficient in adjusting speech rates than C Ss.
Baum, Blumstein, Naeser and Palumbo (1990)	VOT, VD and fricative duration were compared for two subgroups of 8 NAs and 5 FAs. NAs' results indicated articulatory and laryngeal impairments, and FAs also showed evidence of 'subtle phonetic impairments'.
Weismer and Liss (1991a)	Formant trajectory patterns, segmental phenomena, repetitions, movement perseveration and prosodic characteristics were analysed for 4 apraxic speakers. Generally, exaggerated articulatory gestures, misdirected formant trajectories, articulatory perseveration, fragmented groping behaviours and consistency across repetitions of many phenomena were found.
Square-Storer and Apeldoorn (1991)	Duration and amplitude measures were analysed for 3 apraxic speakers. Prosodic and rate measures varied among Ss who had differing loci of lesions.
Baum (1992)	Ten NAs and 8 FAs reduced root syllable duration in two-syllable, but not three-syllable words.
Cohen (1992)	Mean Fo, Fo variability, vocal intensity, number of syllables per second, pause time and intelligibility ratings were compared pre- and post-singing therapy for Ss with 8 NA, apraxia or dysarthria Ss. Number and types of changes varied for each S.
Gandour, Ponglorpisit, Khunadorn, Dechongkit, Boongird and Boonklam (1992a)	VDs were compared among 20 young and old Cs, 14 right hemisphere damaged, 9 FAs and 8 NAs. The phonological contrast was relatively preserved, but a subtle timing deficit was noted in NAs' vowels.
Gandour, Ponglorpisit, Khunadorn, Dechongkit, Boongird and Boonklam (1992b)	VOT was compared among 8 NA, 9 FA, 12 right hemisphere damaged (RHD) and 20 C Thai Ss. Cs showed no overlay; RHDs had a little more overlay than Cs; FAs had more overlay than RHD Ss; NAs had the most overlay.

Baum (1993)	VDs for tense and lax vowels were compared among 10 NAs, 8 FAs and 10 Cs in two different speech rate conditions. FAs and Cs reduced VDs in the fast rate condition, but NAs did not. FAs and Cs did not produce overlapping VDs, but the NAs overlapped tense and lax vowels.
Baum and Ryan (1993)	VOTs were compared among 10 NAs, 7 FAs and 10 Cs in two different speech rate conditions. NAs were similar to Cs but with overlapping VOTs. FAs' and Cs' VOTs were shorter under the fast condition than under the slow condition.
Gandour, Ponglorpisit, Dechongkit, Khunadorn, Boongird and Potisuk (1993)	Tonal coarticulation was measured using Fo among 20 young and old Cs, 12 right hemisphere damaged Ss, 9 FAs and 6 NAs who spoke Thai. Although brain-damaged Ss were more variable in Fo production, no differences in coarticulation were found for aphasia types.
Gandour, Dechongkit, Ponglorpisit, Khunadorn and Boongird (1993)	Intraword timing for 1-, 2- and 3-syllable words were compared among 20 young and old Cs, 14 right hemisphere damaged Ss, 9 FAs and 6 NAs. FAs and NAs were significantly more varied than other Ss.

NAs=Non-fluent Aphasics; FAs= Fluent Aphasics; Cs=Controls; Ss=Subjects

Gandour *et al.* (1989, 1993) observed normal tonal contours but more variable tonal coarticulation in Thai NAs and FAs. Deficits in coarticulation (Ziegler and von Cramon, 1986) and lag in anticipatory coarticulation (Tuller and Story, 1988) have also been observed in the speech of apraxic and NA subjects. Tuller and Story also found a lack of carry-over coarticulation in the speech of FAs.

Students interested in acquired apraxia of speech and aphasias have several challenges in redesigning studies that address the question of motor control of speech. Most of the past research has focused on correct or on-target productions of limited stimuli designed to produce specific measures. Questions concerning the effects of anomic, morphologic and grammatical effects on speech timing and coarticulation when phonetic and phonemic errors are present have yet to be addressed. Only one study (Cohen, 1992) was found which analysed acoustic parameter changes pre- and post-treatment with singing therapy. Unfortunately, subject description and significance of improvement were not clearly delineated in this article. However, acoustic changes, if any, in relation to various types of treatment need to be analysed.

Phonological/phonetic disorders

Acoustic analyses are used to detect developmental differences between phonological/phonetic disordered children and controls, to analyse distortions, substitutions and omissions, and to test hypothesized differences between phonological and phonetic disorders. Ohde and Sharf (1992) and Kent and Read (1992) provide excellent sources for these types of analyses, and students wishing to pursue this type of research should become familiar with the basic information in these texts. Table 2.5 provides a sampling of the acoustic measures that have been applied to phonological/phonetic disorders.

Several studies (Catts and Jensen, 1983; Farmer and Florance, 1977; Glasson, 1984; Tyler and Saxman, 1991; Young and Gilbert, 1988) found VOT to be longer and more variable in phonologically disordered children than in controls, as well as less differentiated with overlaps. However, in one child who perceptually substituted /d/ for a number of phonemes and blends, Maxwell and Weismer (1982) observed VOT differences which indicated that he was consistently differentiating between /d/ target words and words beginning with other sounds. Gierut and Dinnsen (1986) using VOT were able to identify contrastive production in one but not another child who perceptually had the same speech pattern. However, Forrest and Rockman (1988) and Forrest *et al* (1990) found that spectral and aspiration amplitude cues were needed in addition to VOT to further delineate stop production in phonologically disordered children.

As VD is influenced by the intrinsic and extrinsic factors discussed earlier, it can be used to study the speech of children with final sound omission or the open-syllable pattern. Weismer *et al* (1981) and Hambly and Farmer (1982) generally found that older subjects' VDs were appropriate for the omitted final consonants, while some younger subjects did not show a differentiation in their vowel length.

Consonant distortions and substitutions were analysed from spectral patterns, duration measures and formant frequencies. Daniloff *et al* (1980) found that various types of /s/ distortions could be distinguished by their spectra, and Weismer and Elbert (1982) observed more variable /s/ durations in /s/-defective subjects. F2 values and rate of transition generally are implicated in liquid- and glide-defective subjects (Chaney, 1988; Hoffman *et al*, 1983; Huer, 1989; Walton and Pollock, 1993).

Children specifically diagnosed as apraxic were found to have F2s and F3s that differed from control subjects as well as limited F2 movement ratios (Walton and Pollack, 1993) and to be more variable than control and articulatory disordered children (Smith *et al*, 1994). As developmental apraxia rarely occurs (Hall *et al*, 1993) and subtypes of this disorder have been proposed (Crary, 1993), students will be able to raise a number of acoustic questions that can be tested for one or a few subjects. Experimental designs (e.g. de Janette, 1988; Edwards, 1992) are also needed to explore the effects of different conditions on speech motor production in a number of developmentally disordered populations.

Table 2.5. Summary of selected studies examining acoustic parameters in the speech of subjects with phonological/phonetic disorders.

Author(s) (Year)	Findings
Farmer and Florance (1977)	Eleven language-PD children had VOTs (except /d/) and VDs that were significantly longer and more variable than those of age- and sex-matched Cs.
Daniloff, Wilcox and Stephens (1980)	Spectral patterns and durations were compared among 2 Cs, 2 dentalizing, 2 lateralizing and 2 other /s/-defective children. Inter- and intrasubject differences were found in spectral patterns.
Weismer, Dinnsen and Elbert (1981)	VD was measured in 3 boys who omitted word-final stops. The two older boys preserved VD differences which indicated that they were aware of the voicing characteristic of the omitted final stop.
Weismer and Elbert (1982)	Durations of /s/ were compared among 7 adult, 7 normally articulating and 7 /s/-defective Ss. The experimental group had more variable /s/ durations than C groups with the /s/ stop cluster being more variable than the singleton /s/ condition.
Hambly and Farmer (1982)	VDs in the speech of 5 boys with the open syllable were compared with those of sex- and age-matched Cs. VDs were significantly longer for the experimental group only in the single word voiceless condition.
Maxwell and Weismer (1982)	VOT measures were used to analyse /d/ substitutions for 23 phonemes. Voicing distinction, although not perceptible, was found in VOT comparisons.
Hoffman, Stager and Daniloff (1983)	Twelve children who misarticulated /r/ and 5 Cs produced /r/-/w/ contrast sentences. Acoustic analyses showed no difference for F1, duration and amplitude measures. F2 values for /r/ errors were significantly higher than for /w/ in the experimental group.
Catts and Jensen (1983)	VOTs, VDs, consonant closure durations and voicing during consonant closing were compared between 9 PD Ss and 9 Cs. Although individual Ss performed differently, the PD group had less differentiated word-initial VOTs, longer consonant closure durations and less voicing during consonant closure than Cs.
Glasson (1984)	Thirteen duration measures (e.g. VOT, VD, other sounds, word) from sentence repetition were generally longer and more variable for 4 language-phonological/phonetic disordered children than for 3 Cs. Four experimental Ss differed from one another.

Gierut and Dinnsen (1986)	VOTs were compared between 2 PD children. Although initial stop production was perceived as similar in the Ss, VOTs converged in one but not the other subject.
Young and Gilbert (1988)	VOTs were compared between 13 velar fronting articulation disordered Ss and 5 Cs. Experimental Ss generally produced longer /t and k/ VOTs than did Cs. Velar fronting Ss did not increase the VOT for /t and d/ when the target sounds were /k and g/.
de Janette (1988)	F1 and F2 were compared between jaw-free and bite-block conditions of /i,æ, u/ productions among 5 C adults, 5 C children and 5 articulatory disordered children. All Ss produced vowels within normal ranges in both conditions.
Chaney (1988)	F1, F2, F3 and F2 transition rates were compared among 4 correct/w,r,l,j/ producing children, 4 children with developmental w/r and w/l substitutions and 4 w/r misarticulating children. Developmental and experimental groups produced /j/ similarly to the C group but did not differentiate among /w,l,r/ by either formant frequencies or transition rate differences.
Forrest and Rockman (1988)	Fo and F1 at the onset of voicing, burst and aspiration amplitude relative to vowel onset were analysed to disambiguate initial stop consonants produced by 3 language-phonologically disordered children which were not differentiated by VOT.
Huer (1989)	F2 was analysed in a child with w/r substitution over a 70-day treatment period. As the /w/ moved toward /r/, F2 values increased and F2 transition rates decreased.
Forrest, Weismer, Hodge, Dinnsen and Elbert (1990)	Spectral moments were used to analyse /t/ and /k/ in 4 PD children perceived to substitute /t/ for /k/ and 4 C children. One PD child whose /t,k/ was similar to but more variable than those of Cs used appropriate /t,k/ after treatment in which velar-alveolar contrast was not treated. The other 3 PD children who had no acoustic /t,k/ contrast did not acquire /t,k/ contrast after treatment with other target phonemes.
Tyler, Edwards and Saxman (1990)	VOTs were analysed in 4 PD children to determine underlying representations of velar and alveolar stops. When VOT contrasts were adult-like, generalization of the treated contrast was more rapid than when VOT contrasts were unadult-like.
Tyler and Saxman (1991)	VOT contrasts developed in different patterns between 3 PD and 3 normally developing children. Treated Ss' mean VOT for voiced at the time of contrast exceeded adult

	VOT range, and voiceless VOTs in the treated group were more variable than those of C children.
Edwards (1992)	F1 and F2 were compared between 4 PD and 6 C children in control, teeth-clenched and bite-block conditions. Acoustic effects of the bite-block condition were observed for all children.
Walton and Pollock (1993)	F1, F2 and F3 were analysed in perceived vowel and derhotacization errors in five developmental apraxic Ss. Diphthong reduction corresponded with F2 movement ratios of 0.20 or less; tense-lax errors corresponded to F1-F2 coordinates; derhotacization errors corresponded to abnormally high F3 and F2, and F3 were different from that of normal children.
Smith, Marquardt, Cannito, Davis (1994)	F1, F2 and VDs were compared among 1 normally articulating, 1 misarticulating and 1 developmentally apraxic subject from CVC and CVCV productions. The apraxic child was more variable than the other 2 children on all three measures.
McLeod and Isaac (1995)	F1 and F2 for /l/ and /j/ were analysed to demonstrate that 1 child had the underlying representation of these phonemes. The substitution was treated as a motoric rather than as a phonological disorder.

PD=Phonologically Disordered; C=Control; S=Subjects

Hearing impaired

A number of acoustic measures have been used to describe speech patterns of hearing impaired (HI) and deaf individuals. Table 2.6 summarizes studies that provide examples of acoustic measures in this population.

Although Leeper *et al* (1987) and Ryalls and Larouche (1992) did not find signficant differences between HI and control subjects' VOTs, other studies (Brown and Goldberg, 1990; Gilbert and Campbell, 1978; Monsen, 1978) did find significant differences. Further, VOT has been identified as a significant factor in intelligibility of speech for HI speakers (Metz *et al*, 1985; Samar *et al*, 1989). Differences among studies are probably due to types of speech samples, degree of hearing impairment and previous speech training among other variables.

Most of the acoustic research with HI and deaf subjects has focused on vowel production. VD for /i, ɪ/ were more restricted in HI speakers than in controls (Monsen, 1974). Generally, F1 and F2 were more variable and restricted in HI and deaf speakers' vowels than in controls' vowels (Angelocci *et al*, 1964; Monsen, 1976; Rothman, 1976; Ryalls and

Table 2.6. Summary of selected studies examining acoustic parameters in the speech of hearing impaired and deaf subjects.

Author(s) (Year)	Findings
Angelocci, Kopp and Holbrook (1964)	Fo, F1, F2, F3 and amplitude were compared between 18 deaf and 18 C Ss. Fos were higher for the deaf; Fo, F1, F2, F3 and amplitudes were more variable for the deaf.
Monsen (1974)	VDs for /i, IPA/ were compared between 12 severely HI and deaf Ss and 6 Cs in differing consonantal environments. HI and deaf Ss' vowels were more restricted than those of C Ss.
Monsen (1976)	F2 transitions were compared between 6 HI and 6 Cs. F2 transitions in hearing impaired speakers were reduced in both time and frequency as compared with F2s in Cs' speech.
Monsen (1976)	F1 and F2 were compared between 35 deaf and 4 C Ss. Reduced vowel space in deaf speakers was found to be related to a relatively immobile F2 and restricted F1 range.
Rothman (1976)	Formant transitions, coarticulation and neutralization of vowels were compared between 4 adult deaf and 4 C Ss. Formant transitions for the deaf had a slower rate of movement and restricted range; speech of deaf Ss had little coarticulation; vowels of deaf speakers tended to be neutralized.
Monsen (1978)	Intelligibility scores for 67 HI speakers were compared with nine variables. Mean VOT and F2 for specific sounds were highly correlated with intelligibility scores.
Gilbert and Campbell (1978)	VOTs were compared between 9 HI and 9 C speakers only on phonemes which were perceived to be produced correctly. HI speakers did not make as great a differentiation between voiced and voiceless stops as did Cs.
Monsen (1979)	Mean Fo, syllable duration, mean period to period changes in intensity and Fo, spectral energy ration above and below 1000 Hz and intonation contour were compared between 24 HI and 6 child Cs. Intonation contour was the most important characteristic separating experimental and C speakers.
Osberger and Levitt (1979)	Speech waveform modification of relative timing of sentences spoken by 6 deaf children resulted in improved intelligibility.
Oller, Eilers, Bull and Carney (1985)	Vocalizations between 1 deaf infant and 11 hearing infants were compared. Spectrograms were used to illustrate vocalizations between the deaf and C infants.
Metz, Samar, Schiavetti, Sitler and Whitehead (1985)	Segmental, prosodic and hearing ability parameters across 3 measures of speech intelligibility in 20 severely to profoundly HI speakers were compared. Cognate pair VOT

differences and mean sentence duration strongly predicted intelligibility.

Stathopoulos, Duchan, Sonnenmeier and Bruce (1986)	Intonation and timing patterns were compared between 4 female deaf and 4 C speakers during reading. Deaf speakers had a higher and more restricted Fo than Cs. Deaf Ss had longer word duration and pauses than Cs.
Leder, Spitzer, Milner, Flevaris-Phillips, Richardson and Kirchner (1986)	Fo, duration and intensity were compared pre- and post-implant of a single-channel cochlear implant for one adventitiously deaf subject. Post-implant Fo increased for stressed syllables; intensity increased; syllable duration increased for stress.
Osberger (1987)	VD, F1 and F2 were compared in 2 vowels pre- and post-treatment for 2 profoundly HI adolescents. Changes in the measures differed for each subject.
Leeper, Perez and Mencke (1987)	VOTs, VDs and utterance durations were compared between 9 HI and 9 C Ss. VDs and utterance durations were longer and more variable for the HI. VOTs were not significantly different.
Kent, Osberger, Netsell and Hustedde (1987)	Fo levels and contours, formant frequencies of vocalic utterances, and spectral characteristics of fricatives and trills were compared between one normal hearing male and his identical twin who had a bilateral profound hearing loss. Data gathered longitudinally (8, 12 and 15 months) showed differences for all measures.
Carney, Gandour, Petty, Robbins, Myres and Miyamoto (1988)	VOTs were analysed in a Thai speaker with an adventitious, profound sensorineural hearing loss. Categorical production was maintained and only minor articulatory perturbations were found.
Shukla (1989)	F1 and F2 were compared in three vowels between 30 HI and C child and adult Ss. Vowel space was reduced in HI primarily due to lowering of second formant in /i/.
Samar, Metz, Schiavetti, Sitler and Whitehead (1989)	Multiple acoustic, areodynamic and electroglottographic measures of the speech of 40 HI speakers revealed 4 factors with independent relationships to intelligibility including VOT distinctions and pairpeak volume-velocity distinctions for cognate pairs and two factors reflecting production stability of temporal distinctions between cognate pair members.
Brown and Goldberg (1990)	Intelligible utterances of 26 HI children and 15 Cs were compared. VOT was the most critical factor in syllable recognition with consonant durations and vowel formant frequency distributions contributing less to intelligibility.
Ryalls and Larouche (1992)	Syllable duration, VOT, Fo, F1, F2 and F3 were compared on syllables produced by 10 HI and 10 C children. Group

	differences generally did not reach significance although the HI group was more variable.
Economou, Tartter, Chute and Hellman (1992)	Spectrographic analyses of the speech of 1 deaf S following a reimplantation from a single-channel to a multichannel cochlear implant. An increase in Fo for stressed than unstressed syllables, expanded vowel space and improvement in voicing, manner and place of articulation were found.

Larouche, 1992; Shukla, 1989). F2 transition durations are restricted in rate and frequency (Monsen, 1974; 1976).

Fo in HI and deaf speakers was found to be higher than in control subjects (Angelocci *et al*, 1964; Monsen, 1979; Stathopoulos *et al*, 1986). Intonation contours are also different in HI than in control speakers (Monsen, 1976; Stathopoulos *et al*, 1986). Oller *et al* (1985) and Kent *et al* (1987) observed developmental differences in Fo and intonation contours between HI and normal hearing infants.

An exciting area of research has emerged with cochlear implantation for the deaf. Improvement in perception (e.g. Mulder *et al*, 1992; Tyler *et al*, 1992) and, of particular interest here, speech production (Economou *et al*, 1992; Leder *et al*, 1986) should parallel advancements in technical development of implants. Students interested in hearing impairment and acoustics of speech will find this a fertile field for research.

Voice disorders

Acoustic analysis of voice disorders is concerned with fundamental frequency, phonational range, vocal intensity, perturbation (jitter and shimmer), resonance and harmonic-to-noise ratio (H/N). Although early research in voice was generated with the spectrograph, specialized instruments, such as the VisiPitch (Kay Elemetrics Corporation) and PM Pitch Analyzer (Voice Identification, Inc), were developed to measure parameters of voice production. Further, a nasometer can be added to VisiPitch or the Computerized Speech Lab to measure nasalence, and a laryngograph can be attached to assess glottal area (see Chapter 5). In addition, computer programs for acoustic analysis include subroutines and/or extra programs specifically designed to analyse vocal production.

Acoustic research in voice disorders consists of a formidable amount of data. The studies summarized in Table 2.7 expose only the mere tip of the iceberg representing this body of research. Generally, this research describes acoustic characteristics of a particular type of voice disorder, demonstrates the validity of a new technique for measuring specific parameters, and uses acoustic data to compare pre- and post-treatment differences in voice production.

Examples of descriptive studies include nasality (Dickson, 1962), hoarseness (Yangihara, 1967), spastic dysphonia (Wolfe and Bacon, 1976), tremulous voice (Lebrun *et al*, 1982), asthma (Lee *et al*, 1988) and oesophageal speech (Weinberg *et al*, 1980). Rontal *et al* (1975) provided spectrographic illustrations of acoustic characteristics for speakers with nodules, vocal fold paralysis and functional dysphonias, but they stressed the need to supplement acoustic analysis with indirect laryngoscopy due to disorders sharing some acoustic characteristics. Since Rontal *et al*'s warning that observation of the vocal folds should accompany acoustic analysis, endoscopy and videostroboscopy have become fairly common instruments in voice clinics (McFarlane, 1990). However, acoustic analyses can enhance observation of the vocal folds as well as provide pertinent information for functional voice disorders.

Techniques for measuring specific parameters of voice depend on acoustic-perceptual correspondence (Murray *et al*, 1977). Harmonic-to-

Table 2.7. Summary of selected studies of acoustic parameters in the speech of indviduals with voice disorders.

Author(s) (Year)	Findings
Dickson (1962)	Reduction of F1 intensity, intensity of high-frequency harmonics, overall intensity of vowels, extra resonances between vowel formants, resonance just above F1, antiresonance and increase of bandwidth of formants were compared among 20 C Ss, 20 Ss with functional nasality and 20 Ss with cleft palate and nasality. Spectrographic signs of nasality were fewest for the C group, more frequent for the functional group and most frequent for the cleft palate group.
Yangihara (1967)	Vowels produced by 30 Ss with hoarseness included noise components in the main formants, noise components above 3KHz and loss of high-frequency harmonic components.
Rontal, Rontal and Rolnick (1975)	Spectrograms were used to illustrate patterns of vocal disorders in comparison to normal voice production.
Wolfe and Bacon (1976)	Spectrographic comparisons of the speech of 2 spastic dysphonic speakers in which one S's voice was characterized by breathiness by breakdown in formant structure or as the addition of fricative fill superimposed upon resonance bars. The second S's strained-strangle phonation was characterized by widely and irregularly spaced vertical striations.
Murry, Singh and Sargent (1977)	Fo, F1, F2 and amount of periodicity in the glottal waveform were compared with perceptual judgments and airflow for 20 samples of speech from voice disordered Ss. Multi-dimensional analysis indicated that glottal

periodicity, Fo and F2 were discriminating measures for different dimensions.

Weinberg, Horii and Smith (1980)

Speech intensity and long-term averaged spectra were compared between 10 oesophageal and 5 C speakers. Oesophageal speakers had less intense speech and flattened spectral envelopes as compared with C Ss.

Lebrun, Devreux, Rousseau and Darimont (1982)

Tremulous voice characteristics in 1 S are described using narrow and wideband spectrograms. Fo variations, oscillations, vocal arrests and other phenomena are discussed.

Yumoto (1983)

Harmonic/noise (H/N) ratio was used to evaluate 69 Ss with voice disorders and 42 C Ss. H/N ratio was shown to be an effective assessment technique.

Isshiki, Ohkawa and Goto (1985)

Narrow band spectrograms were used to illustrate pre- and post-surgical voice production differences for vowels in Ss with vocal cord stiffness. Generally, Fo was lowered, intensity increased and less noise was noted in some cases.

Robbins, Christensen and Kempster (1986)

VOT and VD were compared among 15 tracheoesophageal (TE), 15 oesophageal (E) and 15 C speakers. TE Ss produced significantly shorter VOTs and longer VDs than Cs.

Lee, Chamberlain, Loudon and Stemple (1988)

VOT, word duration, pause time, total duration, total syllables per breath and average SPL were compared between 16 asthmatic and 10 C Ss. Asthmatics differed from Cs in pause time and syllables per breath.

Gramming and Åkerlund (1988)

Phonetogram comparisons between 37 Ss with non-organic dysphonia and 29 Cs showed that females with voice disorders had significantly lower SPL values for loudest phonation when compared with healthy females, and male dysphonic Ss had significantly higher SPLs than male C Ss in softest phonation.

Sasaki, Okamura and Yumoto (1991)

Section displays of sustained /a/ by 54 voice disordered and 37 Cs were analysed for acoustic energy of voice (V) versus noise (N). Most appropriate filter band widths for the measurements were 22.5Hz (males) and 37.5Hz (females). The N/V ratio correlated significantly with the listener's grading of hoarseness.

Haapanen and Iivonen (1992)

Averaged sound spectra were compared among 4 Ss with a Sanvenero-Rosselli (SR) and 4 Ss with a modified Honig (MH) velopharyngeal flap as well as 4 Cs. Spectra for the MH Ss more closely resemble those of the Cs.

Shoji, Regenbogen, Yu and Blaugrund (1992)	FFT power spectra were compared between 24 Ss with breathy voices and 16 Cs. The Fo of 6 kHz was found to significantly separate breathy from normal voices. Three breathy Ss studied after thyroplasty showed a large drop in the high-frequency power ratio.
Roy and Leeper (1993)	Jitter, shimmer and signal-to-noise ratio (SNR) were compared pre-and post-treatment for 17 Ss with functional dysphonia. Shimmer and SNR were significantly reduced, while jitter differences approached but did not reach significance.
Kitzing and Åkerlund (1993)	Long-time averaged voice spectrograms were used to compare pre- and post-therapy parameters for 174 Ss with functional voice disorders. F1 significantly increased in all Ss; Fo increased in female Ss; quality ratings and spectra parameters were weakly, positively correlated.
Cannito, Ege, Ahmed and Wagner (1994)	Durations in diadokokinetic and trisyllable production were compared between 10 female Ss with spasmodic dysphonia (SD) and 10 matched Cs in three voicing conditions. SD Ss were generally slower than Cs; adductor SD Ss were slower than abductor SD Ss.
McAllister, Sederholm, Sundberg and Gramming (1994)	Pitch and intensity ranges of 60 children's voices were analysed using voice range profiles (VRPs). VRPs differentiated children with chronic hoarseness, nodules and glottal chinks.
Fex, Fex, Shiromoto and Hirano (1994)	Pitch perturbation quotient, normalized noise energy for 1–4 kHz and Fo showed significant improvement in 10 voice disordered Ss pre- and post-accent method voice therapy.
Naranjo, Lara, Rodríguez and García (1994)	Power spectra between 6–10 and 10–16 kHz were compared between 6 dysphonic and 6 C Ss. Power spectra for the dysphonic Ss were significantly higher than those for the C group at both frequency ranges.
Wolfe, Fitch and Cornell (1995)	Jitter, shimmer and harmonic/noise ratio were compared with judged severity of voice problems for 20 normal and 60 voice-disordered Ss. None of the acoustic variables nor any combination was found to be significantly correlated with dysphonia ratings.
de Krom (1995)	Harmonic/noise ratio was found to be the best single predictor of judged breathiness in 78 speakers with normal and voice disorders.

noise ratio (Yumoto, 1983) is a good index of amount of hoarseness in the voice, and Sasaki *et al* (1991) describe another measure that compares the energy of noise with the energy of the voice component (N/V) to estimate the amount of hoarseness. The phonetogram provides a method of analysing vocal sound pressure level (Gramming and Åkerlund, 1988). Degree of breathiness can be estimated from FFT power spectra (Shoji *et al*, 1992).

When acoustic techniques are compared with perceptual judgments of vocal parameters, the results have been mixed. Wolfe, Fitch and Cornell (1995) found no correlation between jitter, shimmer and harmonic/noise ratio and judged severity of voice disorders. However, de Krom (1995) found that harmonic/noise ratio was the best predictor of judged breathiness. Research defining the utility of these acoustic measuring techniques will probably continue to grow with advances in technology.

Clinical rewards for all of this effort not only include improved services to patients, but provide a method for objectively and permanently documenting vocal change. Examples of pre- and post-treatment studies that have shown changes in various disordered populations include vocal cord stiffness (Isshiki *et al*, 1985), velopharyngeal flap surgery (Haapanen and Iivonen, 1992) and functional dysphonia (Kitzing and Åkerlund, 1993; Roy and Leeper, 1993). Acoustic analysis is an ideal merger for clinical and research interests.

Conclusion

The first version of this chapter (Farmer, 1984) ended with the argument that research justified the use of spectrography in every speech-language clinic and that every speech-language student should be trained to use this instrumentation. Unfortunately, the cost of the instrumentation at that time prohibited this ideal state. Fortunately, circumstances have changed. Not only is the instrumentation more powerful and flexible than it was then, but it is also less expensive. Most university laboratories and clinics should definitely be able to assemble a system for teaching and research purposes. As most departments already have personal computers, only minimal hardware and a software package need to be purchased. Students reading this chapter may already have or be planning to purchase their own acoustic analysis system. Once students are trained to use the instrumentation, they will demand that it be a basic professional tool. Increased access to and use of spectrography in clinics and other professional settings by well-trained professionals will be a considerable scientific achievement by our profession. Finally, the Internet contains a number of sources for phonetics, linguistics and other speech and hearing topics. Students will find these sites informative and supportive for acoustic research.

References

Adams MR. Voice onsets and segment durations of normal speakers and beginning stutterers. Journal of Fluency Disorders 1987; 12: 133–39.

Adams SG. Accelerating speech in a case of hypokinetic dysarthria. In Till JA, Yorkston KM, Beukelman DR. (Eds), Motor Speech Disorders: Advances in Assessment and Treatment, pp. 213–28. Baltimore: Paul H. Brookes, 1994.

Agnello J, Wingate ME, Wendell M. Voice onset and termination times of children and adult stutterers. Journal of the Acoustical Society of America 1974; 56: 697.

Angelocci AA, Kopp GA, Holbrook A. The vowel formants of deaf and normal-hearing eleven- to fourteen-year-old boys. Journal of Speech and Hearing Disorders 1964; 29: 156–70.

Ansel BM, Kent RD. Acoustic-phonetic contrasts and intelligibility in the dysarthria associated with mixed cerebral palsy. Journal of Speech and Hearing Research 1992; 35: 296–308.

Armson J, Kalinowski J. Interpreting results of the fluent speech paradigm in stuttering research: difficulties in separating cause from effect. Journal of Speech and Hearing Research 1994; 37: 69–82.

Baken RJ. Clinical Measurement of Speech and Voice. Boston: Little, Brown, 1987.

Baum SR. The influence of word length on syllable duration in aphasia: acoustic analyses. Aphasiology 1992; 6: 501–13.

Baum SR. An acoustic analysis of rate of speech effects on vowel production in aphasia. Brain and Language 1993; 44: 414–30.

Baum SR, Ryan L. Rate of speech effects in aphasia: voice onset time. Brain and Language 1993; 44: 431–45.

Baum SR, Blumstein SE, Naeser MA, Palumbo CL. Temporal dimensions of consonant and vowel production: an acoustic and CT scan analysis of aphasic speech. Brain and Language 1990; 39: 33–56.

Bielamowicz S, Kreiman J, Gerratt BR, Dauer MS, Berke GS. Comparison of voice analysis systems for perturbation measurement. Journal of Speech and Hearing Research 1996; 39: 126–34.

Blumstein SE, Cooper WE, Goodglass H, Statlender S, Gottlieb J. Production deficits in aphasia: a voice-onset-time analysis. Brain and Language 1980; 9: 153–70.

Borden GJ, Kim DH, Spiegler K. Acoustics of stop consonant-vowel relationships during fluent and stuttered utterances. Journal of Fluency Disorders 1987; 12: 175–84.

Brayton ER, Conture EG. Effects of noise and rhythmic stimulation on the speech of stutterers. Journal of Speech and Hearing Research 1978; 21: 285–94.

Brown WS, Goldberg DM. An acoustic study of the intelligible utterances of hearing-impaired speakers. Folia Phoniatrica 1990; 42: 230–38.

Campbell TF, Dollaghan CA. Speaking rate, articulatory speed and linguistic processing in children and adolescents with severe traumatic brain injury. Journal of Speech and Hearing Research 1995; 38: 864–75.

Cannito MP, Ege P, Ahmed F, Wagner S. Diadichokinesis for complex trisyllables in individuals with spasmodic dysphonia and nondisabled subjects. In Till JA, Yorkston KM, Beukelman DR. (Eds), Motor Speech Disorders: Advances in Assessment and Treatment, pp. 91–100. Baltimore: Paul H. Brookes, 1994.

Carney AF, Gandour J, Petty SH, Robbins, AM, Myres W, Miyamoto R. The effect of adventitious deafness on the perception and production of voice onset time in Thai: a case study. Language and Speech 1988; 31: 273–82.

Caruso AJ, Burton EK. Temporal acoustic measures of dysarthria associated with amyotrophic lateral sclerosis. Journal of Speech and Hearing Research 1987; 30: 80–87.

Catts HW, Jensen PJ. Speech timing of phonologically disordered children: voicing contrasts of initial and final stop consonants. Journal of Speech and Hearing Research 1983; 26: 501–10.

Chaney C. Acoustic analysis of correct and misarticulated semivowels. Journal of Speech and Hearing Research 1988; 31: 275–87.

Code C, Ball M. Fricative production in Broca's aphasia: a spectrographic analysis. Journal of Phonetics 1982; 10: 325–31.

Cohen NS. The effect of singing instruction on the speech production of neurologically impaired persons. Journal of Music Therapy 1992; 29: 87–102.

Colcord RD, Adams MR. Voicing duration and vocal SPL changes associated with stuttering reduction during singing. Journal of Speech and Hearing Research 1979; 22: 468–79.

Collins M, Rosenbek JC, Wertz RT. Spectrographic analysis of vowel and word duration in apraxia of speech. Journal of Speech and Hearing Research 1983; 26: 224–30.

Crary MA. Developmental Motor Speech Disorders. San Diego: Singular, 1993.

Daniloff RG, Wilcox K, Stephens MI. An acoustic-articulatory description of children's defective Isl productions. Journal of Communication Disorders 1980; 13: 347–63.

de Janette G. Formant fequencies (F-sub-1, F-sub-2) of jaw-free versus jaw-fixed vowels in normal and articulatory disordered children. Perceptual and Motor Skills 1988; 67: 963–71.

de Krom G. Some spectral correlates of pathological breathy and rough voice quality for different types of vowel fragments. Journal of Speech and Hearing Research 1995; 38: 794–811.

DeNil LF, Brutten GJ. Voice onset times of stuttering and nonstuttering children: the influence of externally and linguistically imposed time pressure. Journal of Fluency Disorders 1991; 16: 143–58.

DeFeo AB, Schaefer CM. Bilateral facial paralysis in a preschool child: oral-facial and articulatory characteristics (a case study). In Berry WR. (Ed.), Clinical Dysarthria, pp. 165–86. San Diego: College-Hill Press, 1983.

Delattre, P. Some factors of vowel duration and their cross-linguistic validity. Journal of the Acoustical Society of America 1962; 34: 1141–42.

Di Simoni FG. Preliminary study of certain timing relationships in the speech of stutterers. Journal of the Acoustical Society of America 1974; 56: 695–96.

Dickson DR. An acoustic study of nasality. Journal of Speech and Hearing Research 1962; 5: 103–11.

Dromey C, Ramig LO, Johnson AB. Phonatory and articulatory changes associated with increased vocal intensity in Parkinson disease: a case study. Journal of Speech and Hearing Research 1995; 38: 751–64.

Duffy JR, Gawle CA. Apraxic speakers' vowel duration in consonant-vowel-consonant syllables. In Rosenbek JC, McNeil MR, Aronson AE. (Eds), Apraxia of Speech: Physiology, Acoustics, Linguistics, Management, pp. 167–96. San Diego: College-Hill Press, 1984.

Economou A, Tartter VC, Chute PM, Hellman SA. Speech changes following reimplantation from a single-channel to a multichannel cochlear implant. Journal of the Acoustical Society of America 1992; 92: 1310–23.

Edwards J. Compensatory speech motor abilities in normal and phonologically disordered children. Journal of Phonetics 1992; 20: 189–207.

Eguchi S, Hirsh IJ. Development of speech sounds in children. Acta Oto-Laryngologica 1969; Suppl. 257: 5–48.

Falck FJ, Lawler PS, Yonovitz A. Effects of stuttering on fundamental frequency. Journal of Fluency Disorders 1985; 10: 123–35.

Farmer A. Stop cognate production patterns in adult athetotic cerebral palsied speakers. Folia Phoniatrica 1977; 29: 154–62.

Farmer A. Voice onset time production in cerebral palsied speakers. Folia Phoniatrica 1980; 32: 267–73.

Farmer A. Spectrography. In Code C, Ball M. (Eds), Instrumentation in Speech-Language Pathology, pp. 21–40. San Diego: College-Hill Press, 1984.

Farmer A, Florance KM. Segmental duration differences: language disordered and normal children. In Andews J, Burns MS. (Eds), Selected Papers in Language Disorders (Vol. 2). Evanston, IL: Institute for Continuing Professional Education, 1977.

Farmer A, Lencione RM. An extraneous vocal behaviour in cerebral palsied speakers. British Journal of Disorders of Communication 1977; 12: 109–18.

Farmer A, Green WB. Differential effects of auditory masking on cerebral palsied speakers. Journal of Phonetics 1978; 6: 127–32.

Farmer A, Brayton ER. Speech characteristics of fluent and nonfluent Down's Syndrome adults. Folia Phoniatrica 1979; 31: 284–90.

Fex B, Fex S, Shiromoto O, Hirano M. Acoustic analysis of functional dysphonia: before and after voice therapy (accent method). Journal of Voice 1994; 8: 163–67.

Forrest K, Rockman BK. Acoustic and perceptual analysis of word-initial stop consonants in phonologically disordered children. Journal of Speech and Hearing Research 1988; 31: 449–59.

Forrest K, Weismer G, Hodge M, Dinnsen D, Elbert M. Statistical analysis of word initial /k/ and /t/ produced by normal and phonologically disordered children. Clinical Linguistics and Phonetics 1990; 4: 327–40.

Freeman FJ, Sands ES, Harris KS. Temporal coordination of phonation and articulation in a case of verbal apraxia: a voice onset time study. Brain and Language 1978; 6: 106–11.

Gandour J, Petty SH, Dardarananda R. Dysprosody in Broca's aphasia: a case study. Brain and Language 1989; 37: 232–57.

Gandour J, Ponglorpisit S, Khunadorn F, Dechongkit S, Boongird S, Boonklam R. Timing characteristics of speech after brain damage: vowel length in Thai. Brain and Language 1992a; 42: 337–45.

Gandour J, Ponglorpisit S, Khunadorn F, Dechongkit S, Boongird P, Boonklam R. Stop voicing in Thai after unilateral brain damage. Aphasiology 1992b; 6: 535–47.

Gandour J, Ponglorpisit S, Dechongkit S, Khunadorn F, Boongird P, Potisuk P. Anticipatory tonal coarticulation in Thai noun compounds after unilateral brain damage. Brain and Language 1993; 45: 1–20.

Gandour J, Dechongkit S, Ponglorpisit S, Khunadorn F, Boongird P. Intraword timing relations in Thai after unilateral brain damage. Brain and Language 1993; 45: 160–79.

Gierut JA, Dinnsen DA. On word-initial voicing: converging sources of evidence in phonologically disordered speech. Language and Speech 1986; 29: 97–114.

Gilbert HR, Campbell MI. Voice onset time in the speech of hearing impaired individuals. Folia Phoniatrica 1978; 30: 67–81

Glasson C. Speech timing in children with history of phonological-phonetic disorders. Seminars in Speech and Language 1984; 5: 85–95.

Gramming P, Åkerlund L. Non-organic dysphonia: II. Phonetograms for normal and pathological voices. Acta Otolaryngologica 1988; 106: 468–76.

Haapanen M-L, Iivonen A. Sound spectra in cleft palate patients with a Sanvenero-Rosselli and modified Honig secondary velopharyngeal flap. Folia Phoniatrica 1992; 44: 291–96.

Hakel ME, Healey EC, Sullivan M. Comparisons of fundamental frequency measures of speakers with dysarthria and hyperfunctional voice disorders. In Till JA, Yorkston KM, Beukelman DR. (Eds), Motor Speech Disorders: Advances in Assessment and Treatment, pp. 193–203. Baltimore: Paul H. Brookes, 1994.

Hall KD, Yairi E. Fundamental frequency, jitter, and shimmer in preschoolers who stutter. Journal of Speech and Hearing Research 1992; 35: 1002–8.

Hall PK, Jordan LS, Robin DA. Developmental Apraxia of Speech: Theory and Clinical Practice. Austin, TX: Pro-ed, 1993.

Hambly RM, Farmer A. An analysis of vowel duration in a group of language disordered children exhibiting the open syllable pattern. Folia Phoniatrica 1982; 34: 65–70.

Harteluis L, Nord L, Buder EH. Acoustic analysis of dysarthria associated with multiple sclerosis. Clinical Linguistics and Phonetics 1995; 9: 95–120.

Healey EC, Adams MR. Speech timing skills of normally fluent and stuttering children and adults. Journal of Fluency Disorders 1981; 6: 233–46.

Healey EC, Gutkin B. Analysis of stutterers' voice onset times and fundamental frequency contours during fluency. Journal of Speech and Hearing Research 1984; 27: 219–25.

Healey EC, Ramig PR. Acoustic measures of stutterers' and non-stutterers' fluency in two speech contexts. Journal of Speech and Hearing Research 1986; 29: 325–31.

Healey EC, Ramig PR. The relationship of stuttering severity and treatment length to temporal measures of stutterers' perceptually fluent speech. Journal of Speech and Hearing Disorders 1989; 4: 313–19.

Hillman RE, Gilbert HR. Voice onset time for voiceless consonants in the fluent reading of stutterers and nonstutterers. Journal of the Acoustical Society of America 1977; 61: 610–11.

Hoffman PR, Stager S, Daniloff RG. Perception and production of misarticulated /r/. Journal of Speech and Hearing Disorders 1983; 48: 210–15.

House AS, Fairbanks G. The influence of consonant environment upon the secondary acoustical characteristics of vowels. Journal of the Acoustical Society of America 1953; 25: 105–13.

Howell P, Vause L. Acoustic analysis and perception of vowels in stuttered speech. Journal of the Acoustical Society of America 1986; 79: 1571–79.

Howell P, Williams M. Acoustic analysis and perception of vowels in childen's and teenagers' stuttered speech. Journal of the Acoustical Society of America 1992; 91: 1697–706.

Huer MB. Acoustic tracking of articulation errors: (r). Journal of Speech and Hearing Disorders 1989; 54: 530–34.

Isshiki N, Ohkawa M, Goto M. Stiffness of the vocal cord in dysphonia – lts assessment and treatment. Acta Otolaryngologica 1985; suppl 419: 167–74.

Itoh M, Sasanuma S. Articulatory movements in apraxia of speech. In Rosenbek JC, McNeil MR, Aronson AE. (Eds), Apraxia of speech: Physiology, acoustics, linguistics. management, pp. 135–166. San Diego: College-Hill Press, 1984.

Jancke L. Variation and duration of voice onset time and phonation in stuttering and nonstuttering adults. Journal of Fluency Disorders 1994; 19: 21–37.

Kent RD. Vocal tract acoustics. Journal of Voice 1993; 7: 97–117.

Kent JF, Kent RD, Rosenbek JC, Weismer G, Martin RE, Sufit RL, Brooks BR. Quantitative description of the dysarthria in women with amyotrophic lateral sclerosis. Journal of Speech and Hearing Research 1992; 35: 723–33.

Kent RD, Rosenbek JC. Prosodic disturbance and neurologic lesion. Brain and Language 1982; 15: 259–91.

Kent RD, Rosenbek JC. Acoustic patterns of apraxia of speech. Journal of Speech and

Hearing Research 1983; 26: 231–49.

Kent RD, Read C. The Acoustic Analysis of Speech. San Diego: Singular Publishing Group, 1992.

Kent RD, Netsell R, Abbs JH. Acoustic characteristics of dysarthria associated with cerebellar disease. Journal of Speech and Hearing Research 1979; 22: 627–48.

Kent RD, Osberger MJ, Netsell R, Hustedde CG. Phonetic development in identical twins differing in auditory function. Journal of Speech and Hearing Disorders 1987; 52: 64–75.

Kent RD, Kent JF, Weismer G, Sufit RL, Brooks BR, Rosenbek JC. Relationships between speech intelligibility and the slope of second formant transitions in dysarthric subjects.Clinical Linguistics & Phonetics 1989; 3: 347–58.

Kitzing P, Åkerlund L. Long-time average spectrograms of dysphonic voices before and after therapy. Folia Phoniatrica 1993; 45: 53–61.

Klich R, May G. Spectrographic study of vowels in stutterers' fluent speech. Journal of Speech and Hearing Disorders 1982; 25: 364–70.

LaPointe LL, Case JL, Duane DD. Perceptual-acoustic speech and voice characteristics of subjects with spasmodic torticollis. In Till JA, Yorkston KM, Beukelman DR (Eds), Motor Speech Disorders: Advances in Assessment and Treatment, pp. 57–64. Baltimore: Paul H. Brookes, 1994.

Lass NJ. (Ed.) Principles of Experimental Phonetics. St. Louis: Mosby, 1996.

Lebrun Y, Devreux F, J-J Rousseau, Darimont P. Tremulous speech: a case report. Folia Phoniatrica 1982; 34: 134–42.

Leder SB, Spitzer JB, Milner P, Flevaris-Phillips C, Richardson F, Kirchner JC. Reacquisition of contrastive stress in an adventitiously deaf speaker using a single channel cochlear implant. Journal of the Acoustical Society of America 1986; 79: 1967–74.

Lee L, Chamberlain LG, Loudon RG, Stemple JC. Speech segment durations produced by healthy and asthmatic subjects. Journal of Speech and Hearing Disorders 1988; 53: 186–93.

Leeper HA, Perez DM, Mencke EO. Influence of utterance length upon temporal measures of syllable production by selected hearing-impaired children. Folia Phoniatrica 1987; 39: 230–43.

Lehiste I. Some acoustic characteristics of dysarthric speech. Bibliotheca Phonetica 1965; 2: 1–124.

Lehiste I. (Ed.) Readings in Acoustic Phonetics. Cambridge, MA: MIT Press, 1967.

Lehiste I. Suprasegmental features of speech. In Lass NJ. (Ed.), Contemporary Issues in Experimental Phonetics, 1–124. New York: Academic Press, 1976.

Lieberman P, Kako E, Friedman J, Tajchman G, Feldman LS, Jiminez EB. Speech production, syntax comprehension, and cognitive deficits in Parkinson's disease. Brain and Language 1992; 43:169–89.

Lisker L, Abramson AS. A cross-language study of voicing in initial stops: acoustical measurements. Word 1964; 20: 384–422.

Ludlow CL, Bassich CJ. The results of acoustic and perceptual assessment of two types of dysarthria. In Berry WR. (Ed.), Clinical Dysarthria, pp. 121–54. San Diego: College-Hill Press, 1983.

Mallard AR, Westbrook JB. Vowel duration in stutterers participating in precision fluency shaping. Journal of Fluency Disorders 1985; 10: 221–28.

Maxwell E, Weismer G. The contribution of phonological, acoustic, and perceptual techniques to the characterization of a misarticulating child's voice contrast for stops. Applied Psycholinguistics 1982; 3: 29–43.

McAllister A, Sederholm E, Sundberg J, Gramming P. Relations between voice range profiles and physiological and perceptual voice characteristics in ten-year-old children. Journal of Voice 1994; 8: 230–39.

McFarlane SC. Videolaryngoendoscopy. Seminars in Speech and Language 1990; 11: 1–59.

McKnight RC, Cullinan WL. Subgroups of stuttering children: speech and voice reaction times, segmental durations, and naming latencies. Journal of Fluency Disorders 1987; 12: 217–33.

McLeod S, Isaac K. Use of spectrographic analyses to evaluate the efficacy of phonological intervention. Clinical Linguistics and Phonetics 1995; 9: 229–34.

McNeil MR, Liss J, Tseng C-H, Kent RD. Effects of speech rate on absolute and relative timing of apraxic and conduction aphasic sentence production. Brain and Language 1990; 38: 135–58.

Metz DE, Conture EG, Caruso A. Voice onset time, frication and aspiration during stutterers' fluent speech. Journal of Speech and Hearing Research 1979; 22: 649–56.

Metz DE, Samar VJ, Schiavetti N, Sitler RW, Whitehead RL. Acoustic dimensions of hearing impaired speakers' intelligibility. Journal of Speech and Hearing Research 1985; 28: 345–55.

Metz DE, Schiavetti N, Sacco PR. Acoustic and psychophysical dimensions of the perceived speech naturalness of non-stutterers and post-treatment stutterers. Journal of Speech and Hearing Disorders 1990; 55: 516–25.

Monsen RB. Durational aspects of vowel production in the speech of deaf children. Journal of Speech and Hearing Research 1974; 17: 386–98.

Monsen RB. Normal and reduced phonological space: the production of English vowels by deaf adolescents. Journal of Phonetics 1976; 4: 189–98.

Monsen RB. Toward measuring how well hearing-impaired children speak. Journal of Speech and Hearing Research 1978; 21: 197–219.

Morris RJ. VOT and dysarthria: a descriptive study. Journal of Communication Disorders 1989; 22: 23–33.

Mulder HE, Van Olphen AF, Bosma A, Smoorenburg GF. Phoneme recognition by deaf individuals using the multichannel nucleus cochlear implant. Acta-Otolaryngolica 1992; 112: 946–55.

Mulligan M, Carpenter J, Riddel J, Delaney MK, Badger G, Krusinski P, Tandan R. Intelligibility and the acoustic characteristics of speech in amyotrophic lateral sclerosis. Journal of Speech and Hearing Research 1994; 37: 496–503.

Murry T, Singh S, Sargent M. Multidimensional classification of abnormal voice qualities. Journal of the Acoustical Society of America 1977; 61: 1630–35.

Naranjo NV, Lara EM, Rodríguez IM, García GC. High-frequency components of normal and dysphonic voices. Journal of Voice 1994; 8: 157–62.

Ohde RN, Sharf DJ. Phonetic Analysis of Normal and Abnormal Speech. New York: Merrill, 1992.

Oller DK, Eilers RE, Bull DH, Carney AE. Prespeech vocalizations of a deaf infant: a comparison with normal metaphonological development. Journal of Speech and Hearing Research 1985; 28: 47–63.

Onslow M, van Doorn J, Newman D. Variability of acoustic segment durations after prolonged - speech treatment for stuttering. Journal of Speech and Hearing Research 1992; 35: 529–36.

Orlikoff RF, Baken RJ. Clinical Speech and Voice Measurement: Laboratory Exercises. San Diego: Singular Publishing Group, 1993.

Osberger MJ. Training effects on vowel production by two profoundly hearing-impaired speakers. Journal of Speech and Hearing Research 1987; 30: 241–51.

Osberger MJ, Levitt H. The effect of timing errors on the intelligibility of deaf children's speech. Journal of the Acoustical Society of America 1979; 66: 1316–24.

Peterson GE, Barney HL. Control methods used in a study of the vowels. The Journal of the Acoustical Society of America 1952; 24: 175–84.

Pindzola RH. Acoustic evidence of abberant velocities in stutterers' fluent speech. Perceptual and Motor Skills 1986; 62: 399–405.

Potter RK, Kopp GA, Kopp HG. Visible Speech. New York: Dover, 1966.

Prosek RA, Montgomery AA, Walden BE, Hawkins DB. Formant frequencies of stuttered and fluent vowels. Journal of Speech and Hearing Research 1987; 30: 301–5.

Ramig PR. Rate changes in the speech of stutterers after therapy. Journal of Fluency Disorders 1984; 9: 285–94.

Ramig LO, Scherer RC, Klasner ER, Titze IR, Horii Y. Acoustic analysis of voice in amyotrophic lateral sclerosis: a longitudinal study. Journal of Speech and Hearing Disorders 1990; 55: 2–14.

Read C, Buder EH, Kent RD. Speech analysis systems: a survey. Journal of Speech and Hearing Research 1990; 33: 363–74.

Read C, Buder EH, Kent RD. Speech analysis systems: an evaluation. Journal of Speech and Hearing Research 1992; 35: 314–32.

Robb MP, Lybolt JT, Price HA. Acoustic measures of stutterers' speech following an intensive therapy program. Journal of Fluency Disorders 1985; 10: 269–79.

Robbins J, Christensen J, Kempster G. Characteristics of speech production after tracheoesophageal puncture: voice onset time and vowel duration. Journal of Speech and Hearing Research 1986; 29: 499–504.

Rontal E, Rontal M, Rolnick MI. Objective evaluation of vocal pathology using voice spectrography. Annals of Otology, Rhinology and Laryngology 1975; 84: 662–71.

Rothman H. An acoustic investigation of consonant-vowel transitions in the speech of deaf adults. Journal of Phonetics 1976; 4: 95–102.

Roy N, Leeper HA. Effects of manual laryngeal musculoskeletal tension reduction technique as a treatment for functional voice disorders: perceptual and acoustic measures. Journal of Voice 1993; 7: 242–49.

Ryalls JH. Note:Intonation in Broca's aphasia. Neuropsychologia 1982; 20: 355–60.

Ryalls JH. Some acoustic aspects of fundamental frequency of CVC utterances in aphasia. Phonetica 1984; 41: 103–11.

Ryalls JH. An acoustic study of vowel production in aphasia. Brain and Language 1986; 29: 48–67.

Ryalls J, Larouche A. Acoustic integrity of speech production in children with moderate and severe hearing impairment. Journal of Speech and Hearing Research 1992; 35: 88–95.

Sacco PR, Metz DE. Changes in stutterers' fundamental frequency contours following therapy. Journal of Fluency Disorders 1987; 12: 1–8.

Samar VJ, Metz DE, Schiavetti N, Sitler RW, Whitehead RL. Articulatory dimensions of hearing-impaired speakers' intelligibility: evidence from time-related aerodynamic, acoustic, and electroglottographic study. Journal of Communication Disorders 1989; 22: 243–64.

Sasaki Y, Okamura H, Yumoto E. Quantitative analysis of hoarseness using a digital sound spectrograph. Journal of Voice 1991; 5: 36–40.

Schwartz MF. Acoustic measures of nasalization and nasality. In Grabb WC, Rosenstein SW, Bzoch KR. (Eds), Cleft Lip and Palate: Surgical, Dental and Speech Aspects. Boston: Little, Brown and Co, 1971.

Seikel JA, Wilcox KA, Davis J. Dysarthria of motor neuron disease: longitudinal measures of segmental durations. Journal of Communication Disorders 1991; 24: 393–409.

Seikel JA, Wilcox KA, Davis J. Dysarthria of motor neuron disease: longitudinal measures of segmental durations: erratum. Journal of Communication Disorders 1992; 25: 210–13.

Shewan CM, Leeper HA, Booth JC. An analysis of voice onset time (VOT) in aphasic and normal speakers. In Rosenbek JC, McNeil MR, Aronson AE. (Eds), Apraxia of Speech: Physiology, Acoustics, Linguistics, Management, pp. 197–220. San Diego: College-Hill Press, 1984.

Shoji K, Regenbogen E, Yu JD, Blaugrund SM. High-frequency power ratio of breathy voice. Laryngoscope 1992; 102.

Shoup JE, Pfeifer LL. Acoustic characteristics of speech sounds. In Lass NJ. (Ed.), Contemporary Issues in Experimental Phonetics, New York: Academic Press, 1976.

Shukla RS. Phonological space in the speech of the hearing impaired. Journal of Communication Disorders 1989; 22: 317–25.

Smith B, Marquardt TP, Cannito MP, Davis BL. Vowel variability in developmental apraxia of speech. In Till JA, Yorkston KM, Beukelman DR. (Eds), Motor Speech Disorders: Advances in Assessment and Treatment, pp. 81–88. Baltimore: Paul H. Brookes, 1994.

Square-Storer PA, Apeldoorn S. An acoustic study of apraxia of speech in patients with different lesion loci. In Moore CA, Yorkston KM, Beukelman DR. (Eds), Dysarthria and Apraxia of Speech: Perspectives on Management, pp. 271–88. Baltimore: Paul H. Brookes, 1991.

Starkweather CW, Meyers M. Duration of subsegments within the inter-vocalic interval in stutterers and non-stutterers. Journal of Fluency Disorders 1979; 4: 205–14.

Stathopoulos ET, Duchan JF, Sonnenmeier RM, Bruce NV. Intonation and pausing in deaf speech. Folia Phoniatrica 1986; 38: 1–12.

Stevens KN, House AS. Development of a quantitative description of vowel articulation. Journal of the Acoustical Society of America 1955; 27: 484–93.

Throneburg RN, Yairi E. Temporal dynamics of repetitions during the early stage of childhood stuttering: an acoustic study. Journal of Speech and Hearing Research 1994; 37: 1067–75.

Tuller B, Story RS. Anticipatory and carryover coarticulation in aphasia: an acoustic study. Cognitive Neuropsychology 1988; 5: 747–71.

Turner GS, Weismer G. Characteristics of speaking rate in dysarthria associated with amyotrophic lateral sclerosis. Journal of Speech and Hearing Research 1993; 36: 1134–44.

Turner GS, Tjaden K, Weismer G. The influence of speaking rate on vowel space and speech intelligibility for individuals with amyotrophic lateral sclerosis. Journal of Speech and Hearing Research 1995; 38: 1001–13.

Tyler A, Saxman JH. Initial voicing contrast acquisition in normal and phonologically disordered children. Applied Psycholinguistics 1991; 12: 453–79.

Tyler A, Edwards M, Saxman J. Acoustic validation of phonological knowledge and its relationship to treatment. Journal of Speech and Hearing Disorders 1990; 55: 251–61.

Tyler RS, Preece JP, Lansing CR, Gantz BJ. Natural vowel perception by patients with the ineraid cochlear implant. Audiology 1992; 31: 228–39.

Umeda N. Vowel duration in American English. Journal of the Acoustical Society of America 1975; 58: 434–45.

Viswanath NS. Global- and local-temporal effects of a stuttering event in the context of a clausal utterance. Journal of Fluency Disorders 1989; 14: 245–69.

Viswanath NS, Neel AT. Part-word repetitions by persons who stutter: fragment types and their articulatory processes. Journal of Speech and Hearing Research 1995; 38: 740–50.

Walton JH, Pollock KE. Acoustic validation of vowel error patterns in developmental apraxia of speech. Clinical Linguistics and Phonetics 1993; 7: 95–111.

Watson BC, Alfonso PJ. A comparison of LRT and VOT values between stutterers and non-stutterers. Journal of Fluency Disorders 1982; 7: 219–41.

Weinberg B, Horri Y, Smith BE. Long-time spectral and intensity characteristics of esophageal speech. Journal of the Acoustical Society of America 1980; 67: 1781–84.

Weismer, G. Acoustic descriptions of dysarthric speech: perceptual correlates and physiological inferences. Seminars in Speech and Language 1984; 5: 293–314.

Weismer G, Elbert M. Temporal characteristics of 'functionally' misarticulated Isl in 4- to 6-year-old children. Journal of Speech and Hearing Research 1982; 25: 30–52.

Weismer G, Liss JM. Reductionism is a dead-end in speech research: perspectives on a new direction. In Moore CA, Yorkston KM, Beukelman DR. (Eds), Dysarthria and Apraxia of Speech: Perspectives on Management, pp. 15–27. Baltimore: Paul H. Brookes, 1991a.

Weismer G, Liss JM. Acoustic/perceptual taxonomies of speech production deficits in motor speech disorders. In Moore CA, Yorkston KM, Beukelman DR. (Eds), Dysarthria and Apraxia of Speech: Perspectives on Management, pp. 245–70. Baltimore: Paul H. Brookes, 1991b.

Weismer G, Martin R, Kent RD, Kent JF. Formant trajectory characteristics of males with amyotrophic lateral sclerosis. Journal of the Acoustical Society of America 1992; 91: 1085–98.

Winkler L, Ramig P. Temporal characteristics in the fluent speech of child stutterers and non-stutterers. Journal of Fluency Disorders 1986; 11: 217–29.

Wolfe VI, Bacon M. Spectrographic comparison of two types of spastic dysphonia. Journal of Speech and Hearing Disorders 1976; 41: 325–32.

Wolfe V, Fitch J, Cornell R. Acoustic prediction of severity in commonly occurring voice problems. Journal of Speech and Hearing Research 1995; 38: 273–79.

Yangihara N. Significance of harmonic changes and noise components in hoarseness. Journal of Speech and Hearing Research 1967; 10: 531–41.

Yaruss JS, Conture EG. F2 transitions during sound/syllable repetitions of children who stutter and predictions of stuttering chronicity. Journal of Speech and Hearing Research 1993; 36: 883–96.

Young EC, Gilbert HR. An analysis of stops produced by normal children and children who exhibit velar fronting. Journal of Phonetics 1988; 16: 243–46.

Yumoto E. The quantitative evaluation of hoarseness: a new harmonics to noise ration method. Archives of Otolaryngology 1983; 109: 48–52.

Zebrowski PM. Duration of the speech disfluencies of beginning stutterers. Journal of Speech and Hearing Research 1991; 34: 483–91.

Zebrowski PM. Duration of sound prolongation and sound/syllable repetition in children who stutter: preliminary observations. Journal of Speech and Hearing Research 1994; 37: 254–63.

Zebrowski PM, Conture EG, Cudahy EA. Acoustic analysis of young stutterers' fluency: preliminary observations. Journal of Fluency Disorders 1985; 110: 173–92.

Ziegler W, von Cramon D. Disturbed coarticulation in apraxia of speech: acoustic evidence. Brain and Language 1986; 29: 34–37.

Zimmerman SA, Sapon SM. Note on vowel duration seen cross-linguistically. Journal of the Acoustical Society of America 1958; 30: 152–53.

Chapter 3
Electromyography

MICHÈLE GENTIL AND WALTER H. MOORE

Introduction to Electromyography

A historical overview

Man has always been interested in the function of skeletal muscles. Aristotle, Galen, Leonardo da Vinci, and Vesalius (the 'father of modern anatomy') all showed great curiosity about the organs of locomotion and power (Singer, 1925). At the end of the eighteenth century, Galvani discovered that skeletal muscles contracted when stimulated electrically and that contracting muscles produce an electrical current or voltage. It was the German physiologist, Du Bois-Reymond, who was the first, in 1851, to measure the electrical activity from a contracting muscle (Dumoulin and Aucremanne, 1959). Yet, the exploitation of Galvani's finding was postponed until the twentieth century when a technique was developed for detecting and recording minute electrical discharges. This technique, known as electromyography (EMG), was developed by neurophysiologists, such as Adrian and Bronk (1929) and Smith (1934). But it was only at the end of World War II, when there was a marked improvement in the technology and electronic apparatus, that EMG began to be used by anatomists, kinesiologists, and clinicians. One of the most important early studies published that led to the general acceptance of EMG was that of Inman, Saunders and Abbot (1944), who investigated the movements of the shoulder region.

EMG is a technique suited to the analysis of skilled movements in general, and of speech movements in particular. It gives the opportunity to study the dynamics of speech production, not only by describing which muscles are contracting and when, but also through revealing the co-ordination of different muscles involved in any one speech gesture. Speech sounds have been described primarily in terms of the position and shapes of the organs of speech, and little attention has been paid to the means by which these were effected. By the 1950s, EMG investigations of speech activity were becoming more common: laryngeal muscles were studied by Faaborg-Andersen (1957), and by Sawashima, Sato, Funasaka and Totsuka (1958); respiratory muscles were investigated by Stetson (1951), and by Draper, Ladefoged and Whitteridge (1959). During the 1960s, EMG was used to study various speech organs, such as the lips (McNeilage 1963; Fromkin, 1966; Lysaught et al, 1961; Öhman, 1967; Öhman et al, 1965), the soft palate (Fritzell, 1963; 1969; Lubker, 1968), the tongue (MacNeilage and Sholes, 1964; Smith and Hirano, 1968), and the larynx (Faaborg-Andersen, 1964; Faaborg-Andersen and Vennard, 1964; Hirano et al, 1967). This pioneering electromyographic research into speech production involved single speech organs only. Then, several speech organs were studied at the same time (Sussman et al, 1973). Gay, Ushijima, Hirose and Cooper (1974) recorded EMG from muscles that control the movements of the lips, tongue and jaw. Folkins and Abbs (1975) studied labial compensation for unpredicted jaw loading: EMG activity was measured from three jaw muscles and one lip muscle. Tuller, Harris and Kelso (1982) and Tuller, Kelso and Harris (1982) observed the transformation of articulation, stress and rate using EMG and acoustic data: one lip muscle, one tongue muscle and three jaw muscles were recorded. Alfonso and Baer (1982) investigated the dynamics of vowel articulation: EMG signals were recorded from one lip muscle, one jaw muscle and two tongue muscles. More recently, much attention has been directed towards the interaction among speech muscles, because one muscle contracts in the context of many other opposing or augmenting forces (Folkins, 1981; Gentil and Gay, 1986; Gentil et al, 1983; Hirose, 1977; Honda et al, 1982; Tuller et al, 1981). Speech motor plasticity in the production of a particular spoken utterance, that is variations among a great number of muscles between several subjects, were also evaluated (Gentil, 1992).

EMG has been applied to the study and assessment of muscle and nerve pathology (Basmajian, 1962; Feinstein, 1945; Weddell et al, 1944), and the clinical significance of EMG as a diagnostic procedure for neuromuscular disorders has long been recognized. In particular, EMG is quite effective for the differentiation of neuropathy from myogenic disorders. EMG has also proved to be very useful in the rehabilitation clinic. Thus, in patients with dyskinesias (e.g. spasmodic torticollis), central palsy, and patients who have suffered stroke and have spasticity, relaxation therapy using EMG techniques enhances their subsequent training and development of improved performance (Andrews, 1964; Basmajian, Kukulka, Narayan and Tabeke, 1975; Brudny, Grynbaum and Korein, 1973; Johnson and Garton, 1973). For a review of biofeedback in medicine and psychotherapy, particularly EMG feedback, see Basmajian (1979) and Inglis, Campbell and Donald (1977). In speech pathology,

EMG is known to provide significant information on the abnormality of the articulatory and phonatory organs at the peripheral neuromuscular level. The application of EMG research and biofeedback to the field of speech disorders is reviewed below.

The physiological basis of electromyography

Motor unit

The structural unit of muscular activity is the muscle fibre which contracts when excited. Contraction is controlled by motoneurones. In 1925, Liddell and Sherrington introduced the term 'motor unit' to describe the smallest functional unit that can be controlled by the nervous system. The motor unit consists of a single motor neuron, its axon, and all the muscle fibres that it innervates. The number of muscle fibres in a motor unit varies from muscle to muscle according to the role they play in motor activity. Muscles requiring delicate adjustments have a small number of muscular fibres for each motor unit, whereas larger muscles requiring gross control have many fibres for each motor unit. For example, the cricothyroid muscle has from 30 to 165 muscular fibres per motor unit (English and Blevins, 1969; Faaborg-Andersen, 1957), and limb muscles have from 400 to 1700 fibres per motor unit (Buchtal, 1961). The range, force or type of movement are determined by the pattern of recruitment and the frequency of firing of different motor units. The motor unit can therefore be considered the elementary unit of behaviour in the motor system.

Neuromuscular junction and propagation of the impulse

The neuromuscular junction is the region where nerve and muscular fibres come into contact. A detailed account of the transmision of nerve impulses at the neuromuscular junction can be found in Eccles (1973), and in Katz (1962, 1966). When the action potential reaches the nerve endings, a transmitter (acetylcholine) is released from the presynaptic element of the junction and floods the postsynaptic membrane of the junction (motor endplate). Acetylcholine depolarizes this membrane and if the depolarization attains enough amplitude it will trigger a muscle action potential (MAP), which will be initiated in the adjacent muscle fibre, which contracts. According to Haines (1932, 1934) a muscle fibre decreases its resting length about 57% on contracting. Contraction of the muscle fibres is seen as electrical activity. Electrical discharges of the muscle fibres are brief and have an amplitude which is measured in microvolts (Basmajian, 1962). The detection and recording of MAPs is what is called EMG. Information about the physiological bases of EMG are to be found in Basmajian (1962), Lippold (1967) and Winter (1989). Concerning speech research especially, see Cooper (1965), Fromkin and Ladefoged (1966), Gay and Harris (1971), Gentil (1990a) and Harris (1981).

Recording and processing of the EMG

With the growing use of the EMG technique, reviews of some of problems and issues that are encountered during the recording of EMG data have been published (Fridlund and Cacioppo, 1986; Turker, 1993). In the same way, Loeb and Gans' book (1986) provides a good introduction to the methods of recording and analysis of EMG signals. Smith (1990) focuses on EMG techniques typically employed in studies of articulatory muscles in speech production. What follows is a brief review of notions relevant to EMG recording and processing.

Electrodes

MAPs are detected by transducers, that is electrodes, placed on the surface of a muscle or inside the muscle tissue. These record the algebraic sum of all MAPs being transmitted along the muscle fibres. Being fundamental components, the electrodes are particularly important, and certain criteria must be satisfied for a good recording. Electrodes are divided into two main classes: surface electrodes, and intramuscular electrodes. The choice between the two types depends on the kind of information needed. Surface electrodes show broad detection of aggregates of motor units that correlate with the global level of contraction of muscles underlying and near the electrodes (Lawrence and De Luca, 1983). Fuglevand, Winter, Patla and Stashuk (1992) mention that detection of MAPs with surface electrodes is influenced by electrode size and spacing. Intramuscular electrodes are preferable (1) when the target muscles are located rather deeply, and (2) for recording the MAPs of small peripheral muscles surrounded by many other muscles. Comparative studies of EMG from facial muscles obtained by surface electrodes on the one hand, and by intramuscular electrodes on the other hand, can be found in Koole, de Jongh and Boering (1991).

Surface pelletized silver–silver chloride electrodes are most commonly used. Surface electrodes detect the EMG signal through skin using a conductive paste or gel, and are used in a paired electrode configuration. All texts on EMG technique recommend careful preparation of the site to which the surface electrodes are to be placed to lower interelectrode impedance to 5–10 KΩ, especially when the EMG signals to be detected are very small. In spite of some disadvantages, the use of surface electrodes seems justified in clinical research and treatment because of the relative ease of application, reduced discomfort to the subject and non-invasive nature. Moreover, miniature surface electrodes can be used for EMG recording from facial muscles.

Among intramuscular electrodes, it is necessary to distinguish needle electrodes from hooked wire electrodes. The needle electrodes used in speech research are of the concentric type and bipolar: two insulated wires are carried in the needle and the region is sampled between their ends; the needle wall acts as an electrostatic shield. Needle electrodes are not really suited to the investigation of speech behaviour. Their rigidity and heavy weight can cause movement artefacts and significant subject discomfort. To circumvent these problems, hooked wire electrodes were developed by Basmajian and Stecko (1962). They are made by passing a loop of very fine insulated wire through a hypodermic needle. The insulation is removed, the wire is cut and the two free ends are folded back over the needle tip. The sterilized needle is inserted into the muscle and then withdrawn, the hooked portion of the wire becomes anchored in the muscle. Hooked wires have become the electrodes of choice for examining speech muscles. However, correct electrode positioning is very difficult and serious placement verification has to be done.

Electrode position and site specification

For surface electrodes in particular, precautions have to be taken concerning the position of the electrode relative to muscle tissue fibre size, location and orientation: a paired electrode placement parallel to the course of the muscle fibres maximizes selectivity. Moreover, it is necessary to be careful with (1) electrode attachment to sites: skinfolds and bony obstructions are to be avoided, (2) EMG activities of straddling muscles. Anatomical and electrophysiological data suggest that even with intramuscular electrodes the probability of recording from a single muscle of the lip in isolation is extremely low (Blair and Smith, 1986).

Accurate location of electrodes requires clear anatomical guidelines together with reliable physiological data on the functions of the muscles under study. No EMG site 'atlas' is available for the facial musculature. Agreement among researchers about electrode placements is absolutely necessary to ensure that findings across studies are comparable. The question of the relation between potentials observed at different electrode sites in the same muscle has been raised in some papers, and noteworthy differences in EMG signals recorded from different points in various muscles involved in speech have been demonstrated (Cooper and Folkins, 1985). Besides, Abbs, Gracco and Blair (1984) indicated that the orbicularis inferior muscle is composed of several functional subdivisions. In the same way, the independent functions of the two heads of the lateral pterygoid muscle were demonstrated (Gentil and Gay, 1986; McNamara, 1973; Tuller, Harris and Gross, 1981). For standardizing electrode placements in orofacial and mandibular muscles, various works have been used: Fridlund and Izard (1983), Gross and Lipke (1979), Hirose (1971), Hirose, Gay and Strome (1971), Isley and Basmajian (1973), Kennedy and Abbs (1979), Leanderson, Persson and Öhman (1971), Möller (1966), O'Dwyer, Quinn, Guitar, Andrews and Neilson (1981).

Amplifiers

The EMG signal is characterized by very small amplitudes measured in microvolts. These must be increased by use of an amplifier. A biological amplifier of certain specifications is required for the recording of the EMG. The major characteristics to take into consideration are the following: input impedance, frequency response, gain and dynamic range, and common mode rejection.

The input impedance (resistance) of a biological amplifier must be sufficiently high so as not to attenuate the EMG signal as it is connected to the input terminals of the amplifier.

The frequency bandwidth of the amplifier should be such as to amplify, without attenuation, all frequencies present in the EMG. The spectrum of the EMG has been widely reported in the literature with a range of 5–2000 Hz. A recommended range for surface electrodes is 10–1000 Hz, and 20–2000 Hz for intramuscular electrodes.

The signal has to be amplified linearly. The larger signals (up to 10 mV) must be amplified as much as the smaller signals (50 μV and below). The dynamic range of the amplifier must be such that the largest EMG signal does not exceed this range.

The human body is a good conductor and acts as an antenna to pick up any electromagnetic radiation. Noise reduction is facilitated by using differential amplifiers to amplify the voltage difference between two points, neither of which is earthed. An identical voltage at both amplifier inputs is a common mode voltage. The ability to eliminate such a signal from the final output is a feature of differential amplifiers. This capability is quantified by the common mode rejection ratio (CMRR), that is the gain of a common mode signal which is expressed in dB. A high CMRR (100 dB or better) is very important to reduce noise (Baken, 1987).

EMG visualization and acquisition

Once an electrical signal is amplified, it must be displayed and recorded. The EMG signal can be seen on an oscilloscope. The appearance of the electromyogram will depend on the size of muscle detected by the electrodes and on the force of contraction. The number of spikes per second of electrical activity is a direct measure of the degree of muscle activation. Normal muscle contraction is the result of the firing of many motor units. The muscle fibres lying between the electrodes belong to different motor units and their firing will be asynchronous. The EMG signal is the sum of the electrical actions and this summation results in an interference pattern. The raw signal is a train of MAPs. Classically, the signal was rectified and integrated (integration is the terminal summation of EMG activity), and recorded on an FM tape recorder for off-line processing. But with today's technology computer digitizing and recording are now quite common. Using a computer requires that signal sampling rates, A/D converter precision and signal gain used to feed the A/D converter, be carefully taken into consideration. There is a danger in undersampling because one cannot know the temporal dynamics of the EMG signal, which may contain valuable information about muscular action. A good rule of thumb is to sample at 4–6 times the highest frequency. Very precise A/D converters allow amplification gain to be such that very weak or very strong muscle actions can be detected precisely. These complex notions cannot be examined in the limited scope of this chapter.

Research and Therapeutic Application of EMG to Speech-Language Disorders

In speech-language disorders, EMG procedures are used (1) for assessing muscle functions, and (2) for biofeedback-based treatment. In both these cases, the EMG technique serves to increase the quantity and quality of information about the patient's functioning. In assessment, such information should help both to identify the critical features that are contributors to the speech disorder, and to determine an appropriate treatment. In treatment, such information is given back to the patient by means of biofeedback methods; the myoelectric signals are translated into audio or visual signals which are very simple to understand, and the patient can use them to improve control of the muscle function. EMG biofeedback has been used to treat voice disorders, dysarthria, apraxia, and stuttering, as outlined below. The discussion that follows will provide some of the research and therapeutic applications of EMG procedures to the understanding and treatment of a variety of speech-language disorders.

Voice and voice disorders

The larynx is a complex structure serving as the gateway to the lower respiratory tract. Evolving from its original function as a purely sphincter organ, it has been adapted to produce sounds in many animals, and speech in man. These activities are accomplished by means of the vocal cords. During quiet respiration the vocal cords remain abducted and move minimally up and down with inspiration and expiration. During phonation the vocal cords are adducted, tensed and lengthened. The midline position of the vocal cords provides resistance to air flow until pressure builds up and then separates the cords. Separation of the cords reduces the pressure and allows them to return to the midline position. This process is repeated, thus producing cord oscillations and voiced sounds. EMG studies have revealed the role of laryngeal muscles during speech (Faaborg-Andersen, 1957, 1964). Hirose (1977) observed a reciprocal activity between the posterior cricoarytenoid muscle, which is active in the production of voiceless sounds, and the interarytenoid muscle, which is inactive for this purpose. This reciprocity was observed for various languages including English (Hirose and Gay, 1972), Danish (Fischer-Jorgensen and Hirose, 1974) and French (Benguerel et al, 1975). Physiological function of the larynx in phonetic control was examined by Fujimura (1979). Numerous investigations have shown increased activity of the cricothyroid muscle with pitch raising (Gay et al, 1972; Hirano and Ohala, 1969; Honda, 1981; Shipp and McGlone, 1971) or decreased cricothyroid activity and increased sternohyoid strap muscle during pitch falls (Erickson et al, 1982). These studies suggest that EMG activity changes the vibratory characteristics of the vocal cords.

In adductor spasmodic dysphonia, the speech is characterized by pitch or voice breaks during vowels, difficulty in initiating voice, and a harsh, strained, effortful voice quality (Ludlow and Connor, 1987). This can be distinguished from abductor spasmodic dysphonia, which is characterized by a breathy voice quality and prolonged voiceless consonants. These disorders are considered a focal dystonia involving the laryngeal musculature (Blitzer et al, 1985, 1988; Ludlow and Connor, 1987). Thus, the two types of spasmodic dysphonia are believed to be due to uncontrolled hypertonia in the thyroarytenoid muscles (Ludlow et al, 1987). Use of botulinum toxin for the treatment of adductor spasmodic dysphonia was first reported in 1987 by Miller, Woodson and Jankovic. Improvements in speech of patients with spasmodic dysphonia have been demonstrated following injection of botulinum toxin into thyroarytenoid muscles with changes in muscle activation patterns (Ludlow et al, 1990). Treatment of abductor laryngeal dystonia by electromyogram guided injections of botulinum toxin into the posterior cricoarytenoid was also successful (Blitzer et al, 1992; Ludlow et al, 1991). Some authors have tried to explain heterogeneity of vocal symptoms in spasmodic dysphonia by means of an analysis of intrinsic laryngeal muscle activity (Watson et al, 1991). Approaches used for treating the symptoms of spasmodic dysphonia have changed over the past few decades as concepts of the disorder have changed. During the 1970s, EMG biofeedback was used to treat these voice disorders. For his treatment of hyperfunctional dysphonia, Lyndes (1975) used visual feedback of the sternohyoid muscle during speech. Prosek, Montgomery, Walden and Schwartz (1978) measured EMG from the cricothyroid region. They gave continuous auditory feedback of EMG below a threshold, and white noise above a threshold. To normalize muscle tension in hyperfunctional voice, by means of feedback, Stemple, Weiler, Whitebead and Komray (1980) measured both prephonatory and phonatory laryngeal area EMG. At present, EMG biofeedback in the remediation of hyperfunctional voice disorders is reserved for certain cases. For example, Allen, Bernstein and Chait (1991) reported results of visual EMG biofeedback training to reduce laryngeal muscle tension in a 9-year-old boy with hyperfunctional dysphonia and vocal nodules.

The pathophysiology of vocal cord paralysis was investigated with laryngeal EMG. This proved to be a safe and effective procedure in the diagnosis of laryngeal neuropathy as distinguished from supranuclear and mechanical disorders of the larynx (Simpson *et al*, 1993). Voice tremor was also studied using the EMG technique (Ardran *et al*, 1966; Koda and Ludlow, 1992; Tomoda *et al*, 1987).

Neurological disorders of speech-language

Dysarthria

Darley, Aronson and Brown (1969) used the collective name of dysarthria for a group of speech disorders resulting from disturbances in muscular control of the speech mechanism resulting from damage to the central or peripheral nervous system. Thus, dysarthric speech results from problems due to weakness, incoordination of the speech musculature or altered muscle tone. Such problems have to be differentiated from problems (1) resulting from impairment of a higher neural centre, devoted to the programming of articulatory movements: these speech disorders being called apraxia of speech, (2) due to impairment in the cerebral hemisphere that has as primary function the processing of the language code: these language disorders being called aphasia. Apraxia and aphasia will be returned to below. Various neurological disorders can be the origin of a dysarthria: for example, cerebral palsy, bulbar palsy, pseudo-bulbar palsy, Parkinsonism, chorea, amyotrophic lateral sclerosis, and cerebellar disorders. A full discussion of the speech characteristics and the neuromechanisms associated with these dysfunctions may be found in Darley, Aronson and Brown (1975). Whatever the aetiology of dysarthria, investigators, such as Hardy (1967), have made wide use of electromyography to understand the physiopathology of these speech symptoms. The primary investigations are reviewed below.

Leanderson, Meyersson and Persson (1971, 1972) compared the EMG activity of lip muscles in patients with Parkinson's disease with that of normal speakers. They observed that the resting activity between utterances was markedly increased up to a sustained hypertonic background activity, and the functional organization of the lip muscles into two antagonistic groups for contrasting speech gesture movements was impaired. Furthermore, the effect of L-dopa treatment on the dysarthric EMG activity was evaluated, and it was found that after medication the tonic hyperactivity was reduced and the reciprocal innervation was re-established. Nakano, Zubick and Tyler (1973) examined the relation between tonic background EMG activity and qualitative features of articulatory movements in Parkinsonian dysarthria. Netsell, Daniel and Celesia (1975), by examining bilateral EMG activity of orbicularis oris superior, noted a weakness in the control signals, which they felt was the origin of the reduced range of articulatory movements in Parkinsonian speech. Moore and Scudder (1989) studied jaw muscle activity in Parkinsonian speakers and often found inappropriate activation. EMG abnormalities of laryngeal muscles were reported in patients with Parkinson's disease in, for example, Guindi, Bannister, Gibson and Payne, 1981; Hirose, 1986; and Hirose, Honda, Sawashima and Yoshioka, 1984.

Few EMG studies have been reported on the speech musculature in cerebellar disease (Gentil, 1990b; Hirose, 1977, 1986; Hirose et al, 1978; Netsell, 1972), or in cerebral palsy (Barlow et al, 1983; Neilson and O'Dwyer, 1981, 1984; O'Dwyer et al, 1983). Physiological deficits in the orofacial system underlying dysarthria in amyotrophic lateral sclerosis (ALS) were observed but a common focus of physiological studies in speech pathology relative to ALS has been to study muscle force characteristics of the orofacial structures (DePaul et al, 1988; Dworkin et al, 1980; Langmore and Lehman, 1994) but very few EMG studies were performed (DePaul and Brooks, 1990; Hirose, 1986).

Dysarthria, with its obvious neuromuscular component, has been treated by EMG biofeedback mostly from the 1970s. Netsell and Cleeland (1973) were among the first to utilize EMG biofeedback with a dysarthric speaker. They trained a patient with Parkinson's disease to decrease excessive activity of the levator labii superioris and reduce lip retraction. The patient was presented with a tone whose frequency was analogous to the voltage recorded from the electrodes and she had to concentrate on lowering this tone. Elsewhere, this method was replicated by Hand, Burns and Ireland (1979) for a Parkinsonian patient who exhibited lip hypertonia and retraction. The authors found a decrease in EMG activity when presented with feedback in both the non-speech and the speech tasks. Netsell and Daniel (1979) used a multiple approach to train a flaccid dysarthric patient to improve his speech; that is, auditory feedback of lip EMG during speech and non-speech tasks, and visual feedback of glottal flow during sustained phonation of vowels. Daniel and Guitar (1978) used a combination of threshold and continuous auditory feedback to recover speech gestures following neural anastomosis. Rubow and Flyn (1980) employed both visual feedback of lip force and auditory feedback of labial EMG to increase lip strength. In other studies, Finley, Niman, Standley and Ender (1976) investigated the effects of frontalis muscle biofeedback on speech and motor tasks in six athetoid cerebral palsy patients. Results revealed reduction in frontalis EMG over the 6-week courses and improvement in both speech and motor functions when pre- and post-treatment scores were compared. A second, more sophisticated, investigation concerning four spastic cerebral palsy children demonstrated the success of EMG biofeedback in improving speech and motor behaviour (Finley *et al*, 1977). Rubow, Rosenbek, Collins and Celesia (1984) also reduced hemifacial spasm and dysarthria by providing auditory feedback of frontalis EMG.

Apraxia of speech

Apraxia of speech is an 'impairment of the capacity to form vocal tract configurations and to move from one sequence to another for volitional speech production, in the absence of motor impairments for other responses of the same musculature' (Rosenbek *et al*, 1984). Investigations concerning apraxia of speech have focused on auditory, perceptual and acoustic manifestations of this disorder (Kent and Rosenbek, 1983). However, the need to observe both movements and muscle activity is important particularly given the classical definition of apraxia of speech which refers to impairments at these levels of system output (Barlow *et al*, 1983; Darley *et al*, 1975). Fromm, Abbs, McNeil and Rosenbek's study (1982) concerning three apraxics indicated various speech muscle abnormalities including antagonistic muscle contraction, continuous undifferentiated EMG activity, and muscle activity shutdown. These authors confirmed that it is impossible to discern the underlying neuromuscular physiopathology without direct observations of physiological variables. They concluded that such an approach allows a characterization of the nature of apraxia of speech with measures that reflect nervous system dysfunction, which could lead to a more concrete and refined understanding of a disorder that has been subject to a notable amount of controversy and ambiguity. In particular, recent works converge on a central finding of motor programming impairment. Ziegler and Von Cramon (1986) identified the basic impairment in apraxia of speech as one of disturbed phase relations of individual speech movements; Kent (1990) suggested that apraxia of speech is 'in part an impairment in the generation of properly timed (phased) motor commands'. Previous works indicated that apraxia of speech resulted from a lack of kinesthetic feedback from the peripheral speech musculature (Luria and Hutton, 1977; Rosenbek *et al*, 1973). These observations suggested that external muscle feedback might be helpful in apraxia disorders. However, biofeedback treatment of apraxia is rarely documented in the literature. McNeil, Prescott and Lemme (1976) trained apraxic or aphasic subjects to decrease frontalis EMG activity in order to increase relaxation. Huffman (1978) found that EMG feedback has clinical utility in the management of apraxic patients.

Aphasia

'Aphasia is a physiologically based inefficiency with verbal symbolic functions. It is caused by damage to the cortical and subcortical structures in the hemisphere dominant for such verbal symbolic behavior' (McNeil, 1984). Thus, aphasia is a reduction in capacity to decode and encode meaningful linguistic elements. Shankweiler, Harris and Taylor (1968) investigated the electromyographic patterns associated with speech production of patients with motor aphasia. However, the authors reported that at the time of testing, the aphasic symptoms were greatly diminished, leaving the articulatory deficit as the major impairment. Lip and tongue muscles were recorded using surface electrodes. Results provided important information about the temporal and spatial organization of defective speech gestures that could not have been obtained with procedures analysing only the acoustic parameters. However, there is a paucity of research and clinical articles relative to the EMG technique applied to understanding and modification of the speech-language disorders of the aphasic patient.

Stuttering

Stuttering is a disorder in which abnormal patterns of speech movements are generated. For a review of major trends in research on speech motor processes in stuttering see Peters and Hulstijn's work (1987), which arose from a conference on speech motor dynamics in stuttering. The precise aetiology of stuttering is unknown. To understand the nature of this disorder and to develop successful therapeutic techniques, it is important to specify the sources in the nervous system that are responsible for the failure of the motor command signals in stutterers' speech. In order to identify the neural sources that produce a motor output, a careful description of that motor output, e.g. movements and muscle activity, is necessary. This is the reason why stuttering has received the greatest attention from researchers exploring EMG correlates of disordered speech-language behaviour. The earliest suggestion that stuttering might be the result of a neuromuscular disorder was provided by Travis (1934) who presented electromyographic data from masseter muscles of 24 adult stutterers and non-stutterers, and showed a basic neurophysiological difference between stutterers and non-stutterers. Later, Williams (1955) found that differences between the two groups' EMG measurements were attributable to the excessive muscular tension and different patterns of jaw movement that accompanied stuttering. Numerous investigators have reported that stuttered speech is associated with excessive levels of muscle activity (Bar *et al*, 1978;

Kalotkin *et al*, 1979; Shapiro, 1980; Van Lieshout *et al*, 1993). Freeman and Ushijima's study (1978) gave evidence of abnormal laryngeal kinesiology in stuttering. They recorded activity from five intrinsic laryngeal muscles, and observed: (1) a high level of muscle activity; and (2) a disruption of abductor-adductor reciprocity. This pattern of disruption of co-ordination could be regarded as a physiological basis of the abnormal laryngeal behaviour in stuttering.

A number of investigations have provided convincing evidence that speech breakdowns in stuttering (disfluencies) are often characterized by abnormal oscillations of EMG activity in the muscles of the jaw, lips and neck (Fibiger, 1971; McClean *et al*, 1984; Platt and Basili, 1973). Smith (1989) found that the spectra of amplitude envelopes of EMGs recorded from jaw, lip and neck muscles could show common frequencies of dominant oscillations during stuttered speech intervals. Denny and Smith (1992) observed similar results in orofacial muscles during stuttered speech and reported that oscillation in the 5–15 Hz band was not present in the fluent speech of these subjects. Thus recordings of orofacial muscles showed that tremor-like oscillations grew greatly during disfluent intervals but that an abnormally high level of oscillatory activity was not present during the fluent speech intervals of stuttering. The question was whether other systems involved in speech, i.e. laryngeal and respiratory systems, were disturbed in the same way in stuttering. Freeman and Ushijima (1978) reported neither qualitative nor quantitative descriptions of oscillation of laryngeal muscle activity associated with stuttering. In Bradylak's investigation, and Smith, Luschei, Denny, Wood, Hirano and Bradylak's (1993) study, spectral analyses of the amplitude envelopes of laryngeal and orofacial EMGs revealed that tremor-like oscillations of EMG activity similar to those observed in orofacial muscles were also present in laryngeal muscles during stuttered speech. Furthermore, tremor-like oscillations appeared to be entrained in some subjects. Further, Caruso, Gracco and Abbs (1987) reported that stutterers responded during their fluent speech to unanticipated perturbations in a different manner from individuals who do not stutter. Specifically, these subtle differences in response to lower lip loads included consistently longer latency values of labial EMG activity and smaller changes in levels of EMG activity. But to understand the underlying process of disfluent speech, investigations of a single domain are inadequate to reveal interactions that define co-ordination of speech movements (Borden and Watson, 1987). Recent research in speech motor behaviour in stuttering is interested in various measures, such as speech reaction time, planning or programming time, the timing of phonatory and articulatory processes and their co-ordination. Surface electromyography, an easy and non-invasive technique, makes it possible to detect the onset of laryngeal and articulatory muscle activity and the timing between them as well as the amplitude level of muscle activity (Peters, 1990).

The various investigations noted above demonstrate some consistent relationship between EMG activity and stutterers' speech. These studies could provide a rationale for the application of EMG biofeedback procedures in the clinical management of stuttering. Guitar (1975) showed decreased EMG activity of four orofacial muscles when subjects were presented with an audio feedback signal. The subjects were trained to reduce muscle activity prior to uttering sentences. Lanyon, Barrington and Newman (1976) gave visual feedback of masseter activity on an oscilloscope or meter display. Results showed virtual elimination of stuttering during feedback with generalization of the treatment effects during no-feedback trials. Hanna, Wilfling and McNeil (1975) used auditory feedback of laryngeal EMG with success, and Moore (1978) showed reductions in stuttering when auditory feedback was provided to stutterers associated with masseter or chin activity. The use of EMG feedback has been shown to be an efficient strategy in the treatment of stuttering. Furthermore, in recent years other types of procedures have been developed. For example, Watson and Dembowski (1990) have recently presented a therapy procedure in which they combined monitoring of respiratory movement with the electroglottographic assessment of vocal fold activity during voice.

Conclusion

There is a great potential for the use of methods now available to us for the study of physiological aspects of speech production. EMG, which has been the focus of this chapter, is such a method that sheds some light on the neuromotor processes. Our knowledge and the application of EMG related to speech and language disorders have greatly increased during the past three decades. EMG analysis of speech disorders is an objective and quantitative procedure of describing the behaviour of the various systems contributing to abnormal speech production. Evaluation of speech muscle activities extends and verifies inferences made using acoustic, aerodynamic or auditory perceptual analyses of speech disorders. EMG measurement is particularly important in assessing motor impairment in disorders such as dysarthria or stuttering. An improved understanding of the nature of physiological aspects of speech deficits related to a specific disorder may lead to the development of treatment approaches that might not otherwise be considered. However, in the attempt to evaluate the clinical relevance of the EMG technique an important question is raised: what are the normal patterns of EMG activation during speech? This question is extremely difficult to answer. The difficulty in defining normal EMG activation patterns in speech is the major impediment to the moving of EMG methodology out of the research laboratories into clinical application. Increased research into basic processes of oral motor system control in speech will enlarge the use of this research tool in the clinic. It is apparent that the EMG technique is not a common procedure used by most speech-language pathologists.

The EMG biofeedback treatment method has received some limited support in the literature. Here, the purpose of the instrumentation is to provide information about parameters directly to the patients who use this information to modify the relevant parameter. Thus, EMG biofeedback has been utilized in remediating a variety of speech and language disorders. Even though the success of EMG biofeedback procedures has been demonstrated, these have been little developed.

The physiological mechanisms underlying oral communication are of primary interest to speech scientists. While the usefulness of applying EMG techniques to speech and language disorders seems obvious, it is clear that investigations into their use and application should continue. The instrumentation is not prohibitively expensive, the measurement techniques are not difficult to learn to use, but the major challenge facing researchers of speech pathology lies in interpreting the data obtained. Basic research that would allow appropriate interpretation of EMG data seems absolutely necessary. This would accelerate the use of EMG as a speech research tool in the clinic.

References

Abbs JH, Gracco VL, Blair C. Functional muscle partitioning during voluntary movement: facial muscle activity for speech. Experimental Neurology 1984; 85: 469–79.

Adrian ED, Bronk DW. The discharge of the impulses in motor nerve fibres. II The frequency of discharge in reflex and voluntary contractions. Journal of Physiology 1929; 67: 119–51.

Alfonso PJ, Baer T. Dynamic of vowel articulation. Language and Speech 1982; 25: 159–73.

Allen KD, Bernstein B, Chait DH. EMG biofeedback treatment of pediatric hyperfunctional dysphonia. Journal of Behavioral Therapy and Experimental Psychiatry 1991; 22: 97–101.

Andrews JM. Neuromuscular re-education of hemiplegic with aid of electromyography. Archives of Physical Medecine and Rehabilitation 1964; 45: 530–32.

Ardran G, Kinsbourne M, Rushworth G. Dysphonia due to tremor. Journal of Neurology, Neurosurgery and Psychiatry 1966; 29: 219–23.

Baken RJ. Clinical Measurement of Speech and Voice. London: Taylor & Francis, 1987.

Bar A, Singer J, Feldman RG. Laryngeal muscle activity during stuttering. Journal of Speech and Hearing Research 1978; 21: 538–62.

Barlow SM, Cole KJ, Abbs JH. A new head-mounted lip jaw movement transduction system for the study of motor speech disorders. Journal of Speech and Hearing Research 1983; 26: 283–88.

Basmajian JV. Muscles Alive. Their Functions Revealed by Electromyography. Baltimore: Williams & Wilkins, 1962.

Basmajian JV. Biofeedback – Principles and Practice for Clinicians. Baltimore: Williams & Wilkins, 1979.

Basmajian JV, Kukulka CG, Narayan MG, Tabeke K. Biofeedback treatment of footdrop after stroke compared with standard rehabilitation technique: effects on voluntary control and strength. Archives of Physical Medicine and Rehabilitation 1975; 56: 231–36.

Basmajian JV, Stecko GA. New bipoolar electrodes for electromyography. Journal of Applied Physiology 1962; 17: 849.

Benguerel AP, Hirose H, Sawashima M, Ushijima T. Laryngeal control in French stops. Fiberoptic acoustic and electromyographic studies. Annual Bulletin of Research Institute of Logopedics and Phoniatrics, University of Tokyo 1975; 10: 81–100.

Blair C, Smith A. EMG recording in human lip muscles: can single muscles be isolated? Journal of Speech and Hearing Research 1986; 29: 256–66.

Blitzer A, Brin MF, Fahn S, Lovelace RE. Clinical and laboratory characteristics of focal laryngeal dystonia: study of 110 cases. Laryngoscope 1988; 98: 636–40.

Blitzer A, Brin MF, Stewart C, Aviv JE, Fahn S. Abductor laryngeal dystonia: a series treated with botulinum toxin. Laryngoscope 1992; 102: 163–67.

Blitzer A, Lovelace RE, Brin MF, Fahn S, Fink ME. Electromyographic findings in focal laryngheal dystonia (spastic dysphonia). Acta Otorhinolaryngologica 1985; 94: 591.

Borden G, Watson B Methodological aspects of simultaneous measurements: limitations and possibilities. In Peters HFM, Hulstijn W. (Eds), Speech Motor Dynamics in Stuttering. Vienna: Springer-Verlag, 1987.

Bradylak S. Spectral analyses of activity of laryngeal and orofacial muscles in stutterers. Journal of Neurology, Neurosurgery and Psychiatry 1993; 56: 1303–11.

Brudny J, Grynbaum BB, Korein J. Spasmodic torticollis: treatment by feedback display of EMG. Archives of Physical Medecine and Rehabilitation 1973; 55: 403–8.

Buchtal F. The general concept of the motor unit. Res Puhl Ass Nerv Ment Dis 1961; 38: 1–30.

Caruso AJ, Gracco VL, Abbs JH. A speech motor control perspective on stuttering: preliminary observations. In Peters HFM, Hulstijn W. (Eds), Speech Motor Dynamics in Stuttering. Vienna: Springer-Verlag, 1987.

Cooper DS, Folkins JW. Comparison of electromyographic signals from different electrode placements in the palatoglossus muscle. Journal of the Acoustical Society of America 1985; 78: 1530–40.

Cooper FS. Research techniques and instrumentation: EMG-ASHA reports 1965; 1: 153–68.

Daniel B, Guitar BV. EMG biofeedback and recovery of facial and speech gestures following neural anastomosis. Journal of Speech and Hearing Disorders 1978; 43: 9–20.

Darley FL, Aronson A, Brown JR. Differential diagnostic patterns of dysarthria. Journal of Speech and Hearing Research 1969; 12: 246–69.

Darley FL, Aronson A, Brown JR. Motor Speech Disorders. Philadelphia: WB Saunders, 1975.

Denny M, Smith A. Gradations in a pattern of neuromuscular activity associated with stuttering. Journal of Speech and Hearing Research 1992; 35: 1216–29.

DePaul R, Abbs JH, Caligiuri M, Gracco VL, Brooks BR. Hypoglossal, trigeminal and facial motoneuron involvement in amyotrophic lateral sclerosis. Neurology 1988; 38: 281–83.

DePaul R, Brooks BR. Differential orofacial muscle impairment in ALS: a longitudinal study, Annual Convention of the American Speech Language Hearing Association, Seattle, 1990.

Draper MH, Ladefoged P, Whitteridge D. Respiratory muscles in speech. Journal of Speech and Hearing Research 1959; 2: 16–27.

Dumoulin J, Aucremanne CH. Précis d' electromyographic. Paris: Maloine, 1959.

Dworkin JP, Aronson AE, Mulder DW. Tongue force in normals and dysarthric patients with amyotrophic lateral sclerosis Journal of Speech and Hearing Research 1980; 23: 828–37.

Eccles JC. The Understanding of the Brain. New York: McGraw-Hill, 1973.

English DT, Blevins CE. Motor units of laryngeal muscles. Archives of Otolaryngology 1969; 89: 778–84.

Erickson D, Baer T, Harris KH. The role of the strap muscles in pitch lowering. Haskins Laboratories, Status Report on Speech Research 1982; 70: 275–84.

Faaborg-Andersen KL. Electromyographic investigation of intrinsic laryngeal muscle in humans. Acta Physiologica Scandinavica 1957; 41: 3–30.

Faaborg-Andersen KL. Electromyography of the laryngeal muscles in man. In Brewer DW. (Ed.), Research Potentials in Voice Physiology, pp.105–23. New York: State University of New York, 1964.

Faaborg-Andersen KL, Vennard W. Electromyography of extrinsic laryngeal muscles during phonation of different vowels. Annals of Otology, Rhinology and Laryngology1964; 73: 248–54.

Feinstein B. The application of electromyography to affections of the facial and the intrinsic laryngeal muscles. Proceedings of the Royal Society of Medicine 1945; 39: 817.

Fibiger S. Stuttering explained as a physiological tremor. Speech Transmission Laboratory Status Report 1971; 2: 1–24.

Finley W, Niman C, Standley J, Ender P. Frontal EMG biofeedback. Training of athetoid cerebral palsy patients. Biofeedback and Self-Regulation 1976; 1: 169–82.

Finley W, Niman C, Standley J, Wansley RA. Electrophysiologic behaviour modification of frontal EMG in cerebral-palsied children. Biofeedback and Self-Regulation 1977; 2: 59–79.

Fischer-Jorgensen E, Hirose H. A preliminary electromyographic study of labial and laryngeal muscles in Danish stop consonant production. Haskins Laboratories, Status Report on Speech Research 1974; 39/40: 231–54.

Folkins JW. Muscle activity for jaw closing during speech. Journal of Speech and Hearing Research 1981; 24: 601–15.

Folkins JW, Abbs JH. Lip and jaw motor control during speech: responses to resistive loading of the jaw. Journal of Speech and Hearing Research 1975; 18: 207–20.

Freeman F, Ushijima T. Laryngeal muscle activity during stuttering. Journal of Speech and Hearing Research 1978; 21: 538–62.

Fridlund AJ, Cacioppo JT. Guidelines for human electromyographic research. Psychophysiology 1986; 23: 567–89.

Fridlund AJ, Izard CE. Electromyographic studies of facial expressions of emotions and patterns of emotion. In Cacioppo JT, Petty RE. (Eds), Social Psychophysiology: A Sourcebook. New York: Guilford Press, 1983.

Fritzell B. An electromyographic study of the movements of the soft palate in speech. Folia Phoniatrica 1963; 15: 307–11.

Fritzell B. The velopharyngeal muscles in speech. An electromyographic and cineradiographic study. Acta Otolaryngologica 1969; Suppl 250: 1–81.

Fromkin VA. Neuromuscular specification of linguistic units. Language and Speech 1966; 9: 170–99.

Fromkin VA, Ladefoged P. Electromyography in speech research. Phonetica 1966; 15: 219–42.

Fromm D, Abbs JH, McNeil MR, Rosenbek JC. Simultaneous perceptual physiological method of studying apraxia of speech. In Brookshire RH. (Ed.), Proceedings of Clinical Aphasiology Conference. Minneapolis: BRK Publishers, 1982.

Fuglevand AJ, Winter DA, Patla AE, Stashuk D. Detection of motor unit action potentials with surface electrodes. Biological Cybernetics 1992; 67: 143–53.

Fujimura O. Physiological function of the larynx in phonetic control. In Hollien H, Hollien P. (Eds), Current Issues in the Phonetic Sciences, pp. 129–63. Amsterdam: John Benjamin, 1979.

Gay T, Harris KS. Some recent developments in the use of electromyography in speech research. Journal of Speech and Hearing Research 1971; 14: 241–46.

Gay T, Hirose H, Strome M, Sawashima M. Electromyography of the intrinsic laryngeal muscles during phonation, Annals of Otology, Rhinology and Laryngology, 1972 81, 401–9.

Gay T, Ushijima T., Hirose H, Cooper F. Effect of speaking rate on labial consonant-vowel articulation. Journal of Phonetics 1974; 2: 47–63.

Gentil M. Organization of the articulatory system: peripheral mechanisms and central coordination. In Hardcastle WJ, Marchal A. (Eds), Speech Production and Speech Modelling, pp. 1–22. Dordrecht, Boston, London: Kluwer Academic Publishers, 1990a.

Gentil M. EMG analysis of speech production of patients with Friedreich disease. Clinical Linguistics and Phonetics 1990b; 4: 107–20.

Gentil M. Variability of motor strategies. Brain and Language 1992; 42: 30–37.

Gentil M, Gay T. Neuromuscular specialization of the mandibular motor system: speech versus non-speech movements. Speech Communication 1986; 5: 69–82.

Gentil M, Gracco VL, Abbs JH. Multiple muscle contributions to labial closures during speech: evidence for intermuscle motor equivalence. Proceedings of the 11th International Congress of Acoustics, Paris vol. 4, pp. 11–14, 1983.

Gross B, Lipke D. A technique for percutaneous lateral pterygoid electromyography. Electromyography and Clinical Neurophysiology 1979; 19: 47–55.

Guindi GM, Bannister R, Gibson WPR, Payne JK. Laryngeal electromyography in multiple system atrophy with autonomic failure. Journal of Neurology, Neurosurgery and Psychiatry 1981; 44: 49–53.

Guitar B. Reduction of stuttering frequency using analog electromyographic feedback. Journal of Speech and Hearing Research 1975; 18: 678–85.

Haines RW. The laws of muscle and tendon growth. Journal of Anatomy 1932; 66: 578–85.

Haines RW. On muscles of full and short action. Journal of Anatomy 1934; 69: 20–24.

Hand CR, Burns MO, Ireland E. Treatment of hypertonicity in muscles of lip retraction. Biofeedback and Self Regulation 1979; 4: 171–81.

Hanna R, Wilfling F, McNeil B. A biofeedback treatment for stuttering. Journal of Speech and Hearing Disorders 1975; 40: 270–73.

Hardy JC. Suggestion for physiological research in dysarthria. Cortex 1967; 3: 128–56.

Harris KH. Electromyography as a technique for laryngeal investigation, Proceedings of the Conference on the Assessment of Vocal Pathology. ASHA Reports 1981; 11: 70–87

Hirano M, Koike Y, Von Leden H. The sternohyoid muscle during phonation. Acta Otolaryngologica 1967; 64: 500–7.

Hirano M, Ohala J. Use of hooked wire electrodes for electromyography of the intrinsic laryngeal muscles. Journal of Speech and Hearing Research 1969; 12: 362–73.

Hirose H. Electromyography of the articulatory muscles. Current instrumentation and technique. Haskins Laboratories Status Report on Speech Research 1971; 25/26: 73–86.

Hirose H. Electromyography of the larynx and other speech organs. In Sawashima M, Cooper FS. (Eds), Dynamic Aspects of Speech Production. Tokyo: University of Tokyo Press, 1977.

Hirose H. Pathophysiology of motor speech disorders. Folia Phoniatrica 1986; 38: 61–88.

Hirose H, Gay T. The activity of the intrinsic laryngeal muscles in voicing control, an electromyographic study. Phonetica 1972; 25: 140–64.

Hirose H, Gay T, Strome M. Electrode insertion techniques for laryngeal electromyography. Journal of the Acoustical Society of America 1971; 50: 1449–50.

Hirose H, Honda K, Sawashima M, Yoshioka H. Laryngeal dynamics in dysarthric speech. Annual Bulletin of Research Institute of Logopedics and Phoniatrics, University of Tokyo 1984; 18: 161–67.

Hirose H, Kiritani S, Ushijima T, Sawashima M. Analysis of abnormal articulatory dynamics in two dysarthric patients. Journal of Speech and Hearing Disorders 1978; 43: 96–105.

Honda K. Relationship between pitch control and vowel articulation, Proceedings of the Conference on Vocal Fold Physiology, Madison, 1981.

Honda K, Baer T, Alfonso PJ. Variability of tongue muscle activities and its implications. Journal of the Acoustical Society of America 1982; 72: S103.

Huffman AL. Biofeedback treatment of orofacial dysfunction: a preliminary study. American Journal of Occupational Therapy 1978; 32: 149–54.

Inglis J, Campbell D, Donald M. Electromyographic biofeedback and neuromuscular rehabilitation. In Kamija (Ed.), Biofeedback and Self-control. Chicago: Aldine, 1977.

Inmann VT, Saunders JB, Abbott LC. Observations on the functions of the shoulder joint. Journal of Bone and Joint Surgery 1944; 26: 1–30.

Isley CL, Basmajian JV. Electromyography of the human cheeks and lips. Anatomical Record 1973; 176: 143–48.

Johnson HE, Garton WH. Muscle reeducation of hemiplegic with aid of electromyograph. Archives of Physical Medicine and Rehabilitation 1973; 54: 320–22.

Kalotkin M, Manschreck T, O'Brien D. Electromyographic tension levels in stutterers and normal speakers. Perceptual and Motor Skills 1979; 49: 109–10.

Katz B. The transmission of impulses from nerve to muscle and the subcellular unit of synaptic action. Proceedings of the Royal Society of London (Biology) 1962; 155: 455–77.

Katz B. Nerve Muscle and Synapse. New York: McGraw-Hill Book, 1966.

Kennedy JG, Abbs JH. Anatomic studies of the perioral motor system: foundations for studies in speech physiology. In Lass NJ. (Ed.), Speech and Language: Advances in Basic Research and Practice, 1. New York: Academic Press, 1979.

Kent RD. The acoustic and physiologic characteristics of neurogically impaired speech movements. In Hardcastle WJ, Marchal A. (Eds), Speech Production and Speech Modelling, pp. 365–401. Dordrecht, Boston, London: Kluwer, 1990.

Kent RD, Rosenbek JC. Acoustic patterns of apraxia of speech. Journal of Speech and Hearing Research 1983; 26: 231–49.

Kobayashi T, Niimi S, Kumada M, Kosakj H, Hirose H. Botulinum toxin treatment for spasmodic dysphonia. Acta Otolaryngologica 1993; 504: 155–57.

Koda J, Ludlow C. An evaluation of laryngeal muscle activation in patients with voice tremor. Otolaryngology and Head and Neck Surgery 1992; 107: 684–96.

Koole P, de Jongh HJ, Boering C. A comparative study of electromyograms of the masseter, temporalis and anterior digastric muscles obtained by surface and intramuscular electrodes. Cranio 1991; 9: 228–40.

Langmore SE, Lehman ME. Physiologic deficits in the orofacial system underlying dysarthria in amyotrophic lateral sclerosis. Journal of Speech and Hearing Research 1994; 37: 28–37.

Lanyon RJ, Barrington CC, Newman AC. Modification of stuttering through EMG biofeedback: a preliminary study, Behavioral Therapy 1976; 7: 96–103.

Lawrence JH, De Luca CJ. Myoelectric signal versus force relationship in different human muscles. Journal of Applied Physiology 1983; 54: 1653–59.

Leanderson R, Meyersson BA, Persson A. Effect of L-dopa on speech in Parkinsonism: an EMF study of labial articulatory function. Journal of Neurology, Neurosurgery and Psychiatry 1971; 34: 679–81.

Leanderson R, Meyersson BA, Persson A. Lip muscle function in Parkinsonian dysarthria. Acta Otolaryngologica 1972; 73: 1–8.

Leanderson R, Persson A, Öhman S. Electromyographic studies of facial muscle activity in speech. Acta Otolaryngologica 1971; 72: 361–69.

Liddell EGT, Sherrington CS. Recruitment and some other feature of reflex inhibition. Proceedings of the Royal Society of London (Biology) 1925; 97: 488–518.

Lippold OCJ. Electromyographic. In Verrables PH, Martin I. (Eds), A Manual of Psychophysiological Methods. New York: John Wiley, 1967.

Loeb GE, Gans C. Electromyography for Experimentalists. Chicago: University of Chicago Press, 1986.

Lou JS, Valls-Sole JV, Toro, C, Hallett M. Facial action myoclonus in patients with olivopontocerebellar atrophy. Movement Disorders 1994: 9: 223–26.

Lubker J. An electromyographic cinefluorographic investigation of velar function during normal speech production. The Cleft Palate Journal 1968; 5: 1–17.

Ludlow CL, Baker M, Naunton R, Hallett M. Intrinsic laryngeal muscle activation in spasmodic dysphonia. In Benecke R, Conrad B, Marsden CD. (Eds), Motor Disturbances, pp. 119–30. Orlando: Academic Press, 1987.

Ludlow CL, Connor NP. Dynamic aspects of phonatory control in spasmodic dysphonia. Journal of Speech and Hearing Research 1987; 30: 197–206.

Ludlow CL, Hallett M, Sedory SE, Fujita M, Naunton RF. The pathophysiology of spasmodic dysphonia and its modification by botulinum toxin. In Berardelli A, Benecke R, Manfredi M, Marsden CD. (Eds), Motor Disturbances. Orlando: Academic Press, 1990.

Ludlow CL, Naunton RF, Terada S, Anderson BJ. Successful treatment of selected cases of abductor spasmodic dysphonia. Otolaryngology and Head and Neck Surgery 1991; 104: 849–55.

Luria AR, Hutton T. Modern assessment of the basic forms of aphasia. Brain and Language 1977; 4: 129–51.

Lyndes KO. The application of biofeedback to functional dysphonia. Journal of Biofeedback 1975; 2: 12–15.

Lysaught G, Rosov RJ, Harris KS. Electromyography as a speech research technique with an application to labial stops. Journal of the Acoustical Society of America 1961; 33: 842.

McClean M, Goldsmith H, Cerf A. Lower lip EMG and displacement during bilabial dysfluencies in adult stutterers. Journal of Speech and Hearing Research 1984; 27: 342–49.

McNamara JA. The independent functions of the two heads of the lateral pterygoid muscle. American Journal of Anatomy 1973; 138: 197–206.

McNeil MR Current concepts in adult aphasia. International Journal of Rehabilitation and Medicine 1984; 6: 128.

McNeil, M, Prescott T, Lemme M. An application of electromyographic biofeedback of aphasia/apraxia treatment. In Brookshire, RH. (Ed.), Proceedings of Clinical Aphasiology Conference. Minneapolis: BRK Publishers, 1976.

MacNeilage PF. Electromyographic and acoustic study of the production of certain final clusters. Journal of the Acoustical Society of America 1963; 35: 461–63.

MacNeilage PF, Sholes GN. An electromyographic study of the tongue during vowel production. Journal of Speech and Hearing Research 1964; 7: 209–32.

Miller RH, Woodson CE, Jankovic J. Botulinum toxin injection of the vocal fold for spasmodic dysphonia. Archives of Otolaryngology and Head and Neck Surgery 1987; 113: 603.

Möller E. The chewing apparatus: an electyromyographic study of the action of the muscles of mastication and its correlation to facial morphology. Acta Physiologica Scandinavica 1966; 69: Suppl 280.

Moore WH. Some effects of progressively lowering electromyographic levels with feedback procedures on the frequency of stuttered verbal behaviours. Journal of Fluency Disorders 1978; 3: 127–38.

Moore, CA, Scudder RR. Coordination of jaw muscle activity in parkinsonian movement: description and response to traditional treatment. In Yorkston KM, Beukelman DR. (Eds), Recent Advances in Clinical Dysarthria. Toronto: Little, Brown and Company, 1989.

Nakano KK, Zubick H, Tyler HR. Speech defects of Parkinsonian patients. Effects of levodopa therapy on speech intelligibility. Neurology 1973; 23: 865–70.

Neilson PD, O'Dwyer NJ. Pathophysiology of dysarthria in cerebral palsy. Journal of Neurology, Neurosurgery and Psychiatry 1981; 107: 684–96.

Neilson PD, O'Dwyer NJ. Reproducibility and variability of speech muscle activity in athetoid dysarthria of cerebral palsy. Journal of Speech and Hearing Research 1984; 27: 502–17.

Netsell R. Lip electromyography in the dysarthrias. Reports of the Annual Convention of the American Speech and Hearing Association, San Francisco, 1972.

Netsell R, Cleeland CS. Modification of lip hypertonia in dysarthria using EMG feedback. Journal of Speech and Hearing Disorders 1973; 38: 131–40.

Netsell R, Daniel B. Dysarthria in adults: physiologic approach to rehabilitation. Archives of Physical Medicine and Rehabilitation 1979; 60: 502–8.

Netsell R, Daniel B, Celesia GC. Acceleration and weakness in Parkinsonian dysarthria. Journal of Speech and Hearing Disorders 1975; 40: 170–78.

O'Dwyer NJ, Neilson PD, Guitar BE, Quinn PT, Andrews G. Control of upper airway structures during nonspeech tasks in normal and cerebral palsied subjects: EMG findings. Journal of Speech and Hearing Research 1983; 26: 162–70.

O'Dwyer NJ, Quinn PT, Guitar BE, Andrews G, Neilson PD. Procedures for verification of electrode placement in EMG studies of orofacial and mandibular muscles. Journal of Speech and Hearing Research 1981; 24; 273–88.

Öhman S. Peripheral motor commands in labial articulation, Speech Transmission Laboratory, Status Report 1967; 4: 30–63.

Öhman S, Leanderson R, Persson A. Electromyographic studies of facial muscles during speech, Speech Transmission Laboratory, Status Report 1965; 3: 1–11.

Peters HFM. Clinical application of speech measurement techniques in the assessment of stuttering. Proceedings of a conference: Assessment of Speech and Voice

Production, Research and clinical applications, NIDCD monograph, Bethesda, 1990; pp. 172–82.

Peters HFM, Hulstijn W. Speech Motor Dynamics in Stuttering. Vienna, New York: Springer-Verlag, 1987.

Platt LJ, Basili A. Jaw tremor during stuttering block. Journal of Communication Disorders 1973; 6: 102–9.

Prosek RA, Montgomery AA, Walden BE, Schwartz DM. EMG biofeedback in the treatment of hyperfunctional voice disorders. Journal of Speech and Hearing Disorders 1978; 43: 282–94.

Rosenbek JC, Kent RD, LaPointe LL. Apraxia of speech. An overview and some perspectives. In Rosenbek JC, McNeil MR, Aronson A. (Eds), Apraxia of Speech: Physiology, Acoustics, Linguistics and Management. San Diego: College Hill Press, 1984.

Rosenbek JC, Wertz RT, Darley FL. Oral sensation and perception in apraxia of speech and aphasia. Journal of Speech and Hearing Research 1973; 16: 22–36.

Rubow RT, Flyn M. Physiologic biofeedback techniques in the treatment of motor speech disorders, Proceedings of Biofeedback Society of America, 1980.

Rubow RT, Rosenbek JC, Collins M, Celesia GC. Reduction in hemifacial spasm and dysarthria following EMG biofeedback. Journal of Speech and Hearing Disorders 1984; 49: 26–33.

Sawashima M., Sato M, Funasaka S, Totsuka G. Electromyographic study of the human larynx and its clinical application. Japanese Journal of Otology 1958; 61: 1357–64.

Shankweiler D, Harris KS, Taylor ML Electromyographic studies of articulation in aphasia. Archives of Physical Medicine and Rehabilitation 1968; 49: 1–8.

Shapiro AI. An electromyographic analysis of the fluent and dysfluent utterances of several types of stutterers. Journal of Fluency Disorders 1980; 5: 203–32.

Shipp T, McGlone RE. Laryngeal dynamics associated with voice frequency changes. Journal of Speech and Hearing Research 1971; 14: 761–68.

Simpson DM, Sternman D, Graves-Wright J, Sanders I. Vocal cord paralysis: clinical and electrophysiologic features. Muscle and Nerve 1993; 16: 952–57.

Singer C. The Evolution of Anatomy. London: Trench, Trubner, 1925.

Smith A. Neural drive to muscles in stuttering. Journal of Speech and Hearing Research 1989; 32: 252–64.

Smith A. Neurophysiological indices of speech production processes, Proceedings of a conference: Assessment of Speech and Voice Production Research and Clinical Applications, NIDCD Monograph, Bethesda, pp. 150–60, 1990.

Smith A, Luschei E, Denny M, Wood J, Hirano M, Bradylak S. Spectral analyses of activity of laryngeal and orofacial muscles in stutterers. Journal of Neurology, Neurosurgery and Psychiatry 1993; 56: 1303–11.

Smith C. Action potentials from single motor units in voluntary contraction. American Journal of Physiology 1934; 108: 629–38.

Smith TS, Hirano M. Experimental investigation of the muscular control of the tongue in speech, Working Papers UCLA 1968; 10: 145–55.

Stemple JC, Weiler E, Whitebead W, Komray R. Electromyographic biofeedback training with patients exhibiting a hyperfunctional voice disorder. Laryngoscope 1980; 90: 471–76.

Stetson RH. Motorphonetics. A Study of Speech Movements in Action. Amsterdam: North Holland Publishers, 1951.

Sussman HM, McNeilage PL, Hanson RJ. Labial and mandibular dynamics during the production of bilabial consonants: preliminary investigation. Journal of Speech and Hearing Research 1973; 16: 397–420.

Tomoda H, Shibasaki H, Kuroda Y, Shin T. Voice tremor: dysregulation of voluntary expiratory muscles. Neurology 1987; 37: 117–22.

Travis LE. Disassociation of the homologous muscle function in stutterers. Archives of Neurology and Psychiatry 1934; 31: 127–33.

Tuller B, Harris KS, Kelso JAS. Stress and rate: differential transformation of articulation. Journal of the Acoustical Society of America 1982; 71: 1534–43.

Tuller B, Harris KS, Gross BD. An electromyographic study of the jaw muscle during speech. Journal of Phonetics 1981; 9: 175–88.

Tuller B, Kelso JAS, Harris KS. Interarticulator phasing as index of temporal regularity in speech. Journal of Experimental Psychology: Human Perception and Performance 1982; 8: 460–72.

Turker KS. Electromyography: some methodological problems and issues. Physical Therapy 1993; 73: 698–710.

Van Lieshout P, Peters HFM, Starkweather CW, Hulstijn W. Physiological differences between stutterers and nonstutterers in perceptually fluent speech: EMG amplitude and duration. Journal of Speech and Hearing Research 1993; 36: 55–63.

Watson BC, Dembowski J. Instrumentation in the evaluation and modification of speech motor control during stuttering therapy. In Peters HFM, Hulstijn W, Starkweather CW. (Eds), Speech Motor Control and Stuttering. Amsterdam: Elsevier Science Publishers, 1990.

Watson BC, Schaefer SD, Freeman FJ, Dembowski J, Kondraske G, Roark R. Laryngeal electromyographic activity in adductor and abductor spasmodic dysphonia. Journal of Speech and Hearing Research 1991; 34: 473–82.

Weddell G, Feinstern B, Pattle RE. The electrical activity of voluntary muscle in man under normal and pathological conditions. Brain 1944; 67: 178–257.

Williams DE. Masseter muscle action potentials in stuttered and non-stuttered speech. Journal of Speech and Hearing Disorders 1955; 20: 242–61.

Winter DA. Biomechanics of Human Movement. New York: John Wiley and Sons, 1989.

Ziegler W, Von Cramon D. Timing deficits in apraxia of speech. European Archives of Psychiatry and Neurological Sciences 1986; 236: 44–49.

Chapter 4
Speech Aerodynamics

DAVID J. ZAJAC AND CAMPBELL C. YATES

Introduction

Speech production involves a series of complex and highly co-ordinated behaviours which include neuromuscular, movement and aerodynamic phenomena. These interrelated events begin with respiration and terminate with the generation of an acoustic speech signal. As Warren (1982) has stated, 'Changes in shape and size of the lower airway produce an air stream which is continuously modified by laryngeal and supralaryngeal structures' (p. 219). This modification of the air stream gives rise to the acoustic events that are perceived as meaningful speech utterances. Anatomic and/or functional anomalies, which may involve the lower airways, the larynx, or the supralaryngeal structures, may adversely affect this process. Aerodynamic assessment methods, therefore, provide valuable information relative to the entire vocal tract. The various air pressures, volumes, flows and resistances associated with respiration, phonation and articulation may be measured and quantitatively documented. This information is vital to our understanding of both normal and deviant speech processes.

Traditionally, the aerodynamics of speech production have been relatively neglected. This is not surprising given the relative ease of capturing the acoustic signal and the implicit assumption that a one-to-one correspondence exists between acoustic and perceptual phenomena. However, with the proliferation of low-cost, commercially available computer-based aerodynamic analysis systems, the practising clinician and/or researcher can no longer afford to ignore this level of analysis.

The purpose of this chapter is to introduce the reader to the aerodynamic assessment of speech production. By design, the focus will be on the assessment of laryngeal and supralaryngeal events as they pertain to speakers with and without palatal clefts. This emphasis was chosen to facilitate the understanding of both normal and deviant speech aerodynamics. Speakers with cleft palate, for example, tend to alter respiratory volumes, intraoral air pressures, rates of nasal airflow and the temporal aspects of these events. Basic principles and assumptions of fluid mechanics and required instrumentation will be discussed as precursors to the clinical application of pressure-flow techniques.

Basic Principles of Fluid Mechanics

Quantitative measurements of pressure and flow rate in human subjects are important to the analysis and understanding of speech production. The geometry of the flow channels and their construction, however, present numerous challenges that are difficult to overcome using the ordinary methods and techniques of fluid mechanics. Foremost among these problems is the difficulty of probe placement to measure dynamic pressures during running speech.

Pressure measurements

Pressure is defined as force per unit area acting perpendicular to a surface, e.g. dynes per square centimetre. In the speech literature, measured pressures are usually expressed in centimetres of water. If the pressure to be measured is associated with air at rest, then the pressure is the same in all directions and orientation of the probe tube is inconsequential (Baken, 1987). The use of a syringe to displace water in a U-tube manometer, with one end open to atmosphere, is an example of static pressure where orientation of the probe tube is insignificant. Under such conditions, the pressure is determined by the height of the stationary column of water and its specific weight, i.e. density multiplied by the acceleration of gravity. The oral pressure generated during occlusion of a bilabial stop consonant is another example of a pressure associated with stagnant flow conditions.

When the pressure to be measured is associated with moving air, the situation becomes more complicated. As shown in Figure 4.1, the spatial orientation of the probe relative to the direction of the airflow is critical. If the opening of the probe is flush with the flow channel wall, the static pressure is sensed. This is the pressure that would be felt if one moved along at the same velocity as the stream of air. The insertion of a pitot tube into the flow such that its opening is perpendicular to the oncoming stream stops the flow and senses both the static and stagnation pressures, the latter may also be called the impact or total pressure. For velocities associated with speech, air may be considered to be an incompressible fluid. For an incompressible flow, the static and stagnation pressures are related to the flow velocity by the Bernoulli equation:

$$P_s = P + (D/2)V^2$$

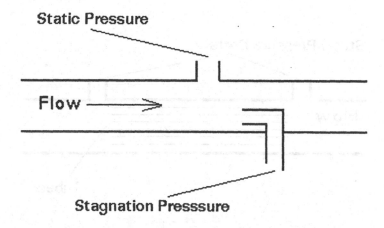

Figure 4.1. Probe alignments to detect static and stagnation pressures in a fluid flow.

where Ps is the stagnation pressure, P is the static pressure, D is the density of air, and V is the velocity. Obviously, a consistent set of units must be used. When air velocity is equal to zero, i.e. when stagnation conditions exist, it is evident from the Bernoulli equation that the static and stagnation pressures are equal.

Other probe designs could be used to measure these pressures but all would require the same orientation of the sensing holes with respect to the flow as shown in Figure 4.1 (Beckwith and Buck, 1961). Although there are probes available that provide direct measurement of air velocity, e.g. hot wires and film devices and thermistors, they too are limited by spatial alignment problems.

In applying these principles to the detection of pressures during running speech, it becomes quite apparent that spatial orientation of the sensing probe is critical to valid pressure measurements. As Baken (1987) has indicated, '. . . at least an approximation of perpendicularity must be obtained if useful pressure measures are to be taken' (p. 244). Determination of intraoral air pressure associated with production of /s/, for example, would result in a spuriously high reading if the opening of the sensing tube was positioned directly in the air stream so that both static and stagnation pressures were detected. Fortunately, there are places in the upper vocal tract where air velocities are very low during certain speech sounds, near stagnation conditions exist, and therefore the pressure is the same in all directions. The oral cavity, oropharynx, and nasopharynx are areas where these conditions may occur during stop-plosive sounds. At these locations, the static and stagnation pressures may be assumed to be equivalent (Zajac and Yates, 1991). To measure pressures associated with these sounds, catheters are inserted through the mouth and/or one of the nasal cavities. As described below,

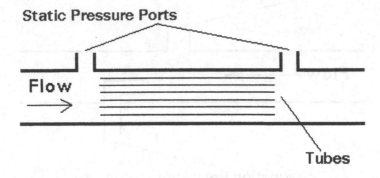

Static Pressure Ports

Flow
→

Tubes

Figure 4.2. Schematic illustration of a tube-type pneumotachograph.

this method is used to estimate the cross sectional area of the velopharyngeal orifice during production of bilabial stop consonants.

Volume flow rates

The requirements for flow rate measurement can be demanding as the
device used must have sufficient sensitivity to give accurate measurements but must not have a significant effect on the performance of the
system being tested. The Fleisch pneumotachograph meets these
requirements and has the added advantage of a linear output. As illustrated in Figure 4.2, the tube-type, Fleisch pneumotachograph provides
a resistance by channelling the flow through a bundle of small diameter
tubes. The pressure taps are positioned so that the measured drop is
independent of the direction of the flow, thereby providing for bidirec-
tional flow measurement.

The design concept of the pneumotachograph is an application of the
Hagen-Poiseuille equation for flow through a circular tube. The pres-
sure-drop is given by the equation:

$$P = 128 \mu \, LQ/\pi D^4$$

where P is the pressure drop, μ is the fluid viscosity, L is the tube length,
Q is the flow rate and D is the tube diameter. Pneumotachographs based
on this principle are available that provide for selection of maximum flow
rate (L/s) and sensitivity (cm H_2O/L/s). As indicated by Baken (1987), the
Fleisch #1 pneumotachograph is suitable for many speech applications.
This pneumotachograph has a maximum useful flow rate of 1.0 L/s, a
resistance of 1.5 cm H_2O/L/s, and dead space of 15 mL.

Screen type pneumotachographs are also available. As described by Rothenberg (1973, 1977), a fine mesh wire screen is used to cover holes placed in the circumference of a face mask. The number of holes is dependent on limiting the pressure drop to approximately 0.3–0.5 cm $H_2O/L/s$. The lower value is recommended for high airflow sounds to minimize speech distortions while the higher value is more suitable for most voiced speech work. As with the tube-type pneumotachograph, the output of the wire screen type is linear.

Both the tube and screen type pneumotachographs require appropriate transducers to convert pressure to electrical signals. They also require the need for heating of the resistive elements to avoid condensation. Although both types of pneumotachographs require a face mask, which may constrict articulatory movements, the circumferentially vented mask has the advantage of permitting the simultaneous acquisition of the acoustic signal, which is relatively undistorted.

A different concept of flow transduction uses a thermistor as the sensing element for measurement of airflow rate (e.g. Ellis *et al*, 1978). Thermistors are best known for their use in temperature measurement. They produce a large, negative change in resistance with temperature. For flow measurement, a heated bead-type thermistor is mounted in the exit tube of a standard anaesthetic mask. For subjects who cannot tolerate the mask, a small under-the-nose device has been used to give approximate indications of nasal airflow during speech.

The output of the thermistor is actually a measure of the air velocity at the point in the tube where the bead is located. Therefore, any difference in the three-dimensional velocity profiles in the exit tube of the mask, either during speech or calibration, will introduce an error in the measurement of flow rate. An advantage of the thermistor system is that it adds very little resistance to the flow regardless of flow direction. For unsteady flow, it also has the advantage of an electrical signal as its output, thus eliminating the need for a pressure transducer.

The 'orifice' equation

Warren and DuBois (1964) first applied hydrokinetic principles to the estimation of velopharyngeal orifice size during speech. The method was based on measurement of pressure loss in a fluid flow. As illustrated in Figure 4.3, if two pressure taps are positioned in a constant area pipe, the static pressure in the water at the two points would be indicated by the heights of the water in the vertical tubes. The difference in the heights of the fluids indicates that there is a pressure loss between the two points. This loss is the result of the viscous nature of the water. For steady flow in a straight pipe, the flow rate is constant and, therefore, the velocity is constant. From the Bernoulli equation it can be shown that the pressure loss is actually a decrease in the stagnation pressure as the

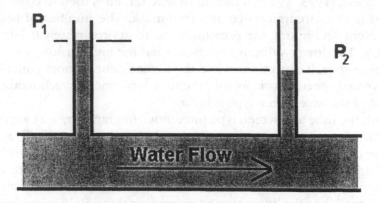

Figure 4.3. Measurement of pressure loss in a fluid flow.

flow moves through the pipe. For air flow, the pressure loss could be measured using a U-tube manometer connected to the two vertical pipes and filled with a liquid such as water or oil.

As the geometry of the upper airways may be described as two relatively large volumes connected by a smaller volume, i.e. the oro- and nasopharynx and the velopharyngeal portal, Warren and DuBois (1964) reasoned that the flow conditions in the large volumes could be considered to be stagnant. For such a flow configuration, the pressure loss created by a high rate of flow through the orifice is nearly equal to the dynamic pressure (ASME, 1959). A simple equation can then be used to estimate the area of the orifice:

$$A = \dot{V}/k[2(p_1 - p_2)/D]^{\frac{1}{2}}$$

where A is orifice area, $\dot{V}$ is the flow rate, k is a dimensionless flow coefficient, p_1 is the upstream stagnation pressure, p_2 is the downstream stagnation pressure, and D is the mass density of air.

Initially, Warren and DuBois (1964) used a small balloon positioned in the oropharynx to indirectly estimate the pressure loss across the velum. This was accomplished by instructing the speaker to breathe through the nose while one nostril was plugged with a cork stopper and the other nostril was connected to a heated pneumotachograph. This manoeuvre effectively detected the pressure drop associated with both the resting velum and the nose. Therefore, during speech any additional pressure drop for a given flow rate was assumed to result from the elevated velum. Differential pressure across the velum was calculated as the difference in breathing from speaking pressures.

Warren (1964) modified the 'pressure-flow' technique by directly measuring differential oral-nasal pressure across the velum. This was done by inserting catheters into the oral and nasal cavities. Figure 4.4 illustrates the placement of the pressure catheters and flow tube relative to the speaker. The nasal cork-catheter effectively created a stagnant column of air that was detected as the downstream pressure. This modification, which interferes only minimally with articulatory movements, eliminated the need to first determine nasal resistance during breathing.

Finally, it must be noted that Warren and DuBois (1964) additionally suggested that 0.65 be used as the value of the flow coefficient. This dimensionless value accounts for differences between the theoretical (laminar) and actual (turbulent) flow conditions in the orifice. From tests of rectangular, thin palate orifices varying in area from 2.4 to 120.4 mm² placed in a model of the upper airway, it was determined that an average value of 0.65 would suffice for the range of areas typically

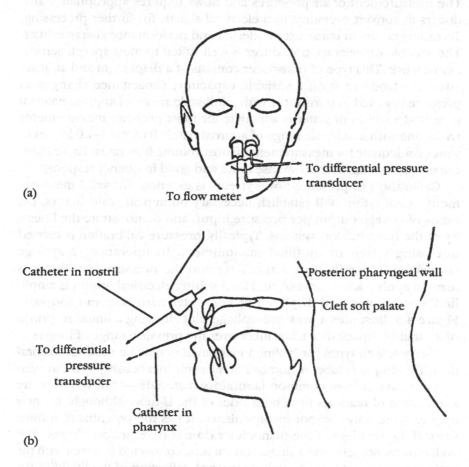

(a)

To differential pressure transducer

To flow meter

Catheter in nostril

Posterior pharyngeal wall

Cleft soft palate

To differential pressure transducer

Catheter in pharynx

(b)

Figure 4.4. The 'pressure-flow' technique. Placement of pressure probes and flow tubes. A, frontal view. B, sagittal view.

encountered in speakers with cleft palates. Although the use of this value has gained widespread acceptance, it should be emphasized that it is only an approximation. Yates *et al* (1990), for example, demonstrated that the value of the flow coefficient is also dependent upon the inlet geometry of the orifice. As stated by Yates *et al* (1990), 'Orifices that create a higher pressure loss for given flow conditions will have a lower value of k, with the opposite being true for orifices that do not produce as much disturbance to the flow' (p.194). When the actual value of the flow coefficient is determined for a given orifice, both model and human studies have demonstrated that the orifice equation provides estimates that are within 5–7% of the known area (e.g. Smith and Weinberg, 1980; Zajac and Yates, 1991).

Instrumentation and calibration

The measurement of air pressures and flows requires appropriate transducers to convert pressures into electrical signals for further processing. Transducers vary in construction, design and performance characteristics. The variable capacitance transducer is well suited to most speech aerodynamic work. This type of transducer consists of a diaphragm and an insulated electrode to form a variable capacitor; capacitance changes as pressure is varied. A transducer with a full-scale range of approximately 0 to ±10–15 inches of water is adequate for most pressure measurements while one with a full-scale range of approximately 0 to ±0.5–1.0 inches of water is adequate for measurement of most volume flow rates. These transducers provide excellent response times and good frequency response.

Calibration of pressure-flow systems is essential for valid measurements. Calibration will establish necessary numerical scale factors, i.e. ratios of voltage output per pressure input, and demonstrate the linearity of the transduction systems. Typically, pressure calibration is carried out using water- or oil-filled manometers. In operation, a syringe connected in parallel to a manometer and the pressure transducer is used to apply a known pressure. The resulting electrical output is amplified, conditioned and displayed by computer hardware and software. Figure 4.5 illustrates a pressure–voltage plot showing a linear response of a variable capacitance transducer over the pressure range of interest.

U-tubes, well types, or inclined manometers may be used for calibration. The simple U-tube manometer is relatively inexpensive — it can even be constructed from common laboratory materials — but requires the summation of readings from both sides of the U-tube. Although this may appear to be only a minor inconvenience, it has the potential to induce error if the two legs of the manometer do not have uniform bores. The well-type manometer has a single vertical tube connected to a well with the scale compensated for the small downward deflection of the liquid in the reservoir. This type of manometer permits the direct reading of pressure.

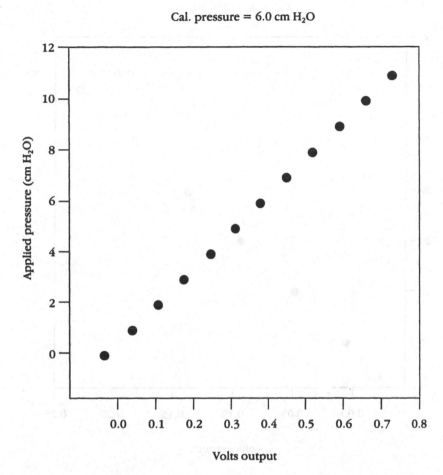

Figure 4.5. Pressure–voltage plot showing a linear response of a pressure transducer.

The inclined manometer is also a well type but provides for greater accuracy in reading the deflection of the liquid. Both types of well manometers are convenient to use but the inclined type has the disadvantage of being much larger in width for a given pressure range when compared with the vertical type.

Calibration of airflow is accomplished with a rotameter as the standard. Rotameters are relatively easy to use in that they provide for either direct or indirect reading of the flow rate, are lightweight, and only require vertical mounting to be accurate. In operation, a captured air supply causes a 'float' to rise in a vertical tube that has a tapered bore. The rise is linear with flow rate. Rotameters are calibrated by the manufacturers. Accuracy of 1% and repeatability of readings of ½% are claimed (Doebelin, 1983). Figure 4.6 illustrates a flow–voltage plot from a pneu-

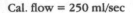

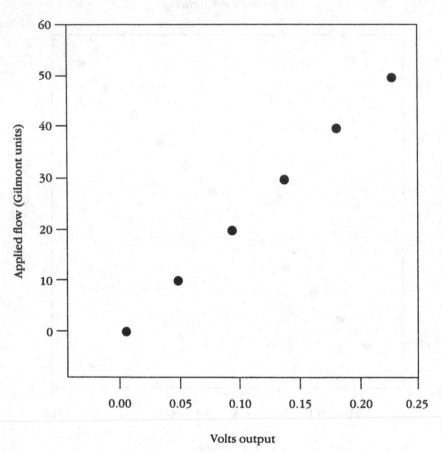

Cal. flow = 250 ml/sec

Note: 40 Gilmont units = 250 ml/sec

Figure 4.6. Pressure–voltage plot showing a linear response of a pneumotachograph and pressure transducer.

motachograph and variable capacitance transducer showing a linear response over the flow range of interest.

Aerodynamics of Normal Speech

Laryngeal function

Voiced speech sounds are produced by subglottic pressure, which causes the rapid opening and closing of the vocal folds and generates a quasi-periodic stream of airflow. This intermittent airflow is responsible for the acoustic excitation of air in the supraglottic vocal tract, which is perceived as the fundamental frequency of voice. Subglottal pressure measurement during speech may be obtained either directly or indirectly. Direct measurement requires the passage of catheters or miniature pressure transducers through the vocal folds (e.g. Koike and Perkins, 1968) or tracheal puncture (e.g. Netsell, 1969). For obvious reasons, the clinical application of either of these methods is not widespread.

Indirect estimation of subglottal pressure is possible by means of the substitution of intraoral air pressure in certain phonetic contexts such as the syllable /pi/ (Smitheran and Hixon, 1981). During oral occlusion of /p/ airflow ceases and pressure momentarily equalizes throughout the vocal tract. A catheter placed in the oral cavity will therefore sense the static pressure present in the trachea. By simultaneously collecting oral airflow during the subsequent vowel, glottal resistance can be estimated. This method, however, assumes airtight velopharyngeal closure in order to maintain stagnation-like flow conditions during the stop segment of the /p/ phoneme.

Early work by Draper *et al* (1959, 1960) indicated that subglottal pressure and glottal airflow remained relatively stable during production of steady-state vowels and equally stressed syllables. Subglottal pressure values for such utterances have been reported to range from approximately 5 to 10 cm H_2O (Holmberg *et al*, 1988; McGlone and Shipp, 1972; Netsell *et al*, 1994; Proctor, 1980; Stathopoulos and Sapienza, 1993). Typical laryngeal airflow values have been reported to range from approximately 100 to 250 mL/s during vowels in isolation (Koike and Hirano, 1968) and in syllables (Holmberg *et al*, 1988; Netsell *et al*, 1994; Putnam *et al*, 1986; Zajac, 1989). Variations among studies are typically due to age and gender of the subjects and differences in measurement techniques.

In practice, laryngeal aerodynamics may be assessed by placing a face mask over the mouth and nose. The mask should be large enough to prevent constriction of mandibular movements during speech. A hole is drilled in the mask to permit the insertion of a catheter into the oral cavity. The exit of the mask is connected to a heated pneumotachograph (Fleisch #1) and differential pressure transducer. The oral catheter is connected to a second differential pressure transducer referenced to atmosphere. Figure 4.7 illustrates the mask and catheter placement relative to the speaker.

Figure 4.8 illustrates a recording of the intraoral air pressure and laryngeal airflow obtained from a 9-year-old boy during repetition of the syllable /pi/ at a self-determined loudness level. The syllable was repeated seven times on continuous exhalation at a rate of approximately two syllables per second. Both pressure and flow data were low-pass filtered at 15 Hz and sampled 100 times per second with 12-bit resolution to an IBM-compatible computer. As shown, the intraoral air pressure peaks —

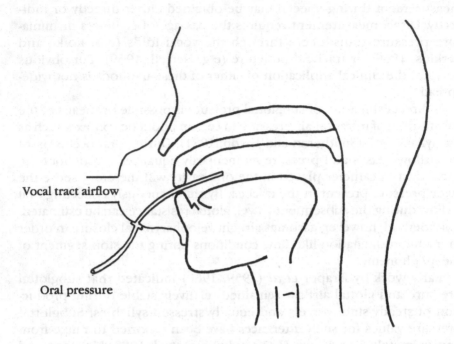

Vocal tract airflow

Oral pressure

Figure 4.7. Method to estimate laryngeal airway resistance.

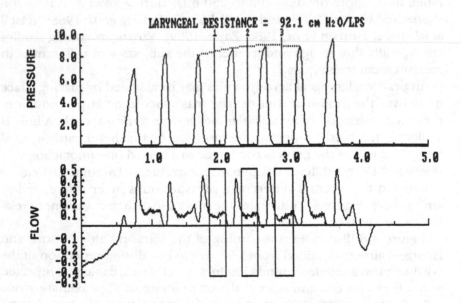

Figure 4.8. Oral air pressure and laryngeal airflow associated with production of /pi/.

which are used to estimate subglottal pressure — became relatively stable at approximately 8 cm of water after the initial syllable.

The airflow record in Figure 4.8 provides detailed information relative to phonation and also to respiration and articulation. All of the following events can be identified: (1) the pre-utterance inspiration gesture; (2) an initial burst of nasal airflow associated with velar elevation at the beginning of speech expiration, i.e. utterance onset nasal emission; (3) the absence of airflow associated with bilabial occlusion during each of the /p/ segments; (4) the abrupt onset of airflow associated with oral release of each /p/; (5) reduced, plateau-like airflow associated with voicing during each of the /i/ segments; and (6) end of utterance respiratory airflow following the last syllable. To estimate subglottal pressure, linear interpolation is carried out between the middle three intraoral air pressure peaks as illustrated by the vertical cursors in the figure. Laryngeal airflow is averaged as indicated by the three rectangular boxes. Laryngeal airway resistance is calculated as pressure divided by flow for each syllable and averaged. Laryngeal resistance for the utterance displayed was 92 cm $H_2O/L/s$. Similar laryngeal resistance values have been reported for other children (Lewis *et al*, 1993; Netsell *et al*, 1994; Zajac, 1995). Smitheran and Hixon (1981) reported average resistance of approximately 35 cm $H_2O/L/s$ for adult speakers. Zajac (1989) reported similar values for adult males, with no significant effect of phonetic context across the vowels /i/, /u/, and /a/. Laryngeal resistance of children appears to be relatively greater than adult values. This is most likely due to the smaller airways of children and the fact that children tend to habitually speak at relatively greater sound pressure levels than adults (Stathopoulus, 1986).

Although Smitheran and Hixon (1981) recommended the measurement of a single flow value at the midpoint of the vowel, we prefer to average the entire plateau-like portion of the vowel in order to obtain a more representative sample of airflow. This may be especially important in cases of respiratory and/or laryngeal pathology (e.g. Finnegan *et al*, 1994). Operationally, the beginning of airflow associated with the vowel is defined as the first flow value where corresponding pressure drops below 0.5 cm H_2O. At this point, intraoral air pressure is essentially atmospheric and lip opening has occurred. This assumption is supported by the data illustrated in Figure 4.9. Oral airflow, electroglottographic (EGG) activity of the vocal folds and oral pressure are shown in the figure. The beginning of airflow associated with oral release of /p/ is identified by the first cursor; the beginning of vocal fold vibration is identified by the second cursor. In essence, the interval between the cursors is a non-acoustic measure of voice onset time, which was approximately 100 ms. As indicated in Figure 4.9, peak airflow for /p/ was approximately 700 mL/s, average airflow for /i/ was approximately

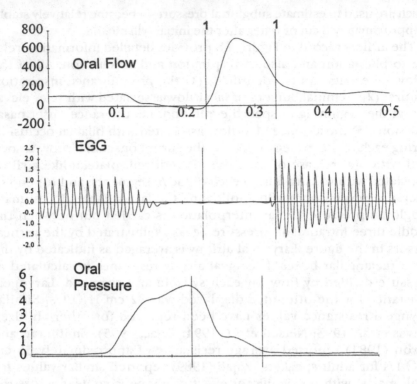

Figure 4.9. Oral airflow, electroglottographic activity, and oral air pressure associated with production of /pi/.

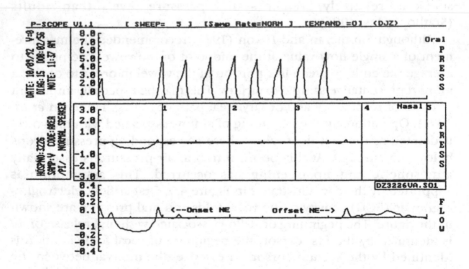

Figure 4.10. Oral and nasal air pressures and nasal airflow associated with production of /pi/.

120 mL/s, and intraoral air pressure at the beginning of voicing was approximately 0.3 cm H_2O.

Supralaryngeal function

Except where otherwise noted, the following examples of upper airway aerodynamics during speech production were obtained from adult speakers using the pressure-flow method as illustrated in Figure 4.4. All utterances were produced at self-determined rate and loudness levels. Examples of consonant-vowel syllables, isolated words and sentences containing various phonemes are illustrated. In all examples, intraoral, nasal and differential air pressures are expressed in centimetres of water, nasal airflow is expressed in litres per second and velopharyngeal orifice area is expressed in square millimetres.

Figure 4.10 illustrates the pressure and flow records of a male speaker during repetition of the syllable /pi/. The magnitude and shape of the intraoral air pressure pulses are strikingly consistent across the eight syllables. Because of the phonetic context, subglottal and intraoral air pressures are considered to be equivalent, at approximately 5–6 cm H_2O. Nasal air pressure and flow are essentially absent, as expected for a non-nasal consonant. Normal onset and offset nasal emissions are evident at the beginning and end of the utterance. Close examination of the second syllable reveals that approximately 40–50 mL/s of nasal airflow was emitted during the beginning of the intraoral pressure pulse. This type of inconsistent nasal airflow may be due to several causes. First, even in the presence of airtight closure, muscular contractions of the velum may displace the nasal volume of air (Lubker and Moll, 1965). As noted by Thompson and Hixon (1979), however, the volume rate of this type of nasal airflow is typically less than 10 mL/s. In a similar manner, nasal airflow may also occur as an artefact from movement of the flow tube. This tends to occur most frequently in phonetic contexts associated with low vowels and extensive mandibular movement. Third, the speaker may have actually relaxed the velum momentarily without affecting the overall acoustic target. Folkins (1986) referred to this type of token-to-token variability as 'flexibility' of the speech motor control system. Finally, there may be a gender bias for such nasal emission. McKerns and Bzoch (1970) reported gender differences in velar anatomy and configuration during speech production. Males apparently achieved velar closure with relatively less contact against the posterior pharyngeal wall than females. This finding suggests that males may be prone to exhibit inconsistent nasal airflow during speech.

The effects of a reduced rate of speaking on velar function are illustrated in Figure 4.11. The speaker produced a series of /pa/ repetitions at approximately two syllables per second as compared with the speaker's rate of approximately 3–4 syllables per second in Figure 4.9. Pulses of nasal airflow are evident throughout the utterance, decreasing in magnitude from the first to the last syllable. The durations and shapes of the intraoral air pressure pulses were also affected. Durations tended to increase with plateaux occurring in the pulses. These effects were caused by the relaxation of the velum after each syllable. In essence, the nasal airflow pulses were the result of multiple end-of-utterance velar gestures. The progressive reduction in the rates of nasal airflow was most likely due to diminishing lung volumes and relaxation pressures during the utterance.

As illustrated in Figure 4.12, aerodynamic characteristics of fricative production are similar to stop-plosives. In this example, an adult female repeated the syllable /si/ five times. To ensure valid pressure measurements associated with moving airflow, one of the following modifications to Figure 4.4 must be made. The oral probe may be curved and held in the mouth at the corner of the lips so that its open end approximates the sagittal plane. Or, the end of the probe may be occluded and static pressure sensing holes drilled in its walls. Either one of these modifications will provide for the required spatial orientation of perpendicularity to airflow. In addition, placement of the probe must be posterior to the alveolar constriction and pressure drop. Although intraoral air pressure during /s/ production is similar in appearance to that generated during stop-plosives, pressure on average is reduced and the duration of the pulse is increased. These changes reflect the continuant nature of fricative production.

The upper airway aerodynamics associated with nasal consonants are complex and dependent upon phonetic context. Figure 4.13 illustrates the pressure-flow characteristics associated with five repetitions of the

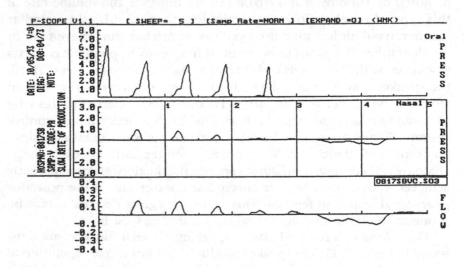

Figure 4.11. Effects of a reduced rate of speaking on velar function.

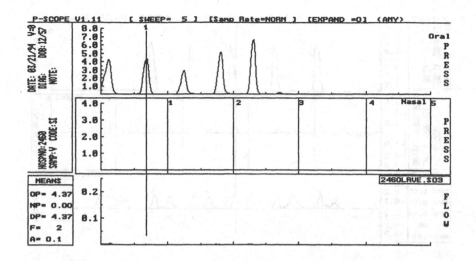

Figure 4.12. Oral and nasal air pressures and nasal airflow associated with production of /si/.

word 'hamper' produced by an adult male. Nasal air pressure and flow are evident throughout the initial syllable of each word. As indicated by the vertical cursor in the third production of 'hamper', nasal airflow was at a maximum during the /m/ segment immediately preceding oral pressure associated with /p/. At this point, the velum had relaxed maximally. The box labelled 'means' in Figure 4.13 indicates the actual values for each parameter at the location of the cursor. As shown, nasal airflow was 208 mL/s and the estimated size of the velar gap was 34.4 mm². Immediately following the nasal consonant, airflow diminished as the velum elevated for production of the oral phone. Table 4.1 presents typical values of intraoral air pressure, nasal airflow and estimated velar orifice size for the /mp/ blend from normal adult speakers (Zajac, 1994).

Figure 4.13 also reveals that the velum had relaxed in anticipation of the nasal consonant beginning with production of the /h/ segment. Indeed, nasal airflow associated with the glottal fricative /h/ was almost of the same magnitude as that associated with /m/. During the vowel /æ/, nasal airflow was reduced to approximately 30 to 40 mL/s. These variations in nasal airflow were the result of changes in both oral and velar configurations. This point is more clearly illustrated in Figure 4.14. The example shows EGG activity, oral airflow and nasal airflow from the same speaker as in Figure 4.13. The oral and nasal airflow records were obtained using a partitioned, circumferentially vented mask. The pair of vertical cursors mark one complete production of 'hamper'. Oral airflow predominated during the voiceless /h/, was reduced in magnitude during voicing associated with /æ/, was essentially absent during the /m/ and stop segment of /p/ and resumed during the release of /p/ and voic-

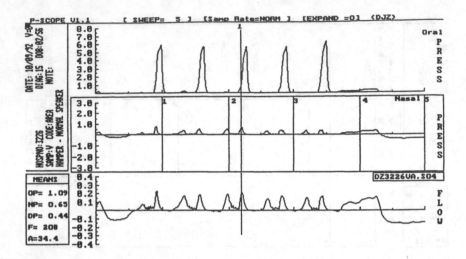

Figure 4.13. Oral and nasal air pressures and nasal airflow associated with production of 'hamper'.

Table 4.1. Means, standard deviations and ranges for intraoral air pressure (IOAP), nasal air flow (NAF), and estimated velar orifice area (VA) for /m/ and /p/ in 'hamper' as a function of gender (M=20, F=21).

	Males			Females		
	M	SD	Range	M	SD	Range
IOAP (cm H$_2$O)						
/m/	1.7	0.9	0.7–3.4	1.2	0.6	0.6–2.5
/p/	6.0	1.6	3.8–9.1	5.0	1.2	2.5–7.8
NAF (mL/s)						
/m/	152	67	47–280	132	34	92–216
/p/	21	22	2–76	9	8	0–30
VA (mm^2)						
/m/	17	9	4–43	22	10	9–2
/p/	1	1	0.1–3	0.5	0.5	0–2

ing associated with /ð/. Inspection of the nasal airflow record reveals the effects of phonetic context on velar function. Initially, the velum was elevated and nasal airflow was absent during /h/. This occurred, most likely, due to the phonetic constraints of the preceding syllable which contained oral phones. The velum relaxed and nasal airflow occurred, however, in anticipation of the nasal consonant after approximately 100 ms. Nasal airflow was reduced during /æ/ and peaked during the /m/ segment. The velum was then elevated and nasal airflow ceased during production of the second syllable.

Although the difficulties of probe alignment have already been noted,

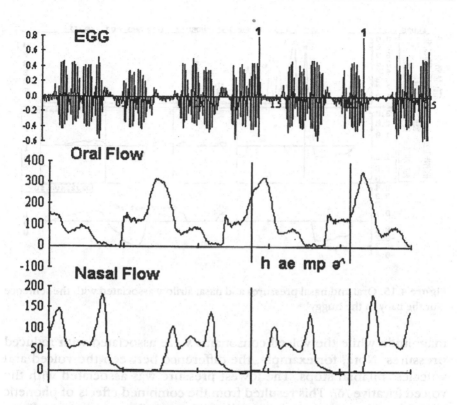

Figure 4.14. Electroglottographic activity, oral airflow and nasal airflow associated with production of 'hamper'.

it is nevertheless possible to record valid pressures associated with all consonant sounds in running speech, regardless of manner of production or place of articulation. To do so, the standard placement of the oral probe as illustrated in Figure 4.4 must be modified so that perpendicularity is maintained in the posterior oropharynx. This may be accomplished most easily by heating a polyethylene tube and then moulding it in place along the buccal-gingival sulcus and around the last posterior molar (Baken, 1987). This procedure permits the valid recording of all oral pressures associated with both moving and stagnation flow conditions. Using this approach, Figure 4.15 illustrates the pressure-flow recordings from an adult male producing the sentence, 'Put the baby in the buggy', with primary stress on the initial word. The most striking feature of the figure is the variability of intraoral air pressures as a function of phonetic context and prosody.

As indicated by Brown *et al* (1973), intraoral air pressure may be influenced by (1) the rate and volume of airflow into the oral cavity; (2) voicing activity; (3) velopharyngeal function; and (4) articulatory constrictions. These effects are evident in Figure 4.15. Pressures associated with the two voiceless stops in the word 'put' were of the greatest

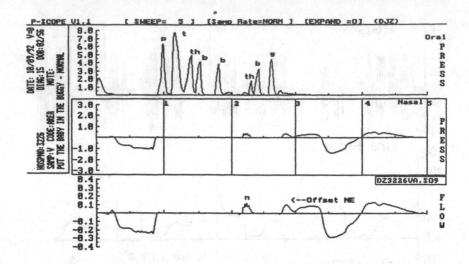

Figure 4.15. Oral and nasal pressures and nasal airflow associated with the sentence 'Put the baby in the buggy'

magnitude while the voiced consonants were associated with reduced pressures. Note, for example, the difference between the voiced and voiceless bilabial stops. The lowest pressure was associated with the voiced fricative /ð/. This resulted from the combined effects of phonetic context and prosody, i.e. /ð/ followed a nasal consonant and was unstressed. Finally, the effects of articulatory constrictions may be seen in the word 'buggy'. Pressure was relatively reduced during the bilabial as compared with the velar stop. This occurred because of a relatively smaller oral volume associated with the velar place of occlusion.

Applications in Speech Pathology

Cleft palate speech

Clinically, it has been recognized that the primary stigmata associated with individuals with cleft palate are hypernasality, nasal air emission, weak pressure consonants and the use of compensatory articulations (e.g. Trost, 1981). Clearly, two of these speech symptoms are aerodynamic by definition. In addition, compensatory articulations, such as the posterior nasal fricative, often have salient aerodynamic characteristics. Pressure-flow assessment, therefore, is particularly suited to individuals with cleft palate.

Figure 4.16 illustrates the pressure-flow recordings from a 12-year-old boy with a repaired bilateral cleft of the lip and palate while repeating the syllable /pi/. Perceptually, the boy's speech was characterized by

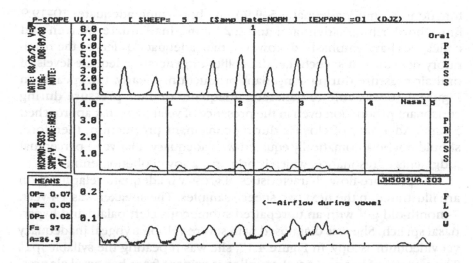

Figure 4.16. Pressure-flow recordings of a speaker with cleft palate and marginal velar function. Productions of /pi/ are shown.

mild hypernasality, which suggested marginal velopharyngeal function. Intraoral air pressures were variable during the utterance, ranging from approximately 2.5 to 5.5 cm H_2O. The lower value is considered to be marginally adequate for speech production, i.e. a minimal subglottal pressure value of 1–2 cm H_2O is required to sustain vibration of the vocal folds (Draper *et al*, 1959, 1960). Although the upper range of oral pressures were adult-like, children and youths typically produce pressures that are relatively higher. The nasal air pressure and flow recordings, however, clearly reveal the speaker's marginal velar function. Consistent nasal emission of air occurred during the bilabial stop and vowel segments, approximately 100 and 40 mL/s, respectively. Typically, nasal airflow during vowel segments is not detected by the pressure-flow method. This is because oral impedance is generally less than nasal impedance, thus shunting most airflow orally. The appearance of nasal airflow during vowels in the speaker suggests the use of increased respiratory effort, compensatory lingual articulation, or both.

Application of the orifice equation to the data in Figure 4.16 reveals that the estimated size of the velar gap was approximately 27 mm² during the indicated vowel segment. This is shown in the means box of the figure. In contrast, the speaker exhibited an estimated gap of approximately 4 mm² at peak pressure of the stop segment immediately before the vowel; pressure at this point in the utterance was approximately 5 cm H_2O. This phonetic variability relative to orifice size highlights an often misunderstood interpretation of Warren *et al's* (1989) categories of velar adequacy. Based upon estimated orifice size, Warren and his colleagues have suggested the following criteria and categories of velar function: <5 mm², adequate; 5–9.9 mm², borderline adequate; 10–19.9 mm², borderline inadequate; and ≥ 20 mm², inadequate. Warren and colleagues have emphasized, however, that 'adequacy' refers to the respiratory demands of speech, i.e. the ability to generate adequate levels of oral air pressure during consonant production. Clearly, the speaker in Figure 4.16 was able to generate 'adequate' oral air pressure during consonant production even in the presence of velar gaps that approached 5 mm². Adequacy of closure during consonant production, therefore, should not be automatically equated with adequacy relative to perceptual judgments of resonance, which is primarily a vowel phenomenon.

The pressure-flow characteristics of grossly inadequate velar function are illustrated in the next two speech samples. The speaker was a 4-year, 7-month-old girl with an unrepaired submucous cleft palate and hypernasal speech. She was diagnosed with severe velopharyngeal inadequacy via videofluoroscopy. In Figure 4.17, she was repeating the syllable /pa/. The severity of her oral-nasal coupling is evident from her nasal air pressure values, which consistently were greater than her oral pressures. At times, nasal airflow during consonant production exceeded 200 mL/s. Valid estimation of the size of the velar gap was not possible due to nasal pressures which exceeded oral pressures.

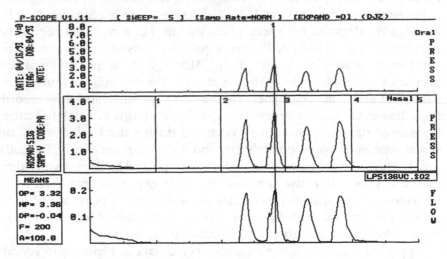

Figure 4.17. Pressure-flow recordings of a speaker with cleft palate and inadequate velar function. Productions of /pa/ are shown.

In Figure 4.18, the same speaker was repeating the word 'hamper'. The most salient feature of these recordings is the complete overlap of oral pressure, nasal pressure and nasal airflow as illustrated by the vertical cursor. In essence, oral-nasal coupling was so complete that the speaker was unable to phonetically distinguish the /m/ from the /p/ segments in the words. Warren *et al* (1989) have shown that this overlap is a distinctive feature of severe velar incompetence. Also demonstrated is the speaker's inability to generate adequate oral pressures, especially after the initial productions when respiratory air volume was presumably depleted.

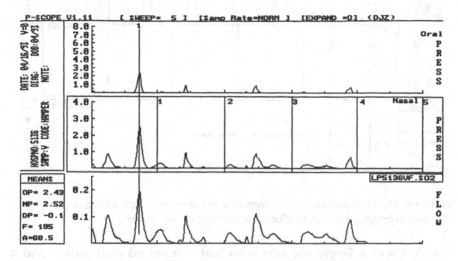

Figure 4.18. Pressure-flow recordings of a speaker with cleft palate and inadequate velar function. Productions of 'hamper' are shown.

Appropriate nasal airflow and resonance can sometimes be compromised by several conditions, including obstruction due to enlarged tonsils and/or adenoids and the effects of secondary surgical procedures. In Figure 4.19, the pressure-flow recordings of 'hamper' from a 10-year-old girl with a repaired cleft plate and a superiorly based pharyngeal flap are illustrated. Perceptually, the girl's speech was characterized by hyponasality. The aerodynamic correlate is clearly seen as a severe reduction in nasal airflow associated with /m/. In addition, anticipatory nasal airflow was entirely absent. Because the patency of the girl's nasal air passages were adequate prior to surgery, it was concluded that her hyponasal resonance was the result of an obstructive pharyngeal flap.

When inappropriate nasal airflow is limited to a single speech sound, usually the /s/, it is referred to as 'phoneme specific nasal emission'. This may occur in the absence of a palatal cleft. In such cases, the misarticulation is presumed to be learned similar to other phonologic processes. If a cleft was present and repaired, the misarticulation is considered to be a retained error pattern. Typically, air is shunted nasally through a narrow velopharyngeal portal by retropositioning of the tongue against the posterior pharyngeal wall. Nasal turbulence is generated which replaces oral frication. Regardless of the aetiology of phoneme specific nasal emission, behavioural intervention is the treatment of choice. In Figure 4.20, an example of a 'posterior nasal fricative' is illustrated. The

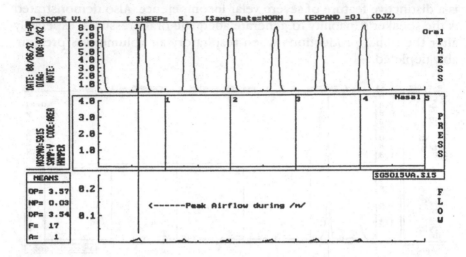

Figure 4.19. Pressure-flow recordings of a speaker with cleft palate, a pharyngeal flap and hyponasal speech. Productions of 'hamper' are shown.

speaker was a 7-year-old boy who had a repaired cleft palate and a pharyngeal flap. Although the pressure-flow recordings are suggestive of severe velar impairment, this pattern occurred only during production of syllables and words containing the /s/ phoneme. This speaker was capable of achieving velar closure, correct lingual placement, and normal oral pressures during production of /s/ after a brief period of behavioural instructions.

The idea that speakers attempt to regulate aerodynamic aspects of speech production in order to maintain some level of constancy was espoused by Warren (1986). He believed that most of the compensatory gestures exhibited by speakers with palatal clefts tended to facilitate the regulation of speech aerodynamics. The use of a nasal grimace, for example, may function to increase both nasal resistance and oral air pressure in a speaker with compromised velar function. McWilliams *et al* (1990) have also noted that some speakers with velopharyngeal inadequacy may use 'generalized laryngeal tension' as a strategy to regulate supralaryngeal airflow. Although conclusive evidence of the existence of an aerodynamic regulating system has yet to be established, many clinical findings support such a notion.

Figure 4.21 illustrates the pressure-flow records of a 7-year-old girl with a repaired bilateral cleft lip and palate repeating the syllable /pi/. Perceptually, she exhibited inconsistent hypernasal resonance and moderate hoarseness. The seven numbered cursors in the figure indicate locations of aerodynamic measurements obtained during the syllables. These are listed at the bottom of the figure. Initially, the girl emitted inappropriate nasal airflow during both consonant and vowel segments. Estimated

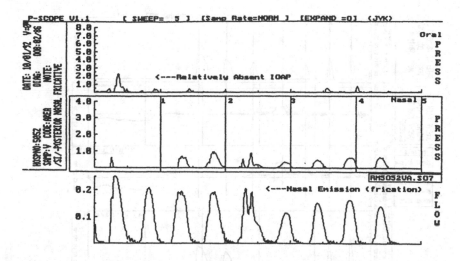

Figure 4.20. Pressure-flow recordings of a speaker with cleft palate, a pharyngeal flap and compensatory articulations. Productions of /si/ are shown.

orifice areas during consonant production, however, were less than 5 mm² during the first and second syllables. During production of the fourth syllable, orifice size increased dramatically to approximately 40 mm² while oral pressure dropped to below 2 cm H_2O. Beginning with the fifth syllable, the girl appeared to use a compensatory strategy as evidenced by a rise in pressure with concomitant decreases in both nasal airflow and estimated orifice size. By production of the sixth syllable, she had achieved essentially airtight velar closure during both consonant and vowel segments. It should be noted that the duration of her intraoral air pressure pulses increased during this process. Warren *et al* (1989) have hypothesized that the use of increased respiratory effort would serve as an effective compensatory strategy in the presence of velar inadequacy. The increases in both amplitude and duration of the air pressure pulses support this hypothesis. Such a strategy, however, may also result in increased laryngeal resistance and perceived hoarseness. Although estimates of glottal resistance were not available for this speaker, it has been our experience that some speakers with velar inadequacy increase laryngeal resistance when attempting to eliminate nasal airflow. Laryngeal resistance, however, does not appear to be affected in speakers with estimated orifice areas that are less than 5 mm² (Lewis *et al*, 1993; Zajac, 1994).

Voice disorders

The incidence of voice disorders in the general population has typically been reported to range from 7 to 10%. Estimates of vocal dysfunction in children have approached 40% in some recent studies (e.g. Powell *et al*,

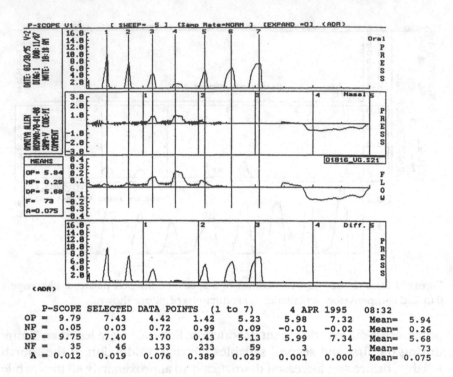

P-SCOPE	SELECTED	DATA POINTS	(1 to 7)		4 APR 1995		08:32	
OP =	9.79	7.43	4.42	1.42	5.23	5.98	7.32	Mean=	5.94
NP =	0.05	0.03	0.72	0.99	0.09	-0.01	-0.02	Mean=	0.26
DP =	9.75	7.40	3.70	0.43	5.13	5.99	7.34	Mean=	5.68
NF =	35	46	133	233	59	3	1	Mean=	73
A =	0.012	0.019	0.076	0.389	0.029	0.001	0.000	Mean=	0.075

Figure 4.21. Pressure-flow recordings of a speaker with cleft palate and inconsistent hypernasality. Productions of /pi/ are shown.

1989). Disorders involving mass lesions and/or neurologic involvement of the laryngeal structures would be expected to produce distinctive changes in laryngeal aerodynamics. The effects of vocal fold nodules, for example, may result in increased subglottal pressures as a result of increased vocal fold mass. Lotz *et al* (1984) reported such a difference between two groups of children, one diagnosed with vocal nodules and a matched control group. The group of children with vocal nodules exhibited significantly greater estimated subglottal pressures, at times exceeding 15 cm H_2O. Although Lotz *et al* (1984) reported some overlap between the groups relative to laryngeal airflow, the vocal nodules group tended to phonate with increased airflow. Although Lotz *et al* (1984) expressed caution regarding cause and effect, they concluded that the chronic use of pressures in excess of 15 cm H_2O was detrimental to acceptable vocal function.

Clinically, we have also observed the effects of organic disorders on laryngeal aerodynamics (Zajac *et al*, 1993). Figure 4.22 illustrates the oral pressure and flow recordings from a 7-year-old girl diagnosed with bilateral vocal nodules and vocal fold paresis. Perceptually, the girl's voice was judged to be moderately harsh and breathy. Average laryngeal airflow during the three /i/ segments marked was 170 mL/s. Airflow was even greater initially in the utterance, especially during the first two syllables. The child's average glottal airflow was at least 70% elevated as compared with the average airflow of the child presented in Figure 4.8. Estimated subglottal pressures averaged 11.2 cm H_2O. Again, these values were substantially higher than the child's in Figure 4.8.

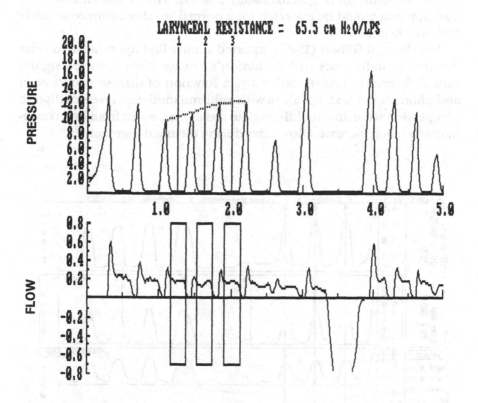

Figure 4.22. Oral air pressure and laryngeal airflow associated with a speaker with bilateral vocal fold nodules and paresis. Productions of /pi/ are shown.

Dysarthria

The defining feature of speakers with dysarthria is muscular weakness of the affected structures during both volitional non-speech tasks and speaking. Figure 4.23 illustrates the pressure-flow records of an adult female with mild mental retardation and dysarthric involvement of the velum while repeating the syllable /si/. Oral examination revealed no evidence of overt palatal clefting. Perceptually, her speech was characterized by extreme hypernasality, weak pressure consonants and turbulent nasal emission accompanied by grimacing during fricative production. Figure 4.23 reveals two striking features. First, the extent of velar impairment is indicated by the extreme magnitude of nasal air pressures and flows. Second, the durations of the /s/ segments are increased approximately two-fold as compared a normal speaker (refer to Figure 4.12 for a comparison). Figure 4.24 shows 'hamper' data from the same speaker. Consistent with severe velar impairment, there is a complete overlap of pressures and flows. In addition, the duration of the nasal airflow pulse associated with /m/ is approximately 250 ms. This is almost twice the duration that would be expected for a normal speaker of approximately 150 ms. (Zajac, 1994).

Hoodin and Gilbert (1989) reported similar findings relative to velar function in individuals with Parkinson's disease. They reported significant differences in nasal airflows as a function of disease progression and phonetic context. Speakers with mild and moderate levels of disease progression were able to differentiate nasal consonants from oral consonants by using increased flow rates during the nasal segments.

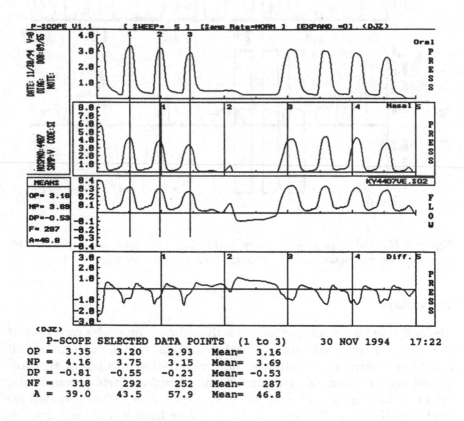

Figure 4.23. Pressure-flow recordings of a speaker with dysarthria and hypernasal speech. Productions of /si/ are shown.

Stuttering

The irregularities associated with stuttering have also been investigated by aerodynamic methods. As reviewed by St Louis (1979), researchers have consistently reported increased intraoral air pressures as the primary characteristic associated with both the fluent and disfluent utterances of speakers who stutter. Fluency enhancing techniques, such as rhythmic pacing via a metronome, were also shown to result in reduced oral pressures of stutterers. Relative to airflow, Adams *et al* (1975) reported that stutterers expended greater volumes of air than non-stutterers during fluent episodes of whispered and normal reading.

Peters and Boves (1988) directly measured subglottal pressure of stutterers and controls using a miniature transducer. The pressure transducer unit was inserted into subjects transnasally and positioned in the posterior laryngeal commissure. Audio and EGG recordings were simultaneously obtained. Peters and Boves (1988) reported that the fluent

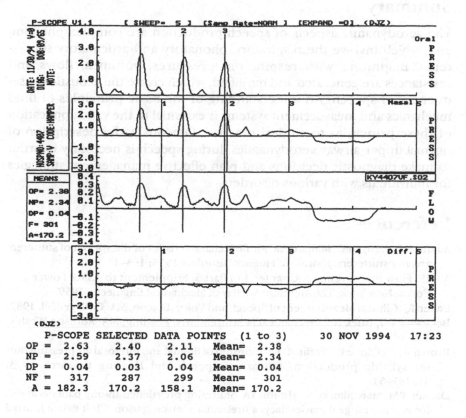

Figure 4.24. Pressure-flow recordings of a speaker with dysarthria and hypernasal speech. Productions of 'hamper' are shown.

utterances of the stutterers differed from those of controls relative to the temporal patterns of subglottal pressure build-up. Specifically, fluent utterances of stutterers tended to show four distinct patterns: (1) monotonically increasing pressure but with at least a 100 ms delay before the start of phonation (for words only beginning with a vowel); (2) non-monotonically increasing pressure before the start of phonation; (3) pressure overshoot, i.e. relatively high pressure that is reduced before phonation; and (4) extremely slow build-up of pressure.

The results of the above studies need to be interpreted with caution. Despite the fact that fluent utterances of stutterers have revealed atypical aerodynamic patterns, cause and effect relationships may still be confounded. Finally, it is interesting to note that Dalston *et al* (1987) commented on the clinical observation that relatively few individuals with cleft palate appeared to stutter. Dalston *et al* (1987) emphasized this apparent paradox because the aerodynamic characteristics of individuals who stutter and of those who have cleft palate are similar.

Summary

The aerodynamic aspects of speech production are complex phenomena, which involve the respiratory, phonatory and articulatory subsystems. Beginning with respiration, pressures, volumes, flows and resistances are generated and modified, which create the acoustic consequences of speech. An understanding of the basic principles of fluid mechanics and measurement systems is essential to the valid application of these principles to clinical practice. Obviously, the description of normal upper airway aerodynamics during speech is necessary in order to make diagnostic decisions and plan effective management strategies for individuals with various disorders.

References

Adams MR, Runyan C, Mallard AR. Air flow characteristics of the speech of stutterers and nonstutterers. Journal of Fluency Disorders 1975; 1: 3–12.

ASME. Flow measurement. Chapter 4 of Part 5. Supplement to ASME Power Test Codes. New York: The American Society of Mechanical Engineers, 1959.

Baken RJ. Clinical Measurement of Speech and Voice. Boston, MA: College-Hill, 1987.

Beckwith TG, Buck NL. Mechanical Measurements. Reading, MA: Addison-Wesley, 1961.

Brown W, McGlone R, Proffit M. Relationship of lingual and intraoral air pressure during syllable production. Journal of Speech and Hearing Research 1973; 16: 141–51.

Dalston RM, Martinkosky SJ, Hinton VA. Stuttering prevalence among patients at risk for velopharyngeal inadequacy: a preliminary investigation. Cleft Palate Journal 1987; 24: 233–329.

Doebelin EO. Measurement Systems: Applications and Design, 3rd Edn. New York: McGraw-Hill, 1983.

Draper M, Ladefoged P, Whitteridge D. Respiratory muscles in speech. Journal of Speech and Hearing Research 1959; 2: 16–27.

Draper M, Ladefoged P, Whitteridge D. Expiratory pressures and air flow during speech. British Medical Journal 1960; 18: 1837–43.

Ellis RE, Flack FC, Curle HJ, Selley WG. A system for the assessment of airflow during speech. British Journal of Disorders of Communication 1978; 13: 31–40

Finnegan E, Luschei E, Barkmeier J, Hoffman H. Sources of error in estimation of laryngeal airway resistance in patients with spasmodic dysphonia. Status and Progress Report, Vol 7. Iowa City, IO: National Center for Voice and Speech, 1994.

Folkins JW. Issues in speech motor control and their relation to the speech of individuals with cleft palate. Cleft Palate Journal 1986; 22: 106–22.

Holmberg E, Hillman R, Perkell J. Glottal airflow and transglottal air pressure measurements for male and female speakers in soft, normal, and loud voice. Journal of the Acoustical Society of America 1988; 84: 511–29.

Hoodin RB, Gilbert HR. Nasal airflows in Parkinsonian speakers. Journal of Communication Disorders 1989; 22: 169–80.

Koike Y, Hirano M. Significance of vocal velocity index. Folia Phoniatrica 1968; 20: 285–96.

Koike Y, Perkins WH. Application of a miniaturized pressure transducer for experimental speech research. Folia Phoniatrica 1968; 20: 360–68.

Lewis JR, Andreassen ML, Leeper HA, McRae MD, Thomas J. Vocal characteristics of children with cleft lip/palate and associated velopharyngeal incompetence. 1993; 22: 113–17

Lotz WK, Netsell R, D'Antonio LL, Chait DH, Brookhouser PE. Aerodynamic evidence of vocal abuse in children with vocal nodules. Paper presented at the Annual Convention of the American Speech-Language-Hearing Association, November, San Francisco, CA, 1984.

Lubker J, Moll K. Simultaneous oral-nasal airflow measurements and cinefluorographic observations during speech production. Cleft Palate Journal 1965; 2: 257–72.

McGlone RE, Shipp T. Comparison of subglottal air pressures associated with /p/ and /b/. Journal of the Acoustical Society of America 1972; 51: 664–65.

McKerns D, Bzoch KR. Variations in velopharyngeal valving: the factor of sex. Cleft Palate Journal 1970; 7: 652–62.

McWilliams BJ, Morris HL, Shelton RL. Cleft Palate Speech, 2nd Edn. Philadelphia, PA: BC Decker, 1990.

Netsell R. Subglottal and intraoral air pressures during the intervocalic contrast of /t/ and /d/. Phonetica 1969; 20: 68–73.

Netsell R, Lotz WK, Peters JE, Schulte L. Developmental patterns of laryngeal and respiratory function for speech production. Journal of Voice 1994; 8: 123–31.

Peters HFM, Boves L. Coordination of aerodynamic and phonatory processes in fluent speech utterances of stutterers. Journal of Speech and Hearing Research 1988; 31: 352–61.

Powell M, Filter MD, Williams B. A longitudinal study of the prevalence of voice disorders in children from a rural school division. Journal of Communication Disorders 1989; 22: 375–82.

Proctor D. The upper respiratory tract. In Fishman A. (Ed), Assessment of Pulmonary Function. New York: McGraw-Hill, 1980.

Putnam A, Shelton R, Kastner C. Intraoral air pressure and oral airflow under different bleed and bite-block conditions. Journal of Speech and Hearing Research 1986; 29: 37–49.

Rothenberg M. A new inverse-filtering technique for deriving the glottal air flow wave-
    form during voicing. Journal of the Acoustical Society of America 1973; 53:
    1632–45.
Rothenberg M. Measurement of airflow in speech. Journal of Speech and Hearing
    Research 1977; 20: 155–76.
Smith BE, Weinberg B. Prediction of velopharyngeal orifice area: a re-examination of
    model experimentation. Cleft Palate Journal 1980; 17: 277–82.
Smitheran J, Hixon T. A clinical method for estimating laryngeal airway resistance
    during vowel production. Journal of Speech and Hearing Disorders 1981; 46:
    138–46.
St Louis K. Linguistic and motor aspects of stuttering. In Lass N. (Ed.), Speech and
    Language: Advances in Basic Research and Practice. New York: Academic Press,
    1979.
Stathopoulos ET. Relationship between intraroal air pressure and vocal intensity in
    children. Journal of Speech and Hearing Research 1986; 29: 71–74.
Stathopoulos ET, Sapienza C. Respiratory and laryngeal measures of children during
    vocal intensity variation. Journal of the Acoustical Society of America 1993; 94:
    2531–43.
Thompson AE, Hixon TJ. Nasal air flow during normal speech production. Cleft
    Palate Journal 1979; 16: 412–20.
Trost JE. Articulatory additions to the classical description of the speech of persons
    with cleft palate. Cleft Palate Journal 1981; 18: 193–203.
Warren DW. Velopharyngeal orifice size and upper pharyngeal pressure-flow pat-
    terns in cleft palate speech: a preliminary study. Plastic and Reconstructive
    Surgery 1964; 34: 15–26.
Warren DW. Aerodynamics of Speech. In Lass N, McReynolds L, Northern J, Yoder D.
    (Eds), Speech, Language, and Hearing, Volume 1, Normal Processes.
    Philadelphia, PA: WB Saunders, 1982.
Warren DW. Compensatory speech behaviors in cleft palate: a regulation/control
    phenomenon. Cleft Palate Journal 1986; 23: 251–60.
Warren DW, DuBois A. A pressure-flow technique for measuring velopharyngeal ori-
    fice area during continuous speech. Cleft Palate Journal 1964; 1: 52–71.
Warren DW, Dalston R, Morr K, Hairfield W. The speech regulating system: temporal
    and aerodynamic responses to velopharyngeal inadequacy. Journal of Speech and
    Hearing Research 1989; 32: 566–75.
Yates CC, McWilliams BJ, Vallino LD. The pressure-flow method: some fundamental
    concepts. Cleft Palate Journal 1990; 27: 193–98.
Zajac DJ. Effects of respiratory effort and induced oronasal coupling on laryngeal
    aerodynamic and oscillatory behaviors. PhD thesis, University of Pittsburgh,
    Pittsburgh, PA, 1989.
Zajac DJ. Gender differences in velopharyngeal timing characteristics. Poster present-
    ed at the Annual Meeting of the American Speech-Language-Hearing Association,
    November, New Orleans, LA, 1994.
Zajac DJ. Laryngeal airway resistance in children with cleft palate and adequate
    velopharyngeal function. Cleft Palate-Craniofacial Journal 1995; 32: 138–44.
Zajac DJ, Yates CC. Accuracy of the pressure-flow method in estimating induced
    velopharyngeal orifice area: effects of the flow coefficient. Journal of Speech and
    Hearing Research 1991; 34: 1073–78.
Zajac DJ, Farkas Z, Dindzans LJ, Stool SE. Aerodynamic and larygographic assessment
    of pediatric vocal function. Pediatric Pulmonology 1993; 15: 44–51.

Chapter 5
Electrolaryngography

EVELYN ABBERTON AND ADRIAN FOURCIN

Introduction

It is of considerable theoretical interest and practical value to be able to monitor, measure and display aspects of larynx activity in both normal and disordered speech. In this chapter we provide an introduction to a simple method of doing so, that does not interfere with speech production: the electrolaryngograph (or simply 'laryngograph') is a non-invasive device that has become a standard tool in the Voice Clinic as well as in teaching and research laboratories all over the world. It is used to provide qualitative and quantitative information on vocal fold vibration, and also as the basis of PC-based interactive voice therapy. In these ways it complements and enriches the clinician's perceptual assessments of a client's voice difficulties and progress in therapy (Fourcin *et al*, 1995).

Although an ordinary listener perceives speech as a whole, for the phonetician and speech-and-language pathologist and therapist it can be studied in terms of separate but interacting components from each of the points of view of speech production, acoustics and perception. Thus, in acoustic terms, the physical form of voiced speech (the most frequent and most energetic speech sounds) depends on a quasi-periodic sound from the vibrating vocal folds in the larynx. This laryngeal tone, rich in harmonics, is called voice, and its production is known as phonation; this component is filtered by the vocal tract due to the changing configurations and, therefore, resonances of the supra-glottal cavities produced by the movements and muscular tension of the articulators. Although phonation and resonance interact, the characteristics of each may be separated conceptually, perceptually and experimentally, and one or the other may be selectively impaired. Thus, to consider two extreme conditions, in glossectomy, phonation and intonation are preserved, and in laryngectomy, although the normal source of speech is lost, articulatory capability is essentially intact.

From a perceptual point of view the laryngeal excitation components of speech are vitally related to both intelligibility and acceptability, through the segmental phonological voiced–voiceless contrast and through the non-segmental prosodic and paralinguistic systems of phonation type and tone and intonation. A speaker with the irregular and intermittent phonation and reduced fundamental frequency range associated with laryngitis is not so easily understood as when his or her larynx is adequately lubricated and vibrating normally. An adult male using falsetto voice is not so socially acceptable as his fellows with normal vocal fold vibration in an appropriate fundamental frequency range (Carlson, 1995); and foreigners may err socially as well as linguistically when they use an inappropriate intonation pattern or phonation type. Type and rate of vocal fold vibration provide the essential skeletal foundations of normal speech communication.

Type of vibration is responsible for vocal register; for a particular speaker a given vibration type (phonation type) is typically associated with a particular fundamental frequency range (Hollien, 1974). Rate of vibration (fundamental frequency) is the major correlate of the pitch patterns of the linguistic prosodic systems of tone and intonation. In tone languages (e.g. Chinese) the relative pitch height or contour with which a word is spoken changes the dictionary meaning of that word (Pike, 1948); speakers of tone languages suffer a particularly severe communication handicap when the ability to perceive or produce pitch variations is impaired (Fok Chan, 1984; Yiu *et al*, 1994). The pitch patterns of intonation perform grammatical (prosodic) and attitudinal (paralinguistic) functions similar to those of punctuation in written language, but the number of contrasts involved is far greater. Relative pitch height, and direction and location of pitch changes need to be taken into account. It has been shown that both phonation type and fundamental frequency patterning contribute importantly to perceived personal voice quality (Abberton and Fourcin, 1978), normal individuals in age-, sex-, and accent-matched groups being easily identified even when no supraglottal resonance information is available. These experiments, with natural and synthetic stimuli, demonstrate the important indexical (speaker-identifying) role that laryngeal speech components play.

The importance of larynx activity as the framework for speech is also shown by the young child's early ability to perceive and produce basic patterns of phonation and the basic tone and/or intonation contrasts of the native language well before the full range of segmental phonological contrasts and phonotactic patterning is controlled. It has frequently been observed that before the first birthday a child already shows language-specific pitch patterns, and Crystal (1979) suggests that by two-and-a-half years of age the tone system of a tone language has been learned, and the major intonation contrasts in an intonation language.

As yet, there are hardly any reliable quantitative studies of this stage of language acquisition but an example of very early prosodic interaction between a mother and her baby has been studied by Fourcin (1978) using spectrographic techniques to measure the fundamental frequency contours and ranges of the mother's and baby's utterances during mutual imitation.

It is not surprising that larynx vibration pattern, fundamental frequency range and intonation are disordered in many speech and language pathologies, developmental and acquired, with a range of aetiologies. For example, laryngeal patterning problems may be associated with impaired hearing (Whetnall and Fry, 1964; Abberton *et al*, 1985; Abberton *et al*, 1991), emotional or psychiatric difficulties (Leff and Abberton, 1981; Greene, 1980), or hormonal imbalance (Van Gelder, 1974), as well as those conditions with an obvious anatomical focus in the laryngeal assembly itself such as paralysis, inflammation or growths benign or malignant. The (dys)function of intonation in the speech of people with interactional, pragmatic difficulties or with dysphasia provides an example of the importance of control of larynx function at the higher, central levels of speech organization. The phonatory and pitch characteristics of the voices of speakers with difficulties of either central or peripheral origin often pose considerable descriptive and therapeutic challenges, and electrolaryngography provides a convenient way of obtaining both qualitative and quantitative information on vocal fold vibration and its linguistic use, as well as providing a clinical tool for interactive visual feedback therapy.

Operation and Output of the Electrolaryngograph

Electrolaryngography is a non-invasive technique based on the monitoring of the varying electrical admittance of the vibrating vocal folds by means of two gold-plated guard ring electrodes superficially applied to the skin of the neck on each wing of the thyroid cartilage. The notion of electrical impedance monitoring, which is basic to the design of the electrolaryngograph, was introduced by Fabre (1957) in his 'glottograph', but its implementation in the present device is quite different. These differences, the operation of the electrolaryngograph and its output waveform, Lx, have been described in detail in Fourcin and Abberton (1971), and Fourcin (1974, 1982, 1993). Here, it is sufficient to emphasize that Lx provides information about the closed phase of the vocal fold vibratory cycle. High-speed photography (Fourcin, 1974) confirms that the waveform is positive going for increasing vocal fold closure and that each peak corresponds to maximum contact between the folds; the leading edge of the waveform gives a precise indication of the beginning of the closure phase because closure normally occurs much more rapidly than opening. This interpretation of the Lx waveform has also been confirmed by Gilbert *et al* (1984) using direct vocal fold contact monitoring techniques; and by Noscoe *et al* (1983) using ultra-short pulse X-radiography ('X-flash' technique). The Lx waveform does not give explicit information about glottal aperture size and, for this reason, is called a laryngograph rather than a glottograph. (A true glottograph gives information about the glottis, which is the volume between the vocal folds.) The term electrolaryngography (ELG) may be used to distinguish the monitoring technique it makes possible from the radiographic method of enhancing soft laryngeal tissue images, which is known as laryngography (Landman, 1970).

Lx waveforms

Vocal fold vibration is a complex three-dimensional motion. The horizontal opening and closing movements of the vocal folds to and from the mid-line are familiar from views in the laryngoscope mirror and introductory textbook illustrations, but the less well described vertical component of the vibratory cycle is extremely important in the effective production of voice. Just prior to phonation the vocal folds are approximated by the rotation of the arytenoid cartilages, and as the pulmonic egressive air stream passing up the trachea flows it increases in velocity and sucks the vocal folds together, very rapidly, from the bottom upwards — an example of the Bernoulli effect. The folds then peel apart more slowly, again from the bottom upwards (as subglottal air pressure builds up), and air flows into the vocal tract. In the normal voice this cycle is repeated with great regularity, over a range of frequencies dependent on the length and tension of the speaker's vocal folds: an adult man may have a fundamental frequency range of about 80–200 Hz, and an adult woman a range from 140 Hz to 310 Hz, in conversational speech. In citation forms, expressive reading or excitement this range is extended. For the greater part of these ranges the speaker will use 'normal' or 'modal' voice, or vocal register. At the top end of his range a speaker may, on occasion, use the falsetto register, produced with thin, stretched vocal folds with a much-reduced vertical component in the vibration. At the lowest part of his range, a speaker will typically have the creaky register available. This type of voice is produced with thick, slack folds, some long closure phases and a low air-flow rate.

Figure 5.1 shows speech and Lx waveforms for three phonation types or registers, each being produced by a male adult and taken from the vowel in the word 'vast'. In each example, the upper waveform, Sp, is for the acoustic output from a microphone (positive pressure upward) and the lower waveform, Lx, is from the simultaneous output from a standard laryngograph (vocal fold closure upward). In Figure 5.1a, the acoustic waveform (Sp) has a well-defined periodicity, with the typical damped complex oscillation in each period that is the result of the

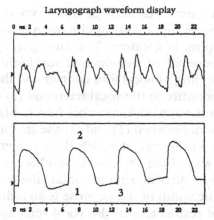

(a) Normal voice quality

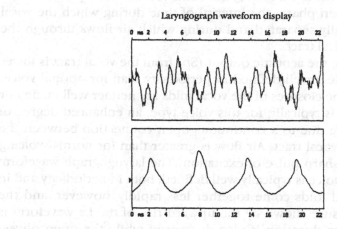

(b) Breathy voice quality

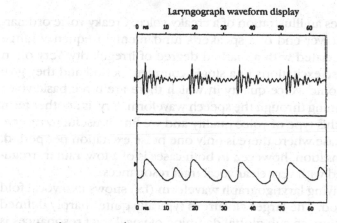

(c) Creaky voice quality

Figure 5.1. Important voice quality types.

response of the acoustic resonances of the vocal tract to a sharply defined pressure pulse input. During the open phase (defined below), the acoustic damping is greatest. The laryngograph waveform (Lx) shows a regular sequence of well-defined vocal fold closures: (1) indicates the very beginning of vocal fold contact and the start of the input pulse of acoustic pressure to the vocal tract; and (2) marks the point on Lx that corresponds to maximum vocal fold contact and the end of substantial excitation. Between (1) and (2) the steepness of the Lx waveform is a measure of the rate at which the speaker's vocal folds have closed and hence also of the sharpness (and higher frequency content) of acoustic excitation. After maximum contact the vocal folds more gradually peel apart. The width of the Lx pulse is an indication of the extent to which the main resonances of the vocal tract are isolated from the trachea during each vocal fold cycle. Point (3) has been placed in the middle of the open phase: the interval of time during which the vocal folds are maximally separated and during which air flows through the glottis into the vocal tract.

In Figure 5.1b, the acoustic output (Sp) from the vocal tract is lower in intensity and less well defined in periodicity than for normal voice. This is because the closures of the vocal folds are neither well made nor complete. There is typically, for this voice type, an enhanced degree of acoustic damping due to a continuous open connection between the trachea and the vocal tract. Air flow is greater than for normal voicing and there is no sharp pulse of excitation. The laryngograph waveform (Lx) for breathy voice is typically well defined, both in periodicity and in shape. The vocal folds come together less rapidly, however, and the steepness of closure shown by the upward rise of the Lx waveform is reduced. Closure duration is also decreased while the open phase, during which the vocal folds are separated completely, is very substantially increased.

Figure 5.1c gives an illustration of a creaky voice. Creaky voice ordinarily occurs at the lower end of a speaker's fundamental frequency range and is always associated with a marked degree of irregularity. Very often there are two pulse excitations in a single complete period and they give rise to a 'diplophonic' voice quality in which there are three basic voice pitch patterns running through the speech waveform. 'Fry' is another term used to describe this type of voice quality and we find it useful to reserve this term for the case where there is only one pulse excitation per period. The dominant sensation, however, in both cases is of a low, rather irregular pitch associated with very clear vocal tract resonances.

The accompanying laryngograph waveform (Lx) shows two vocal fold closures per period. The larger closure is typically quite sharply defined and of long duration, so sub-glottal damping of vocal tract resonances is minimized. The smaller closure in each cycle is less well defined both in rapidity of closure and amplitude and may disappear and return during even a brief sequence of vibratory cycles; it is often not linked to an evident acoustic response.

In summary, for a modal or 'chest' voice, the rapid closing phase produced by the Bernoulli effect is clearly different from the slower opening phase of the vibratory cycle as the folds peel apart. In falsetto, opening and closing rates are more nearly equal and the waveform more like that of a simple, sinusoidal, vibration. In creaky voice, closure is rapid but opening extremely slow; cycles of alternating large and small duration and amplitude also occur. Each of these three types of vibration may be accompanied by audible friction or breathiness, produced either by a longer open phase for each cycle or by incomplete antero-posterior closure of the vocal folds. In the former case, closing and opening rates will be more nearly equal.

The output from the laryngograph can be recorded and stored using conventional tape or DAT recorders. Typically, the acoustic speech signal is recorded using a microphone on one channel, and the laryngograph signal simultaneously on the other. Multi-channel recorders allow the capture of further speech production signals at the same time. Lx can be displayed live, or from recordings, on an oscilloscope. Increasingly, however, clinicians are using PC-based interfaces, with display facilities and analyses provided by their own, or commercially available, software. The manufacturers of the electrolaryngograph, Laryngograph Ltd, produce a suite of PC programs called PCLX, which perform a range of analyses based on the Lx waveform via a PC interface derived from a Laryngograph Processor. One of the programs, PCWave, allows the joint capture and display of speech and Lx waveforms.

Direct Examination and Visualization of Laryngeal Vibration

The detailed patterns relating to, for example, laryngeal air velocity or glottal area variation as functions of time are not open to simple visual examination, nor are their parameters available to the speaker on the basis of introspection as are certain gross articulatory gestures. Auditory analysis of voice quality and intonation patterns is a skill that for many people is learned only after a painstaking apprenticeship. Several methods are available for examining vocal fold vibration but they all either depend on complex electronic processing of the acoustic speech signal or interfere with speech production (Fourcin and Abberton, 1971). Classic indirect laryngoscopy, for example, involving the insertion of a mirror into the pharynx and the protrusion of the tongue, prevents more than an artificial vowel sound being produced. The flexible nasendoscope has decreased patient discomfort during laryngeal examination but the tongue is still protruded and normal speech not possible. The speed of vocal fold vibration produces only a blurred image of the superficial surface, in the laryngoscope mirror, unless a stroboscopic light source is used. Little or nothing is seen of the vertical component of vocal fold vibration. High-speed photography is possible but costly and, as it involves endoscopy, prevents examination of normally produced speech.

Stroboscopy is now beginning to be more routinely used in the ENT or Voice Clinic and to be combined with video recording (Hirano and Bless, 1993). Stroboscopy does not show the fine details of one cycle of vocal fold vibration but shows a pattern over a sequence of several cycles by making vibration appear to occur in slow motion. The larynx is illuminated by intermittent flashes of light, which are either synchronous with the vibratory cycles of the vocal folds (occurring at the same part of the vibratory cycle each time), or slightly delayed from flash to flash. The source of the trigger signals for the light flashes is the speaker's voice. When the flashes occur at the same frequency as that of the vocal fold vibration at an identical point in successive vibratory cycles, a frozen image of the vocal folds can be seen. A slow-motion effect is produced when the flashes occur at frequencies slightly different from the frequency of vocal fold vibration (each successive flash occurring slightly later in the vibratory cycle than the previous flash). The occurrence of these staged flashes is controlled by the examiner: it may be difficult to obtain clear views of irregular, pathological vocal fold vibration.

The clinician will be observing the following features:

1.   Symmetry of amplitude of vibration of the vocal folds.
2.   Phase of vibration.
3.   The mucosal wave.
4.   Periodicity of vibration.
5.   Presence or absence of glottal closure.
6.   The appearance of the edges of the folds.

A recent development introduced by McGlashan and de Cunha (Fourcin *et al*, 1997) uses the electrolaryngograph to control the light flashes automatically.

Figure 5.2a shows eight effectively instantaneous views of the vibrating vocal folds taken with a rigid endoscope looking down towards them from the pharynx. The arytenoids are at the top of each picture. The light source has been switched on under the control of a PC for only 5 micro seconds for each shot. The laryngograph waveform, Lx, has been used both to trigger each pulse of light and also to provide a reliable measure of the period of time for one complete open-closure sequence, Tx. This value of Tx has been automatically divided so that the eight photographs are equally spaced through the larynx cycle. The triggering point on the Lx waveform associated with each individual photograph is shown directly underneath it. The phonation frequency was 200 Hz.

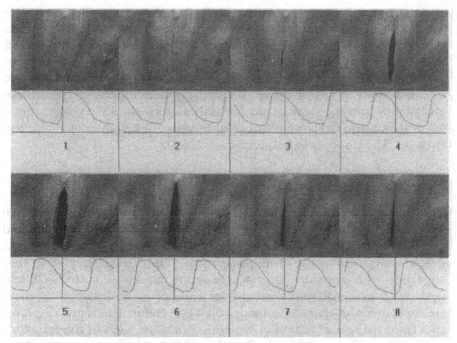

(a)Normal

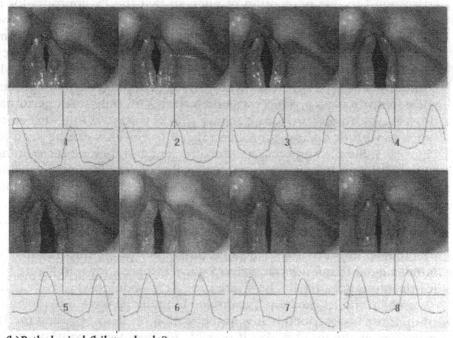

(b)Pathological (bilateral sulci)

Figure 5.2. Stroboscopic views of the vibrating vocal folds. The laryngo-stroboscopic method has been developed by Julian McGlashan and Darryl de Cunha in collaboration with Laryngograph Ltd; and this figure is included by courtesy of Mr Julian McGlashan.

In Figure 5.2b, the patient is a professional singer and comedienne with a congenital abnormality of the vocal folds in which the epithelium is attached to the underlying ligament. This condition allied with a degree of work-induced vocal fold abuse has given a pathological breathy and hoarse voice quality. The vocal folds never completely close in this sequence and the lack of correspondence between minimum glottal area and the peak of closure indicated by the Lx waveform indicates an abnormal degree of vocal fold contact below their viewable top surfaces. The phonation frequency was 208 Hz.

Fundamental Frequency Monitoring

The rate of vibration of the vocal folds is continually changing in normal speech. This fundamental frequency, Fx, variation is rule-governed and provides the major physical correlate of the prosodic and paralinguistic pitch systems of tone and intonation. The electrolaryngograph, together with another programme from the PCLX suite, PCPitch, provides a maximally accurate way of monitoring and displaying these patterns in a non-transient manner on a PC screen. The visual display is of a trace rising and falling in sympathy with the pitch of the speaker's voice. These contours are displayed on a logarithmic (octave) scale to correspond to our perception of pitch so that the Fx contours for a high-pitched voice appear higher up the screen than those for a low voice but the pattern for each is the same. As the derivation of Fx from Lx is accomplished in real time, the display of fundamental frequency that is provided shows cycle-by-cycle variation as well as overall contour. Thus, gaps appear for voiceless segments, and normal, regular, vocal fold vibration produces a smooth trace with only small perturbations for voiced obstruent consonants. Creaky voice and other irregular types of vibration show a broken ragged trace. This can be seen in Figure 5.3. Simple and accurate measurement and therapeutic training of 'voice pitch' become possible when the Lx waveform is available directly in the clinic or, if only measurement is required, from a suitable tape recording. Direct access to the moment-by-moment movement of the vocal folds eliminates the need to rely on uncertain measurement based on the acoustic signal and can give real-time feedback to the user of reliable information of intonation shape, range and regularity. Fundamental frequency traces derived from Lx are shown in Figure 5.3 for the utterances 'ha ‚llo, how `are you?', 'I'm `fine'.

Both Lx and Fx can be of great value in remedial work and the basis of their use is described below in the section on therapy. Using the Lx waveform as the input makes it possible to show these contours without any averaging as opposed to classic methods of speech signal analysis for example, Noll, (1967). In this way, small closure-to-closure variations can be clearly seen.

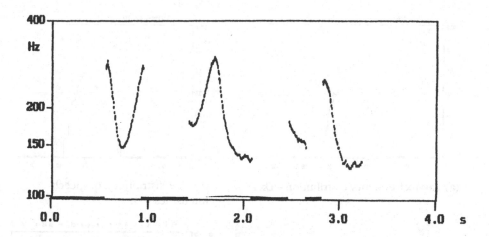

Figure 5.3. Cycle-by-cycle fundamental frequency contours — Fx.

Quantitative Description of Vocal Fold Vibration Using Electrolaryngograph Recordings and the PCPitch Program

As the electrolaryngograph signal, Lx, can be recorded on a tape-recorder or direct to computer memory, large amounts of data from spontaneous speech or reading can thus be collected and conveniently stored. Fundamental frequency information from a large sample of speech can be summarized, in a compact visual representation, by the use of a statistical analysis of the probability distribution of larynx periods. The resulting fundamental frequency range distributions correspond well with our auditory impression of wide or narrow pitch ranges, and the clearly visible modes or peaks (corresponding to a speaker's preferred fundamental frequency) correspond with our perception of high and low voices (Abberton, 1976; Fourcin and Abberton, 1976). Figure 5.4 shows some PC-based measures related to normal voice range and regularity and intensity.

In Figure 5.4a, a normal adult male reading a standard text has been recorded on a two channel DAT recorder with Sp, the acoustic signal, on the left channel and Lx, the accompanying laryngograph output, on the right channel. This Dx1 analysis uses only the Tx, larynx period, measurements made from the detection of successive peaks in the Lx waveform. The graph shows the probability of larynx vibrations over the range of frequencies normally linked with voice production. Here, the range is well defined and there is a clear modal (most prominent) frequency.

The same Lx recorded information has been used in Figure 5.4c to give an analysis of the degree of regularity in the speaker's vocal fold

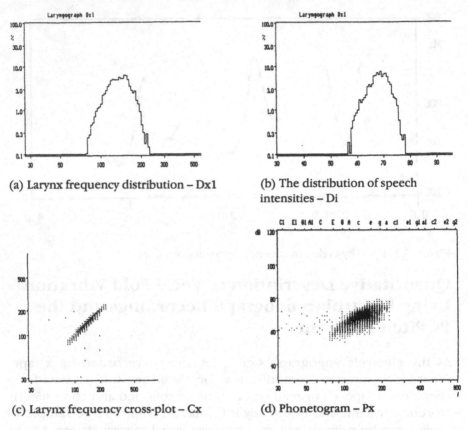

(a) Larynx frequency distribution – Dx1

(b) The distribution of speech intensities – Di

(c) Larynx frequency cross-plot – Cx

(d) Phonetogram – Px

Figure 5.4. Quantitative measurements of normal voice and speech.

vibration sequences. This has been done by taking the Lx periods in successive pairs and simply plotting the period of the first member of each pair against the period of the second — all through the complete recording. In this way, any irregularity shows up as a plotted point, which is not on the main diagonal.

Figure 5.4b shows the distribution of speech intensities, Di. This sample is an important indicator of phonatory control and, just as in the case of the phonetogram, (d), the combined use of Sp and Lx makes it feasible to measure the peak acoustic intensity in each vocal fold cycle by using the Lx closure to define the momentary peak of acoustic activity. Here, only the acoustic information is plotted and this shows, for this speaker, a well-defined range with no abnormality.

The phonetogram (Figure 5.4d) classically shows the range of acoustic intensities in the speaking or singing voice plotted against their corresponding vocal fold frequencies. Px, in this figure, has been obtained by making use of the Sp and simultaneously recorded Lx signals so that the larynx synchronous peak intensity of the acoustic waveform is plotted against the Fx value for that particular larynx cycle. This technique gives an accurate measure of Fx and it also makes it possible to obtain instantaneous measures of peak speech intensity, even in a relatively noisy clinic.

Other voice parameter measurements are also available with the PCLX programs. An important correlate of perceived breathiness is provided by the relative durations of the open and closed phases of the vocal fold vibratory cycle. The variation with time of this measure is illustrated in Figure 5.8(d).

Another graphical representation of quality of phonation is provided by Qx plots (Figure 5.5). Qx is the ratio of closed phase duration to the duration of the total larynx period, and relates to the quality of excitation of the vocal tract provided by the vibrating vocal folds. The longer the closed phase, the 'better' the voice, in the sense that it is perceived as being well projected. The analysis in Figure 5.5a is based on a 2-minute sample of read speech using material familiar to the speaker, a normal 40-year-old. The range of Qx (expressed here as a percentage of the corresponding Lx period) is typical and is shown by the distribution of filled circles. The size of each little circle corresponds to the number of larynx periods which had that level of Qx for that value of Fx.

In Figure 5.5b, the speaker is also reading a passage that is well known to her and is of the same age with Dx1 and Cx very similar to those for the normal speaker above. She is a heavy smoker and has Reinke's Oedema, however, and her poor Qx range is associated with a very breathy voice. This analysis is of real diagnostic and therapeutic value since it so clearly presents an essential dimension of voice quality which is not otherwise readily quantified.

Electrolaryngography in Speech Pathology

It has always been the aim of the electrolaryngography work originating from University College London to provide basic information not only on normal phonatory processes and fundamental frequency patterning and their relationships with perceived voice quality and 'tone of voice', but also on a range of voice production and perception disorders; a further aim has been to develop associated practical methods of therapy for the reduction of these disorders. Fourcin (1982) points out that (1) in the assessment of vocal pathology it is essential to produce evaluations that relate to voice production; and that (2) the electrolaryngograph is well suited to this purpose as its output is directly related to the events in the cycle of vocal fold vibration (the closing and closed phases), which are most important to the production of speech sounds: the vocal tract receives maximum excitation when it is isolated from the sub-glottal cavities by the closed vocal folds. Disorders of phonation will most likely be associated with the closing and closed phases of vocal fold

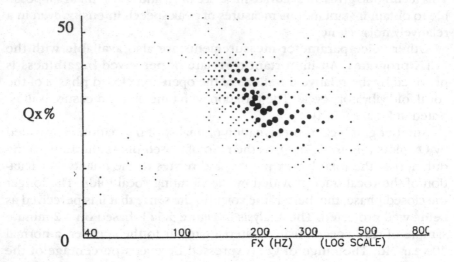

(a) Normal

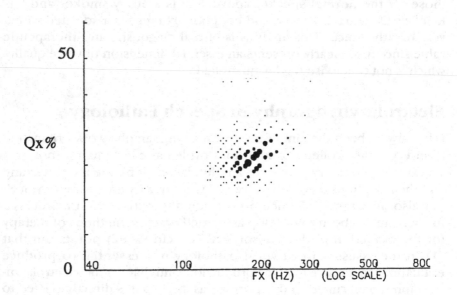

(b) Pathological

Figure 5.5. Closed phase plotted against fundamental frequency – Qx v Fx.

vibration. The measures referred to in the previous section are thus well suited to the evaluation of pathological vocal fold vibration.

Abnormal Lx

A voice with an abnormal excitation may be characterized physically by irregular or otherwise imperfect vocal fold vibration throughout an utterance, or by only short sections of abnormal or inadequate vibration which nevertheless auditorily colour the speech continually. These points of inadequacy typically occur at major pitch changes (nuclear tones, for example) or in association with certain oral articulations, such as the lingua-velar adjustments needed for velar consonants. In both these cases, the aerodynamics of laryngeal air flow are disturbed and the speaker cannot produce regular vocal fold vibration.

Normal vocal folds are of equal mass and stiffness and their mucous covering provides viscosity. These physical features may be disturbed in a variety of pathological conditions: mass can be increased on one fold by a growth such as a polyp or a carcinoma; stiffness asymmetry results from unilateral paralysis; and viscosity is altered in infections such as laryngitis, or when the folds are abnormally dry for other reasons. Figure 5.6 illustrates an effect on Lx waveforms of a pathological condition. In normal phonation the lower surfaces of the vibrating vocal folds come into contact first. The peak of contact is achieved when the upper surfaces are in evident close contact and by then the lower surfaces are already separated. For the pathological condition shown in Figure 5.2b this normal sequence of events has not applied. The Lx waveform in Figure 5.6a, taken from a DAT recording of this speaker, shows minor but important closure irregularities. In addition to the variability in closure amplitude, three of the closing phases, on the left of each peak, show a small indentation. This is often an indication of an inadequacy of lower surface contact (and is found in other conditions, for example in laryngitis when the lower surfaces are more affected than the upper).

In Figure 5.6b, the Sp and Lx waveforms are taken from the word 'make', in the same recording, immediately at the beginning of the devoicing associated with the voiceless [k]. In normal speech production, the [k] closure in the vocal tract for this word is linked with a laryngeal adduction of the vocal folds so as to inhibit the continuation of voicing. For this speaker, the deformity of the opposing vocal folds has led to an unusual increase in contact as a transient result of this manoeuvre — and a quite abnormal Lx waveform.

Abnormal Lx waveforms have been presented and discussed in a number of studies. The first such study (Fourcin and Abberton, 1971) illustrated typical waveforms from speakers with unilateral vocal fold paralysis, ventricular vibration and laryngitis, and the observation was made, for the first time, that phonation is not necessarily consistently

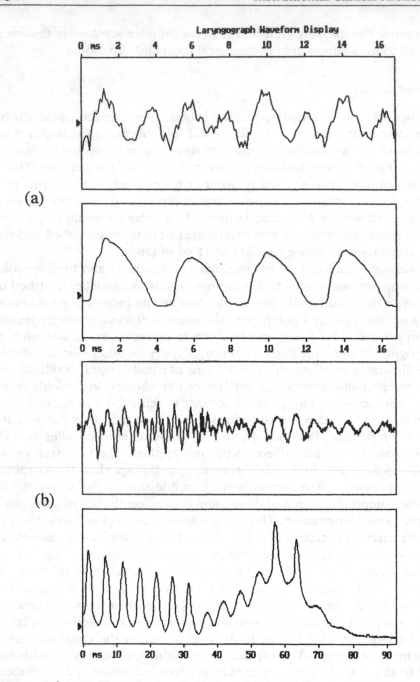

Figure 5.6. Sp and Lx examples of pathological voice quality.

and uniformly impaired in a pathological condition, and that a failure found repeatedly in one part of an intonation pattern may not be found elsewhere. Fourcin and Abberton (1976) show Lx waveforms with the corresponding pressure-time speech waveforms from speakers with unilateral paralysis, a pedunculate polyp (pre- and post-operatively) and from a normal speaker who had had an intramuscular injection of atropine to produce artificially dry vocal folds. In all the pairs of waveforms the simplicity of the Lx waveform compared with the complexity of the acoustic waveform allows the nature of the physical impairment of vocal fold vibration to be seen and interpreted in physical terms (Fourcin and Abberton, 1976, p. 118). Wechsler (1976a,b, 1977) studied vocal fold vibration before, during and after treatment for 20 speakers with inflammatory conditions or disorders of muscular control. Voice quality was assessed with the help of standard qualitative laryngologists' and speech therapists' judgments and patients' opinions, and of Lx waveforms. Fourcin (1982) interprets normal Lx waveform shapes in terms of the five features listed below, and points out that in pathology the Lx waveform can usefully be interpreted with reference to these five features to derive an indication of the nature and degree of the impairment. The five features have clear perceptual correlates.

1. Uniform Lx peaks are likely to be associated with a correspondingly uniform acoustic output, and perceived smooth voice quality.
2. Sharply defined Lx contact implies good acoustic excitation of the vocal tract.
3. Long closure duration (contact plus separation) is likely to be associated with well-defined, relatively undamped formants. Features 2 and 3 relate to the perception of a strong, well-projected voice.
4. Regular sharply defined contact periodicity will give a well-defined percept of pitch.
5. Progressive change in sharply defined Lx period lengths will be associated with a smoothly changing voice pitch.

The relationship between perceptual and phonetic categories and physical, quantitative correlates is discussed and illustrated with particular reference to laryngographic assessment of phonation in Fourcin (1993), and (Fourcin et al, 1997).

It is important to realise that there is no unique relationship between a pathological Lx waveform and a given anatomical or physiological condition. ELG-based measures help to make more precise *quantitative* descriptions of a disorder, as do physical interpretations of the waveform in terms of mass, tension, symmetry and conductivity. All these contributions to our understanding supplement, but do not replace, visual examination by laryngoscopy. Stroboscopic laryngoscopy (see above) is becoming more widespread in Britain and the possibility of controlling the illumination of the larynx by laryngograph-based phasing of the light flashes allows the clinician to observe anatomical details and abnormalities of motion in an increasingly precise manner. This can obviously help in planning surgery and voice therapy (Fourcin *et al*, 1995; Fourcin *et al*, 1997) (see Figure 5.2).

Abnormalities of Fundamental Frequency

It is important from a theoretical point of view as well as from a clinical standpoint to realize that the laryngeal (and, incidentally, supra-glottal) components of a perceived voice quality do not depend only on consistent or 'long-term' settings of the speech apparatus. The dynamic features associated with changing fundamental frequency interact with variations in phonation type and play an essential role in giving the characteristic auditory colour to a voice. The following fundamental frequency characteristics may be impaired: (1) smoothness of Fx contour; (2) Fx contour shape; (3) Fx range; and (4) distribution of frequencies within the overall Fx range. The use of the characteristic pitch patterns, the intonation, of a language also play a vital role in the perception of voice quality: a good example is provided by the common assessment of an impaired voice as being 'monotonous'. Vocal monotony is a complex percept. It may, as the term suggests, be related to a narrow pitch range (but very rarely a true monotone), and also to constant loudness or quietness; however, it may be the case that a perceptually monotonous voice has a normal pitch range but a limited, stereotyped use of intonation patterns (Abberton *et al*, 1991) and it is this linguistic deficit rather than a pure production problem that is responsible for the 'monotonous' label. The combined use of linguistic patterning and physical measures provides insights into the nature of the perceived voice.

The derivation of Fx from Lx is accomplished in real time and on a cycle-to-cycle basis with no averaging. Thus, every detail of the timing of successive vocal fold closures can be examined. Fourcin and Abberton (1971), Abberton and Fourcin (1978), Abberton *et al* (1989) and Fourcin (1993) show typical Fx contours for English intonation patterns from a normal speaker: the Fx traces are smooth, reflecting regular vocal fold vibration, and show clearly defined changes associated with the words of greatest pragmatic importance in the utterances. The only departures from smooth contours are, as described above, for gaps in the Fx traces for voiceless consonants, and a broken trace for the normal brief use of creaky voice at low fundamental frequencies. In Fx traces from speakers with laryngeal or auditory processing problems, on the other hand, the regularity may be disturbed in predictable ways. In cases of extreme mechanical abnormality, regular symmetrical vibration is impossible, broken traces are produced throughout, and no clear perception of pitch changes is produced. Often, however, vibration may become irregular or cease altogether only at certain points, particularly at major pitch changes. When a voiced obstruent consonant is produced, the normal momentary lowering of fundamental frequency may be replaced by a cessation of voicing. Although stretches of Fx remain regular the disturbed portions are sufficient to give an impression of continuous abnormality, because of our auditory sensitivity to random variation in the timing characteristics of vocal fold vibration. Fourcin (1982) gives Fx traces for an utterance including a high falling nuclear tone and a voiced velar plosive from the same speaker (1) with normal vocal folds and (2) following an intramuscular injection of atropine. The disturbances described above as well as the stretches of normal vibration are clearly seen.

A great deal of ELG work has been carried out on the description, measurement and remediation of abnormal Lx and Fx patterning in hearing-impaired speakers. The original work (with adults) and the relevant fundamental frequency and linguistic parameters are described and illustrated in Fourcin and Abberton (1971) and Abberton and Fourcin (1975). Because of the lack of adequate auditory monitoring, deaf and deafened speakers are likely to have abnormal voices with defects in the areas of Fx patterning listed above. Regularity of vibration and Fx contour choice and shape are typically two major areas of difficulty; phonation may be in falsetto or creaky registers (intermittently or consistently) and contrastive use of pitch changes lacking or reduced. (See Fourcin and Abberton (1971); Abberton and Fourcin (1972, 1975) and Abberton et al (1977) for illustrations.) Wirz and Anthony (1979) show Fx traces for deaf children illustrating improvement in vocal fold regularity through interactive ELG based training, and also improvements in overall Fx levels and the beginnings of intonation control — all features that had previously been monitored and improved in adults as described in the publications referred to above. King and Parker (1980) similarly describe the use of of ELG techniques when considering the importance of prosodic features in speech work with deaf children.

Demographic trends make it likely that, in future, speech and language therapists will increasingly work with older people who have hearing problems.

Recent ELG work with deaf speakers has concentrated on the provision of perceptual ability for voice pitch-based aspects of speech, and improvements in their control of speech production, for very profoundly, or totally, deafened adults (Abberton et al, 1985; Ball, 1991). Voice quality and intonation are essentially invisible features of speech for people who must rely on lip reading for speech perception. Such is the case for people who are so very profoundly deaf that they cannot make use of even the best conventional amplifying hearing aids, or who are totally deaf. For totally deaf speakers, cochlear implants providing electrical stimulation to the auditory nerve can restore useful speech perceptual ability (Rosen et al, 1981; Rosen, 1997). For the far greater numbers of very profoundly deaf speakers, cost-effective acoustic hearing aids based on clarification rather than simple amplification of speech are being developed (Fourcin, 1990). In principle, these speech pattern element aids can provide a single feature (such as voice pitch) or a combination of features (e.g. pitch + frication) depending on the remaining receptive abilities of the user. They are essentially complementary to lipreading, providing information that is invisible to supplement information, such as place of articulation, which can often be seen on the face of the speaker. The electrolaryngograph is being used to help in the design of these aids and in the perceptual and productive speech rehabilitation of users. Speech pattern element aids make use of miniaturized computer technology, and algorithms known as neural nets. The first, and arguably the most important, speech element to be presented via these aids is voice pitch and the neural net programs needed are based on ELG data.

Users of any hearing aid must be helped to make best use of the unfamiliar sound they receive. This is particularly so for profoundly deaf users, and interactive visual displays of the sort described in the next section can be of great value in speech production as well as speech perception work. Here, again, is an example of the speech and language therapist's use of the interplay of physical and linguistic features in pathology and therapy: both regularity of vocal fold vibration and the use of the contrastive pitch and rhythm patterns of intonation contribute importantly to perceived normal or abnormal voice quality and are essential parameters to work with in assessment and therapy.

Fundamental frequency range and distribution of frequencies within that range are important indices of vocal performance, and they are capable of compact quantitative expression using Fx histograms suitable for inclusion in case notes. The effects of pathology can be clearly seen. In a normal speaker the Fx probability distribution is clearly defined with prominent modes (Abberton, 1976; Fourcin, 1982). The loss of the high or low ends of a speaker's range with, for example, inadequate vocal fold lubrication and impaired viscosity are easily visible (Fourcin, 1982), as are the extension of the low frequency end on the distribution and the the lack of peaks seen, for example, with prolonged smoking (Abberton, 1976). The effects of surgery or therapy can be clearly indicated in this way: Fourcin (1982) and Abberton *et al* (1977) show the extension of Fx range produced by deaf adults after work with an interactive Fx display. Ball, Faulkner and Fourcin (1990) and Toffin *et al* (1995) show similar immediate effects for a profoundly deaf speaker with and without self-monitoring provided by a speech pattern element hearing aid of the sort described above. Fourcin and Abberton (1976) and Wechsler (1977) show histograms for patients before treatment for laryngeal disorders either by surgery or speech therapy. The Lx waveform provides an excellent basis for this sort of analysis, because the beginning of each closure is indicated with a greater precision than is at present possible with other methods of analysis, and the simple form of the Lx waveform lends itself to real time analysis in which a simple algorithm identifies the start of onset for each vocal fold closure (Fourcin and Abberton, 1976; Fourcin, 1982).

Figure 5.7 shows ELG-based measures for speakers with disorders of laryngeal control. In Figure 5.7a, Dx1, as in Figure 5.4, is based on the use of the Lx waveform and this, as before, has made it possible to show features of the phonation which are otherwise difficult to observe. The main part of the Dx1 plot indicates a useful voice range with a well-defined mode (and the asymmetrical shape that we have learned to associate with a young(ish) woman). At the low end of the frequency range the secondary peaks are ordinarily indicative of creak or irregularity.

The Cx plot in Figure 5.7b shows strikingly that the speech sample is not entirely normal in regard to its regularity of vocal fold vibration. Pairs of closure cycles are far from uniformly similar.

The intensity distribution in Figure 5.7c has two striking features. First it is rather narrow, indicating a narrow range of intensity control. Second, Di1 has an unusual low frequency tail. In the second order, Di2 distribution which is not shown here (but which, like Dx2 is part of the standard Laryngograph Ltd package), the plotting only of those pairs of successive intensities that fall into the same intensity range eliminates the contribution of irregular, shimmer type, variations from cycle to cycle and this low frequency tail disappears.

Just as it is possible to plot pairs of Dx that show both the events in the sample which are irregular and those which are consistent, so also is it feasible to plot a pair of phonetograms that show, in Px1, all the samples and, in Px2, only those which are pairwise regular (Figure 5.7d). For normal speech, the difference between these analyses is not striking. For this mildly pathological sample, however, the comparison confirms the previous results in showing a marked difference, with the low-frequency points eliminated in Px2.

Clinical Applications of Electrolaryngography

The previous sections have shown how the electrolaryngograph can contribute to our knowledge of the definition of vocal pathology and its perceptual effects. The ELG work has always been explicitly oriented towards clinical therapeutic applications as well as the theoretical in the study of pathological speech perception and production. Although, therefore, it is rather artificial to describe the work under separate pathology and clinical headings, as the techniques and findings we have described are now widely employed abroad as well as in the UK, it is worth commenting on the main clinical speech and language therapy applications of electrolaryngography.

The earliest therapy with ELG using interactive feedback techniques

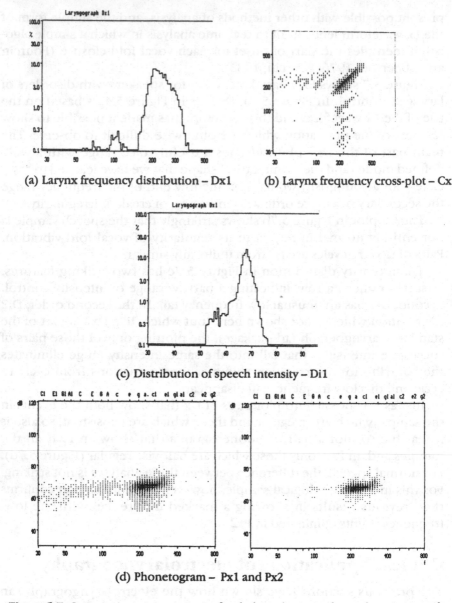

(a) Larynx frequency distribution – Dx1   (b) Larynx frequency cross-plot – Cx

(c) Distribution of speech intensity – Di1

(d) Phonetogram – Px1 and Px2

Figure 5.7. Quantitative measurements of pathological voice and speech — an example.

with a dynamic display of Lx or Fx was with profoundly deaf adults (Abberton *et al*,1977). It is clear that with phonetically and linguistically informed guidance these speakers can benefit from the visual informa-tion derived directly from their vocal folds to learn new patterns of laryn-geal control and to monitor their speech in new ways. Subsequent studies showed that young children and adolescents can also benefit from the technique. Fourcin (1980) describes some results obtained with children showing how their perception of a basic intonation contrast improved as a result of linguistically oriented production work of this sort. The enhancement of perception as well as production is essential for the maintenance of new speech skills, no matter what pathology is involved. Abnormal vocal fold vibration is a common problem for hearing-impaired speakers and, along with intonation patterning, is a focus of attention in therapy with laryngograph techniques. Dysphonia in normally hearing speakers with laryngeal problems provides a range of conditions open to investigation, description and remediation using the PCLX software package. Once again, the clinical focus is on the interaction of perception and production in bringing about voice improvement as speakers become aware of what they are doing and what they sound like by having their attention drawn to dynamic visual displays related to perceptually and productively salient features.

Therapy for Speech Perception and Production based on ELG

Dynamic displays of Lx or Fx on VDUs/PC screens form the basis of highly effective interactive programmes of therapy based on reinforcing or error-correcting visual feedback (Fourcin and Abberton, 1971, Fourcin *et al*, 1993). The same displays can also be used for foreign language learning and teaching (van Wieringen and Abberton, 1994). They are motivating for both the voice patient and foreign language learner and often produce improvements not possible with other techniques (Carlson, 1995). Attention can be drawn to the key speech elements that are being worked on, and then the practice technique is essentially that of pattern matching: a model pattern – Lx waveform, or Fx contour – is displayed on the screen and the speaker compares his or her output (also on the screen, below the model) with the target, and the therapist and patient consider the match. Feedback can thus be correcting or reinforcing. It is worth emphasizing that perception as well as production can be worked on with visual pattern presentation; indeed, focusing and 'tuning' the user's hearing must typically precede production practice, to help establish auditory and linguistic awareness of voice quality and intonation (Abberton *et al*, 1985). This association of heard and seen patterns lays the foundation for future self-monitoring by hearing alone after interactive speech production work with the displays has established new knowledge and skills. Observation of Lx is used to establish or change vocal fold vibration type (register), and Fx contours for work on pitch height and range, and intonation. In association with a microphone, input Fx traces can be modulated by intensity (Fourcin and Abberton, 1995) to indicate rhythmic stresses using a thickening of the trace; a patterned indication of voiceless frication can also be presented for plosive bursts and fricative consonants, particularly sibilants.

Important factors that make for successful 'biofeedback' therapy of this kind are as follow:

1.   The visual feedback provided is patterned: speakers are not simply given binary 'yes' or 'no' information about the correctness of their utterances: they can see where and in what way they have gone wrong. A balance is struck in the patterns presented between showing excessive detail (as would be the case with a raw speech waveform or conventional spectrogram, Figure 5.8a), and over-simplification (such as smoothing Fx contours) which obscures perceptually important detail. Thus, ELG displays of fundamental frequency show cycle-by-cycle variation giving a clear visual indication of the smooth, regular vocal fold vibration associated with clear, modal phonation (Figure 5.8b), but also showing a broken, ragged trace if vocal fold vibration is irregular and associated with creaky voice or excessive use of glottal stops and 'hard attack'. Rhythmic structure is indicated by thickened parts of the Fx trace.

2.   The visual patterns are not transitory and feedback is immediate, with the patterns appearing on the screen as the speaker produces them. At the appropriate stage in therapy, as a means of encouraging auditory rather than visual appraisal of the utterance, delayed feedback is possible by the provision of a 'hide' facility allowing the patterns to appear only after the speaker has made an auditory judgment on their acceptability. The traces and waveforms produced can be stored so that later discussion is facilitated, comparisons can be made and progress monitored. Storage can be on disk and printout.

3.   For effective visual feedback the patterns must correspond in a straightforward manner to our auditory perception. Thus, for fundamental frequency, the trace rises and falls in sympathy with the pitch of the voice, and a logarithmic (octave) scale is used to conform with our auditory perception of pitch: speakers with high or low voices (and correspondingly very different average fundamental frequencies) will produce contours of the same shape – but higher or lower on the screen – corresponding in a natural and simple way to our normal experience of intonation patterns and 'tone of voice'. Acoustic auditory targets are thus provided rather than articulatory instruction (Abberton *et al*, 1976).

4.   An important practical advantage when working in schools and clinics is that ELG-based displays are impervious to ambient acoustic noise. Thus, they are accurate and uncontaminated, even in noisy surroundings. Nevertheless, a microphone input can be used for obtaining Fx from 'difficult' necks, and is needed for the display of frication information. Lx, of course, is not available from a microphone-based device.

5.   The success of interactive therapy using visual feedback depends on the use of accurate displays showing appropriate, but avoiding irrelevant, detail; patterns must be linguistically and communicatively relevant, and used in a graded programme of work based on phonetic and linguistic knowledge of speech production and phonological patterning in the language concerned, as becomes possible with the structured use of the speech pattern elements shown in Figure 5.8a,b. Very young children may respond to a 'games' approach in the early stages of therapy but care must be taken in such cases that un-speech-like utterances are not encouraged or rewarded.

The wide-band spectrogram shown in Figure 5.8c is for the utterance 'speech norms' spoken by a man. As is normal for this type of analysis, a rather complex picture is given, which contains a great deal of useful information. This information is, however, embedded in a sea of detail. Structured training, in which, for example, the aim is to work on frication or voice pitch or nasality alone, is not readily possible.

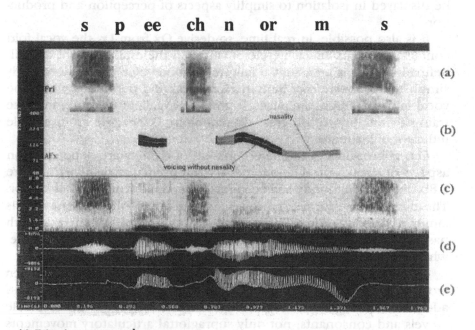

(a) Frication pattern elements
(b) Loudness, pitch and nasality pattern element in a composite display
(c) Wide band speech spectrogram
(d) Speech pressure waveform, Sp
(e) laryngograph waveform, Lx

Figure 5.8. Speech pattern element displays for the utterance 'speech norms'.

The print in Figure 5.8a,b is from a real-time display of a limited number of speech pattern elements. The upper part shows a sequence of blocks, vertically in frequency and horizontally in time, each one of which corresponds to frication in one of the speech sounds in the utterance. Within each of these blocks, the darkness of the trace represents the intensity of the frication and the position of this darkness in the block corresponds to its frequency. Using this part of the display alone, attention can easily be directed to the control of timing and of the nature of fricative contrasts in the absence of confusing details.

In practical terms, our hearing for the sounds of speech is very different from their representation given in a spectrogram and the pattern display in Figure 5.8b takes this into account. This region of the real-time display shows contours for the fundamental frequency of the voiced sounds. These contours also carry information about important aspects of the phonetic quality of these sounds. Loudness is shown by using the intensity of the voiced sound to change the thickness of the contour. Nasality is shown by changing its colour from dark blue to red (dark to light shading in the figure). Any one of these speech components could be displayed in isolation to simplify aspects of perception and production.

It is also possible, in real time, to derive Qx from Lx, the vocal fold contact waveform. In each cycle of vibration the establishment of well-defined contact is an essential feature of good voice production. Qx is simply the proportion of time in each vocal fold period for which the vocal folds are in good contact. It gives an excellent measure, in some training situations, of progress. In pathology, Qx, can be an invaluable indicator of inadequacy.

Our approaches to the determination of nasality are dependent on aspects of speech production and, for the particular display in Figure 5.8b, the information has been directly obtained from a nasal sensor. The output wave form from this sensor is one of the options in this family of displays. When this is done it is interesting to note that each nasal 'pulse' indeed occurs during the corresponding Lx open phase, when the pressure on the wall of the nose is greatest.

The therapist's knowledge of speech production is essential when working with Lx: laryngeal and vocal tract components interact and adequate excitation of the vocal tract is needed to produce acceptable vowels and consonants; not only supraglottal articulatory movements are important. Knowledge of vocal fold activity in the production of different phonation types supports the interpretation of changing Lx waveform shape and this knowledge is expanding with the increasing use of stroboscopy. Phonological knowledge, particularly suprasegmental, is essential for the insightful use of Fx: voiced-voiceless contrasts are clearly seen as is the importance of duration differences to English rhythm and intelligibility (Fourcin and Abberton, 1971). Intonation control and improvement are achieved by teaching and learning simple rules. In English, for example, these include the correct, context-determined placement of the major pitch change in a groups of words – the nuclear tone – and the shape of that pitch contour: rising, falling, falling-rising, rising-falling (O'Connor and Arnold,1973; Cruttenden, 1986). Intonation rules of this kind have important paralinguistic as well as linguistic functions and therefore are important for both intelligibility and social acceptability. The approach to teaching and learning is essentially a cognitive one rather than an attempt to teach only situation-based repertoires of fixed utterances. The emphasis is on patterns and rules for their shape and use together with the enhancement of self-monitoring.

Conclusion

We have tried to outline, in a simple way, a method of monitoring, assessing and measuring vocal fold vibration in speech, and the principles of a type of therapy that it makes possible. The approach is highly effective and often brings about improvements that were not possible with other techniques. The principles and techniques we have described were developed at University College London, and have now become quite widespread in Britain and around the world. One of the aims of the original work was to reduce the voice problems of hearing-impaired speakers (Fourcin and Abberton, 1971). This has continued and been developed in cochlear stimulation (Rosen, 1997) and the design of speech pattern element hearing aids (Fourcin, 1990). The approach is also used with a wide range of voice difficulties in normally hearing people and, in principle, is suitable for use by anyone with problems of phonation, rhythm, pitch control or intonation. Many challenging developmental, pathological and therapeutic studies still remain to be done, and ELG provides the possibility of adding quantitative information to the investigator's qualitative evaluation. External pressures in clinical practice, such as audits, as well as the move towards client-centred therapy techniques mean that interactive computer-based displays of speech patterns are likely to become widespread, and with the development of CALL (Computer Assisted Language Learning) techniques, self-study packages may well become available involving computer appraisal of the speaker's utterance and automatic routeing to the next appropriate exercise. However, in the therapeutic situation, interactive displays of the sort we have described are likely to be an increasingly valuable support and tool but not as a replacement for guidance by an interacting clinician.

References

Abberton E. A laryngographic study of voice quality. PhD thesis, University of London, London, 1976.

Abberton E, Fourcin AJ. Laryngographic analysis and intonation. British Journal of Disorders of Communication 1972; 7: 24–29.

Abberton E, Fourcin AJ. Visual feedback and the acquisition of intonation. In Lenneberg E, Lenneberg E. (Eds), Foundations of Language Development, a Multidisciplinary Approach. Vol.2, pp. 157–165. New York: Academic Press, 1975.

Abberton E, Fourcin AJ. Intonation and speaker identification. Language and Speech 1978; 21: 305–18.

Abberton E, Ashby MG, Fourcin AJ. Speech patterns in the teaching of pronunciation. In Lindblom B, Nordstrom P-E. (Eds), Fonetik och Uttalspedagogik, pp. 67–76. Stockholm: University of Stockholm, 1976.

Abberton E, Parker A, Fourcin AJ. Speech improvement in deaf adults using laryngograph dislays. In Pickett JM. (Ed.), Papers from the Research Conference on Speech Analysing Aids for the Deaf, pp. 172–88. Washington, DC: Gallaudet College, 1977.

Abberton E, Fourcin AJ, Rosen SM, Howard DM, Douek EE, Moore BCJ. Speech perceptual and productive rehabilitation. In Schindler RA, Merzenich MM. (Eds), Cochlear Implants, pp. 527–38. New York: Raven Press, 1985.

Abberton E, Fourcin AJ, Howard DM. Laryngographic assessment of normal voice: a tutorial. Clinical Linguistics and Phonetics 1989; 3: 281–96.

Abberton E, Fourcin AJ, Hazan V. Fundamental frequency range and the development of intonation in a group of profoundly deaf chidren. Proceedings, XII International Conference of Phonetic Sciences, Vol.5, pp. 142–45. Aix-en-Provence: University of Provence Press, 1991.

Ball V. Computer-based tools for asessment and remediation of speech. European Journal of Disorders of Communication 1991; 26: 95–114.

Ball, V, Faulkner A, Fourcin AJ. The effects of two different speech-coding strategies on voice fundamental frequency control in deafened adults. British Journal of Audiology 1990; 24: 393–409.

Carlson E. Electrolaryngography in the assessment and treatment of incomplete mutation (puberphonia) in adults. European Journal of Disorders of Communication 1995; 30: 140–48.

Cruttenden A. Intonation. Cambridge: Cambridge University Press, 1986.

Crystal D. Prosodic development. In Fletcher P, Garman M. (Eds), Language Acquisition: Studies in First Language Development, pp. 33–48. Cambridge: Cambridge University Press, 1979.

Fabre P. Un procédé électrique percutané d'inscription de l'accolement glottique au cours de la phonation: glottographie de haute fréquence. premiers résultats. Bulletin de l'Académie Nationale de Médécine 1957; 141: 69–99.

Fok Chan AYY. The teaching of tones to children with profound hearing impairment. British Journal of Disorders of Communication 1984; 19: 225–36.

Fourcin AJ. Laryngographic examination of vocal fold vibration. In Wyke B. (Ed.), Ventilatory and Phonatory Control Mechanisms, pp. 315–333. London: Oxford University Press, 1974.

Fourcin AJ. Acoustic patterns and speech acquisition. In Waterson N, Snow C. (Eds), The Development of Communication, pp. 47–72. London: John Wiley, 1978.

Fourcin AJ. Speech pattern audiometry. In Beagley HA. (Ed.), Auditory Investigation: The Scientific and Technological Basis, pp. 170–208. Oxford: Clarendon Press, 1980.

Fourcin AJ. Laryngographic assessment of phonatory function. In Ludlow CK. (Ed.),

Proceedings of the Conference on the Assessment of Vocal Pathology, ASHA Reports, vol. 11, pp. 116–27. Rockville, Maryland, USA: ASHA, 1982

Fourcin AJ. Prospects for speech pattern element aids. Acta Otolaryngol (Stockholm) 1990; suppl 469: 257–67.

Fourcin AJ. Normal and pathological speech: phonetic, acoustic and laryngographic aspects. In Singh W, Soutar DS. (Eds), Functional Surgery of the Pharynx and Larynx, pp. 31-54. Oxford: Butterworth Heinemann, 1993.

Fourcin AJ, Abberton E. First applications of a new laryngograph. Medical and Biological Illustration 1971; 21: 172–82. [Reprinted, Volta Review 1972; 74: 161–76; reprinted in Pickett JM, Levitt H, Houde RA. (Eds), Sensory Aids for the Hearing Impaired. New York: John Wiley, 1980.]

Fourcin AJ, Abberton E. The laryngograph and Voiscope in speech therapy. In Loebell E. (Ed.), Proceedings of the XVI International Congress of Logopaedics and Phoniatrics, pp. 116–22. Basel: S. Karger, 1976.

Fourcin AJ, Abberton E. Speech pattern elements in assessment, training and prosthetic provision. In Plant G, Spens K-E. (Eds), Profound Deafness and Speech Communication, pp. 492–509. London: Whurr, 1995.

Fourcin AJ, Abberton E, Ball V. Voice and intonation – analysis, presentation and training. In Elsendoorn BAG, Coninx F. (Eds), Interactive Learning Technology for the Deaf, pp. 137–50. Berlin: Springer-Verlag, 1993.

Fourcin AJ, McGlashan J, Huckvale M. The generation and reception of speech. In Gleeson M. (Ed.), Scott Brown's Otolaryngology Vol 1, pp. 1/14/1–1/14/27. London: Butterworth Heinemann, 1997.

Fourcin AJ, Abberton E, Miller D, Howells D. Laryngograph: speech pattern element tools for therapy, training and assessment. European Journal of Disorders of Communication 1995; 30: 101–15.

Gilbert HR, Potter CR, Hoodin R. Laryngograph as a measure of vocal fold contact area. Journal of Speech and Hearing Research 1984; 27: 173–78.

Greene M. The Voice and its Disorders, 3rd edn. London: Pitman Medical, 1980.

Hirano M, Bless D. Videostroboscopy of the Larynx. London: Whurr, 1993.

Hollien H. On vocal registers. Journal of Phonetics 1974; 2: 125–44.

Kelman AW, Gordon MT, Morton FM, Simpson IC. Comparison of methods for assessing vocal function. Folia Phoniatrica 1981; 33: 51–65.

King A, Parker A. The relevance of prosodic features to speech work with hearing impaired children. In Jones FM. (Ed.), Language Disability in Children, pp. 179-201. Lancaster: MTP Press, 1980.

Landman GHM. Laryngography and Cinelaryngography. Amsterdam: Excerpta Medica Foundation, 1970.

Leff J, Abberton E. Voice pitch measurements in schizophrenia and depression. Psychological Medicine 1981; 11: 849–52.

Noll MA. Cepstrum pitch determination. Journal of the Acoustical Society of America 1967; 41: 293–309.

Noscoe NJ, Fourcin AJ, Brown NJ, Berry RJ. Examination of vocal fold movement by ultra-short pulse X-radiography. British Journal of Radiography 1983; 56: 641–45.

O'Connor JD, Arnold GF. Intonation of Colloquial English London: Longman, 2nd Edn. 1973.

Pike KL. Tone Languages. Michigan: University of Michigan Publications in Linguistics, 1948.

Rosen SM. Cochlear implants. In Stephens D. (Ed.), Scott Brown's Otolaryngology Vol. 2, 2/15/1–2/15/20. London: Butterworths, 1997.

Rosen SM, Fourcin AJ, Moore BCJ. Voice pitch as an aid to lip-reading, Nature 1981; 291: 5811, 150–52.

Toffin C, Spens K-E, Smith K, Powell R, Lente P, Fourcin A, Faulkner A, Dahlqvist M, Fresnel-Elbaz E, Coninx F, Beijk C, Agelfors E, Abberton E. Voice production as a function of analytic perception with a speech pattern element hearing aid. Proceedings of the XIII International Congress of Phonetic Sciences 1995; 3: 206–9.

Van Gelder L. Psychosomatic aspects of endocrine disorders of the voice. Journal of Communication Disorders 1974; 7: 257–62.

Van Wieringen M, Abberton E. The use of computerised visual representations in L2 acquisition of intonation: a pilot study. Speech, Hearing and Language Department of Phonetics and Linguistics. University College, London. 1994; 8: 245–58.

Wechsler E. Laryngographic study of voice disorders, speech and hearing: work in progress. Department of Phonetics and Linguistics, University College London, 1976a. pp. 12–29 .

Wechlser E. The use of the laryngograph in the study of some patients with voice disorders. MSc thesis, University of London, London, 1976b.

Wechsler E. Laryngographic study of voice disorders. British Journal of Disorders of Communication 1977; 12: 9–22.

Whetnall E, Fry DB. The Deaf Child. London: William Heinemann Medical Books, 1964.

Wirz S, Anthony J. The use of the Voiscope in improving the speech of profoundly deaf children. British Journal of Disorders of Communication 1979; 14: 137–52.

Yiu EM-L, van Hasselt CA, Williams SR, Woo JKS. Speech intelligibility in tone language (Chinese) laryngectomy speakers. European Journal of Disorders of Communication 1994; 29: 339–48.

Chapter 6
Electropalatography and its Clinical Applications

WILLIAM J. HARDCASTLE AND FIONA GIBBON

Introduction

The tongue is an important organ for the production of speech and it is of both theoretical and practical interest to the phonetician and speech/language therapist to record details of tongue activity in both normal and pathological speech. The technique of electropalatography (EPG) is designed to record details of the timing and location of tongue contacts with the hard palate during continuous speech. It has evolved from older techniques of palatography, which recorded locations of lingual contact for isolated sounds (e.g. Abercrombie, 1957). This was done usually by spraying the surface of the roof of the mouth with a dry black powder (e.g. a mixture of charcoal and chocolate) and photographing the area of 'wipe off' after tongue contact for the sound had occurred. Unlike these earlier techniques of palatography, EPG records dynamic aspects of contact as they occur during connected speech, and so is potentially very useful as a clinical and research tool.

At present there are three commercially available systems of EPG: a Japanese system marketed by the Rion Corporation (Fujimura *et al*, 1973); a British system developed at the University of Reading (Hardcastle *et al*, 1989b, 1991a; Jones and Hardcastle, 1995) and an American Palatometer system (described in Fletcher *et al*, 1975; Fletcher, 1983) marketed by Kay Elemetrics Corporation. All three commercial systems use an artificial palate made usually of acrylic and moulded to fit the roof of the mouth. Tongue contact is recorded by electrodes located on the surface of the artificial palate. Varying degrees of contact occur for all English lingual obstruents such as /t, d, k, g, s, z, ʃ, ʒ, tʃ, dʒ/, the palatal approximant /j/, nasals /n, ŋ/, lateral /l/, relatively close vowels such as /i, ɪ, e/ and diphthongs with a close vowel component such as /eɪ, aɪ, ɔɪ/. There is usually little contact with back vowels and diphthongs e.g. /u, ʊ, aʊ, əʊ, ɔ/ and open vowels such as /ɑ, æ, ɒ/.

149

There are important differences between the three systems in the placement of electrodes. The Reading EPG3 system places 62 electrodes according to strictly defined anatomical landmarks, such as the junction between the hard and soft palates (see Figure 6.1 and further details in Hardcastle *et al*, 1991a) to enable comparisons in lingual contact patterns to be made between different subjects. The Japanese system, on the other hand, uses palates that contain 64 electrodes, and selects the best fit for an individual's palate from a set of standard templates which are meant to cover at least the majority of different palate sizes and shapes (Figure 6.2). One consequence of the latter scheme is that electrodes may not be placed sufficiently far back on the hard palate to detect contact for velar sounds. Palates manufactured for use with the Kay Palatometer are thinner and more flexible than those made for the other two systems. These polyester palates do not have retention wires, but instead fit snugly over the inner and outer surfaces of the upper teeth. The number of electrodes in the palates manufactured for use with the Kay Palatometer vary (up to 96 compared with 62 in the Reading system) and different configurations of electrode placement can be adopted for different experimental purposes. For example, to investigate the effects of context on lingual consonants, a 3.0 mm grid pattern was used (Dagenais *et al*, 1994c). A concentration of electrodes on the alveolar ridge can facilitate the detection of very fine differences in tongue palate contact patterns for sounds produced in this region, and the Reading and some configurations of the Kay palates adopt this arrangement.

EPG has become well established in many experimental phonetics laboratories and speech therapy clinics throughout the world as a safe and convenient technique for use in the investigation of an important aspect of tongue activity. The wide applicability of the technique and its usefulness as a tool in phonetic descriptive work is reflected in the range of phenomena that has been researched in recent years. Areas include: the articulatory characterization of lingual fricative production (Wolf *et al*, 1976; Hardcastle and Clark, 1981; Hoole *et al*, 1989, 1993); aspects of lingual articulation and coarticulation in a variety of languages including English (Butcher, 1989; Byrd, 1996; Dagenais *et al*, 1994c; Hardcastle, 1994, 1995; Hardcastle and Roach, 1977; Wright and Kerswill, 1989), German (Butcher and Weiher, 1976; Kohler, 1976), Japanese (Miyawaki *et al*, 1974), Catalan (Recasens, 1984b, c, 1989; Recasens *et al*, 1993, 1995), French (Marchal, 1988); Italian (Farnetani, 1990; Farnetani *et al*, 1985; Recasens *et al*, 1993) and Greek (Nicolaidis, 1994); articulatory dynamics of egressive and implosive stops in Shona (Hardcastle and Brasington, 1978); dental and alveolar stops in Kimvita Swahili (Hayward *et al*, 1989); palatalization and palatal consonants in Estonian (Eek, 1973), Catalan (Recasens, 1984a; Recasens *et al*, 1993) and Japanese (Matsuno, 1989); symmetry of lingual gestures in English

(Hamlet *et al*, 1986), in Japanese (Hiki and Imaizumi, 1974), in French (Marchal and Espesser, 1989) and in Italian (Farnetani, 1988); 'emphatic' consonants in Sudanese colloquial Arabic (Ahmed, 1984); 'force of articulation' in French (Marchal *et al*, 1980); 'vocalized' /l/ in English (Hardcastle and Barry, 1985); articulatory correlates of voicing (Dagenais *et al*, 1994c; Farnetani, 1989; Palmer, 1973); general lingual articulatory dynamics (Recasens, 1989); timing in /kl/ clusters (Hardcastle, 1985; Gibbon *et al*, 1993a); and articulatory correlates of rate variation (Byrd and Tan, 1996).

In speech pathology also, the technique has been useful both in the assessment and treatment of speech disorders (see Nicolaidis *et al*, 1993, for a recent bibliography). Among the numerous different types of speech pathologies that have been investigated with the technique are the following: structural abnormalities of the vocal tract, including cleft palate (Fletcher, 1985; Gibbon and Hardcastle, 1989; Hardcastle *et al*, 1989a; Michi *et al*, 1986; Whitehill *et al*, 1995, 1996; Yamashita *et al*, 1992); occlusal disorders (Itoh *et al*, 1980; Suzuki, 1989); glossectomy (Barry and Timmermann, 1985 Fletcher, 1988; Imai and Michi, 1992);

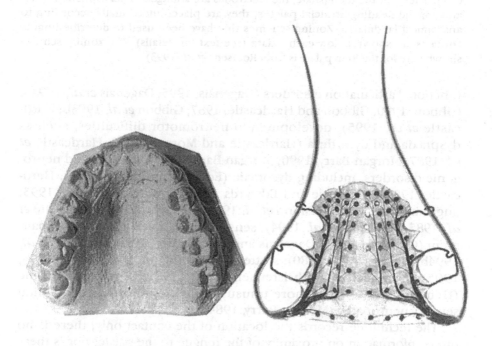

Figure 6.1. Photograph of artificial palate used in the Reading EPG system, shown here with a plaster impression of the upper palate and teeth. The subject is a child aged 13 years.

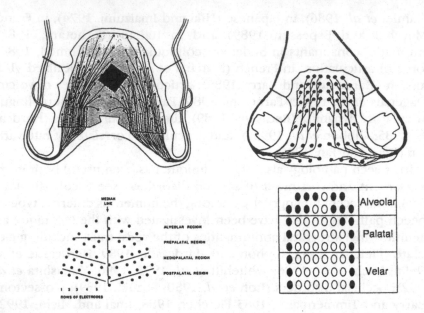

Figure 6.2. Electrode configuration for the Rion (left) and the Reading (right) artificial palates. For the Rion palate, the electrodes are arranged in hemispheric curves, and for the Reading artificial palates, they are placed individually according to anatomical landmarks. Zoning schemes that have been used to describe lingual contacts are shown below each palate (see text for details). The zoning scheme shown here for the Rion palate is from Recasens *et al* (1993).

functional articulation disorders (Dagenais, 1995; Dagenais *et al*, 1994a; Gibbon, 1990; Gibbon and Hardcastle, 1987; Gibbon *et al*, 1993b; Hardcastle *et al*, 1995); developmental neuromotor difficulties, such as dyspraxia and dysarthria (Hardcastle and Morgan, 1982; Hardcastle *et al*, 1987; Morgan Barry, 1990; Morgan Barry, 1995a, b); acquired neurogenic disorders, including dyspraxia (Edwards and Miller, 1989; Hardcastle, 1987; Hardcastle and Edwards 1992; Howard and Varley, 1995; Sugishita *et al*, 1987; Washino *et al*, 1981), and dysarthria (Hardcastle *et al*, 1985; Goldstein *et al*, 1994); sensory losses, such as hearing impairment (Crawford, 1995; Dagenais and Critz-Crosby, 1991; Dagenais *et al*, 1994b; Fletcher *et al*, 1980); stuttering (Harrington, 1987; Wood, 1993, 1995); laryngectomy (Christensen *et al*, 1992); Down's Syndrome (Hamilton, 1993); and more unusual conditions such as congenital sensory neuropathy (Morgan Barry, 1984).

The technique records the location of the contact only; there is no direct information on proximity of the tongue to the palate; nor is there any way of inferring directly which part of the tongue is producing the particular contact pattern. This must be deduced from the shape of the subject's palate, the location and timing of the contact patterns themselves, and a knowledge of the anatomy and physiology of the tongue. Another difficulty in interpreting the contact patterns in terms of tongue movement arises from the fact that the electrodes are discrete points on the surface of the artificial palate, and continuous lingual contact cannot be assumed when two adjacent electrodes are contacted. This is particularly relevant in the lateral parts of the palate, where, on occasions, all side electrodes may register the presence of full contact, but the anatomical seal along the sides of the palate may not, in fact, be complete. There may also be cases where incomplete velar contact is registered on the palate while there is complete closure further back than the most posterior row of electrodes.

Because of these limitations, it is advisable to adopt a multi-channel approach to the investigation of lingual activity and to supplement EPG data with information from, for example, movement tracking devices e.g. electromagnetic transduction systems (for example the Articulograph, Schönle *et al*, 1989), aerodynamic data for example pressure/flow variations and an audio signal representation. Much of the current work on EPG adopts this multi-channel approach (e.g. Hardcastle and Marchal, 1990; Hardcastle *et al*, 1989b; Hoole *et al*, 1989, 1993).

In this chapter, the technique of EPG is first described in some detail. In the second part an EPG-based classification of speech error patterns is outlined, followed by a description of the clinical applications of the technique in the assessment, diagnosis and remediation of a range of different types of speech disorders.

Description of the Reading EPG3 Technique

As mentioned above, an essential component of the EPG system is an artificial palate. Figure 6.2 shows a comparison between artificial palates manufactured for use with the Japanese Rion and the British Reading EPG systems. The artificial palate is made from an accurate model of the subject's upper palate and teeth and contains the electrodes, which register lingual contact. Different types of palate manufacture are reviewed in Hardcastle, Gibbon and Nicolaidis (1991b). It is obviously important that the palate should interfere as little as possible with normal speech production. It should therefore be as thin as possible (1.5 mm seems adequate for most purposes) but at the same time robust enough to tolerate frequent use and retain its shape accurately. Edges of the palate are smoothed so as to avoid any sharp areas, particularly at the anatomical junction between hard and soft palate. An exact fit is essential and the palate should not move even when considerable pressure is exerted at the posterior edge, as may happen, for example, during the closure for a velar stop. Speakers are advised that wearing the palate for at least a 2-hour period of continuous use prior to a recording allows them to become accustomed to the feel of the device in the mouth. Initially, increased salivation may occur but this quickly decreases (see further details in Hardcastle *et al*, 1989b).

The type of hardware used varies with the different systems but in general the principles of operation are similar. The Reading EPG3 system is designed to operate in conjunction with an IBM personal computer or a similar compatible computer. For this particular system, the computer controls the acquisition of the lingual-palatal contact data, together with the acoustic signal from a microphone, and also provides various data displays and analysis programmes. Hard copies of these displays and of other processed data are available when a suitable printer is connected to the computer. In operation, the subject wears the acrylic palate (see Figure 6.3), and holds an electrode providing a small sinusoidal signal. The electrodes are then scanned by the electronic circuits, and lingual-palatal contact is identified by the presence of this signal on a given electrode. The patterns of contact are then transmitted to the computer for storage and display. The three main parts of the system, that is the multiplexers, EPG unit and interface card are described in detail in Hardcastle, Gibbon and Jones (1991a).

The connections from the acrylic palate are plugged into a multiplexer unit, which is worn around the neck and which also has an

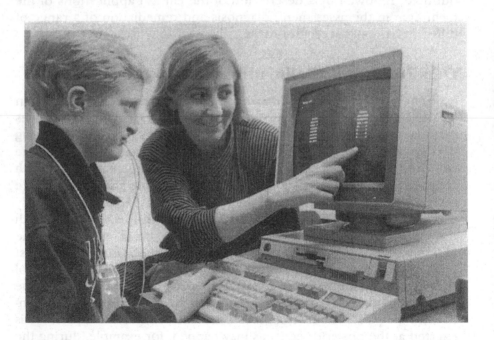

Figure 6.3. Photograph of EPG set-up showing the client and therapist looking at the computer monitor. The screen shows the feedback mode in EPG3. To the right there is a single palatogram which is static and displays a (normal) target /t/. On the left of the screen there is a palatogram which is a real-time dynamic display, and here gives the client's current attempt to copy the target pattern.

output for the hand-held signal electrode. The multiplexer contains circuits that scan the electrodes and send amplified signals to the main EPG unit where they are detected and identified. The electrodes are scanned in groups of four in order to increase the scanning rate. The time to detect the presence of a signal is 200 microseconds, which allows all 62 electrodes to be scanned in 3.2 milliseconds. This implies a maximum data rate in the order of 300 EPG patterns (or frames) per second. In practice, data rates of 100 or 200 frames per second are used (100 in the case of EPG3), which are considered sufficient to resolve most dynamic movements of the tongue in detail.

The EPG3 main unit contains the timing circuits that control the scanning of the palate electrodes, and the signal detection circuits. The signals from the multiplexer are amplified, and the peaks are detected, and compared with a pre-set reference level to determine if a contact is made. The reference level is set to discriminate against a background level of unwanted signals which are due to capacitive coupling from the subject's palate, and from conduction through saliva. Adjustment of the reference level is provided on the front panel to cater for some variation in the conductivity of an individual's saliva. Optocoupling systems ensure that the speaker is protected from any possible leakage currents from the computer and peripherals (see details in Hardcastle *et al*, 1991a).

An interface card in the computer's expansion bus enables sampling of both the lingual-palatal contact patterns and the acoustic signal from the microphone. The sampling rate for the acoustic signal is 10 000 samples/s, thus allowing a bandwidth of approximately 5 kHz. This bandwidth gives an acceptable quality of speech output when played back, and when displayed with the EPG patterns on the computer screen, allows features of the acoustic signal and the EPG patterns to be directly correlated. The system samples the data to computer RAM memory (not to hard disk) and therefore the recording duration is determined by the RAM available. This means that, in general, sample lengths are restricted to 10 s or less.

Two different modes of operation are possible: an analysis mode and a feedback mode. In the analysis mode, recorded data are displayed, as shown in Figure 6.4. The EPG pattern (top left) occurs at the point in the acoustic signal identified by the position of the left-hand cursor. The cursor can be moved along the waveform and the corresponding EPG patterns observed. The two cursors together are used to select a portion of the acoustic trace which can then be expanded, measured for duration or played back through a loudspeaker. The small window on the top right of the display shows a spectral slice taken at the position of the right-hand cursor (i.e. during the aspiration in velar [kʰ] production). This display gives a plot of amplitude against frequency, and the small cursor in this window allows the frequency of points in the spectrum to

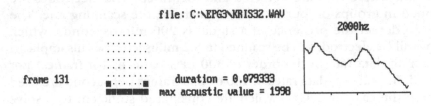

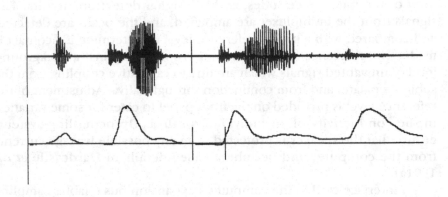

Figure 6.4. EPG3 screen display of the utterance 'kitkat'. The velar pattern indicated by the left-hand cursor position shows assimilated /t/ in the [tk] sequence (see text for further details of the display).

be measured. The feedback mode provides a real-time display of lingual contacts and is used in speech therapy to modify lingual contact patterns (see Figure 6.3 and further below).

It is possible also to obtain a three-dimensional representation of the palate with electrodes shown in actual spatial relationships to each other (Jones and Hardcastle, 1995). For this representation, XYZ coordinates of each electrode position on the palate are first obtained either with the aid of a Reflex Microscope (Speculand *et al*, 1988) or by manual measurement with a depth gauge. Figure 6.5 shows a 3D representation of electrodes on a 'wire-frame' display in surface and side views. A schematic representation of the actual shape of the palate as well as spacing between electrodes can be seen on such a display. The left-hand cursor is positioned during the initial velar closure in the word 'cock-tail'.

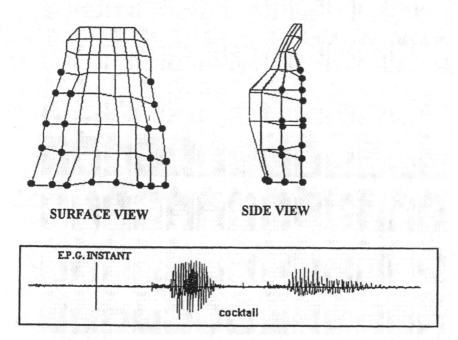

Figure 6.5. 3D representation of electrodes on a 'wire-frame' display. The electrodes are located at the wire intersections, with contacted electrodes indicated by filled black circles.

Printouts of palatal lingual patterns are available for selected stretches of speech. Figure 6.6 shows a printout for the word 'tactics' (palatograms are numbered and read from left to right). The range of spatial and temporal detail can readily be seen in such a printout. The individual schematic palate diagrams are at 10 ms intervals, and contact is indicated by zeros along the eight horizontal rows. The printout begins with complete closure for /t/, shown as a horse-shoe shaped configuration with complete contact down both sides of the palate and across the alveolar ridge (rows 1 and 2 from the top). The closure is released at frame 60 and the /æ/ vowel continues until velar closure at frame 82. A brief period of double alveolar-velar closure ensues (frames 94–96) as the /t/ gesture overlaps with the /k/. The velar is then released

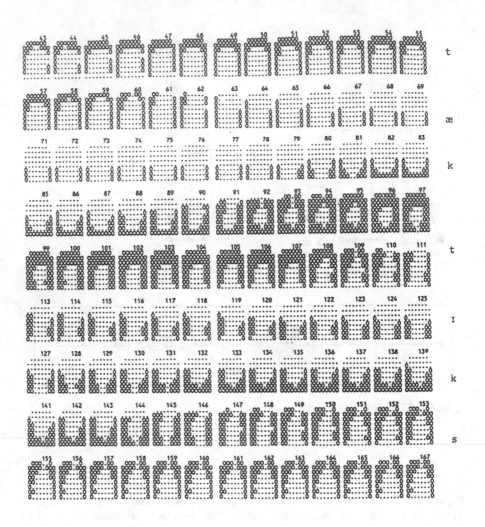

Figure 6.6. Full EPG printout of the word 'tactics' produced by a normal speaker. The top of individual palatograms represents the alveolar region, and the bottom the junction between the hard and soft palates. The sampling interval is 10 ms (see text for full details).

(frame 97) followed by the /t/ (frame 109). The contact for the /ɪ/ is more extensive at the sides than for /æ/ indicating the closer vowel. The second /k/ (frames 132–143) has noticeably more palatal contact than the first, due to the influence of the preceding vowel. Finally, the second /k/ is released into a narrowed groove configuration for the /s/.

From contact information such as this it is possible to identify a limited number of specific patterns that appear to characterize particular speech targets (see Figure 6.7). These are idealized static patterns that have been found to occur at particular characteristic phases (e.g. at the midpoint of the closure phase for a plosive) during production of various speech sounds. Pattern 1 (the alveolar stop pattern) typically occurs during the closure phase of alveolar plosives and nasals when produced in words as citation forms. It is characterized by contact along the lateral margins of the palate and complete closure across the first two or three rows. Pattern 2, occurring during the closure phase of velar plosives and nasals in the environment of back open sounds, has minimal contact along the margins of the palate and complete contact across the most posterior row. One can assume there is some contact also on the soft palate although this is not registered with conventional EPG. In Pattern 3 (a palatal stop pattern) there is more extensive lateral contact than in Pattern 2, some contact even extending as far forward as rows 2 or 3. Central contact occurs in the posterior two or three rows. This pattern occurs during the closure phase of velar plosives and nasals in the environment of close front vowels (e.g. in 'key'). Pattern 4 (the double alveolar-velar pattern) occurs during velar-alveolar or alveolar-velar consonant sequences, such as in the word 'tactics' (see Figure 6.6) or 'catkin'. The alveolar grooved pattern (Pattern 5) is typical of the stricture during an /s/ or /z/. Contact is complete along both lateral margins and there is a narrow grooved configuration in the anterior two or three rows. The amount of side contact varies with the phonetic context (e.g. there is more side contact when /s/ is followed by a close front vowel, such as in 'see'). Pattern 6 is typical of stricture during /ʃ/ or /ʒ/ and in comparison with /s/ or /z/ has a wider and more posteriorly placed groove. Pattern 7 (the 'apical' pattern) occurs during an /l/ in an open or back vowel environment and is characterized by minimal anterior, central contact. One can assume from the amount of contact, that it is the tip of the tongue making contact with the alveolar ridge in this case.

With reference to these idealized citation-form patterns, actual contact patterns that occur during normal spontaneous speech can be described. For example, the lingual gesture for a phoneme target /t/ is frequently produced with incomplete closure across the alveolar region, and for the target /k/ (Pattern 2) there is frequently incomplete closure in the posterior rows.

Although the full palatal contact data, such as in Figure 6.6, are useful for many descriptive purposes, it is frequently convenient to quantify the contact patterns by extracting relevant parameters from the full data. Typical data reduction procedures are reviewed below.

Data Reduction and Numerical Indices

A number of different procedures have been developed for analysing EPG patterns. These include measurements of 'place of articulation',

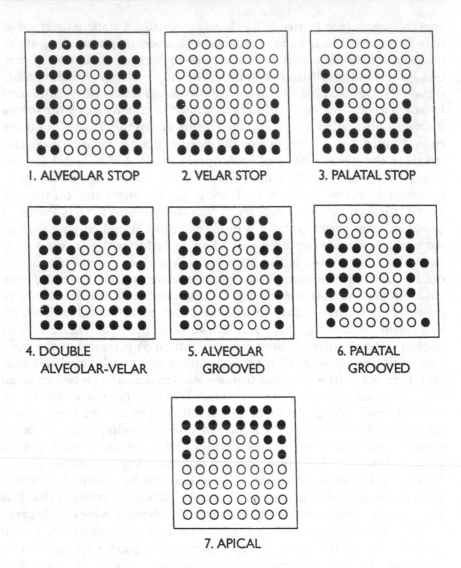

1. ALVEOLAR STOP   2. VELAR STOP   3. PALATAL STOP

4. DOUBLE
   ALVEOLAR-VELAR

5. ALVEOLAR
   GROOVED

6. PALATAL
   GROOVED

7. APICAL

Figure 6.7. Idealized EPG contact patterns found in normal speech (see text for descriptions of each pattern).

dynamic profile displays, frequency of contact and numerical indices based on specific frames during production of speech sounds. 'Place of articulation' measures are usually obtained for individual speech sounds such as, for example, fricatives. A specific frame during production of the speech sound is selected (for example the frame showing maximum lingual contact) and various measures can be made from this frame. Such measures have included medial groove width (Fletcher, 1985), length and location of constriction, back gradient (defined as the change in number of contacted electrodes per row over the range from the point of maximum

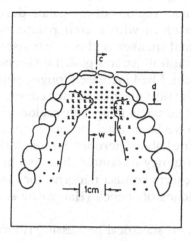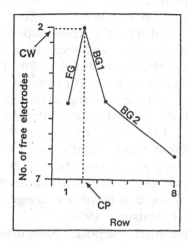

Fletcher (1985)

• - electrode location

x - contacted electrode

w - medial groove width
     (minimum)

c - medial groove centre
     (lateral)

d - distance from incisor
     ((posterior)

Hoole et al (1989), Hardcastle and Clark (1981).

For fricatives /s/ and /ʃ/.

CP - 1st local minimum in free electrode vector in first four rows.

CW - number of free electrodes at point of maximum constriction.

BG1 - change in number of free electrodes per row over range from CP to 1.5 rows behind.

BG2 - as BG1, but range 1.5 behind CP to 4.5 rows behind.

FG - Gradient over range one row in front of CP.

Figure 6.8. Place of articulation measures for alveolar fricatives. The left-hand diagram shows the layout of electrodes on the artificial palate and measures used by Fletcher (1985). The right-hand illustration shows a graph plotting the number of free electrodes (y axis) for each row (x axis) and gives details of measures used by Hoole et al (1989) and Hardcastle and Clark (1981).

constriction to 1.5 rows behind the constriction, see Hoole et al, 1989). Figure 6.8 illustrates some of these place of articulation measures.

Contact profiles take account of dynamic changes in contact patterns over time and may be shown as graphs where EPG frame numbers are plotted against the total number of activated contacts in a specific region of the palate (Hardcastle *et al*, 1991b). Figure 6.9 illustrates the dynamic changes that occurred in different contact regions of the palate during the production of three words by a child with a cleft palate, and compares these with those from a normal speaker. A phonetic transcription is given below each graph. The graph illustrates global differences in contact patterns. For example, this child had increased tongue palate contact in the velar region during production of labial sounds compared with the normal speaker. Percent total contacts in specific regions (see Byrd, 1994, 1996; Byrd *et al*, 1995) have been used, as has contact in different regions of the palate for identifiable reference points during VCV sequences (Butcher, 1989). Frequency of contact has also been found to be a useful indication of long-term contact patterns, for example those that occur over longer stretches of speech (Hardcastle *et al*, 1991b; Matsuno, 1989).

For many purposes, particularly when statistical processing is envisaged, it is desirable to represent specific contact patterns in terms of a single numerical index. A number of such indices have been developed illustrating different aspects of the EPG contact pattern, and these are summarized in Table 6.1. One index, the coarticulatory index, has been found to be particularly useful for representing contextual influences of surrounding vowels on the place of articulation of lingual stops and fricatives. Figure 6.10 shows two EPG sequences and the method of calculating the coarticulation index.

Clinical Applications of EPG

Over the past 20 years there has been a rapid expansion in the number of studies concerning the clinical applications of EPG (see above and Nicolaidis *et al*, 1993, for a review). One explanation for the increasing popularity of EPG is that the technique assists in two fundamental clinical activities, namely assessment and therapy. As an assessment procedure, EPG has revealed many types of error patterns, which capture both spatial and temporal aspects of abnormal articulatory behaviour. It has also shown that different speech disorders tend to exhibit characteristic EPG error 'profiles' or clusters of patterns. For example, spatial distortions are frequently found in speakers with cleft palate (Gibbon and Hardcastle, 1989; Hardcastle *et al*, 1989a; Whitehill *et al*, 1995; Yamashita *et al*, 1992), whereas speakers with acquired apraxia show predominantly (but not exclusively) temporal or serial ordering difficulties (Hardcastle, 1987; Hardcastle and Edwards, 1992).

An EPG error classification gives an additional dimension to the assessment process, and this supplements information from other diagnostic procedures, in particular auditory-based analyses and other instrumental measures. Studies have interpreted error patterns in the light of the current knowledge-base, and this has generated new insights

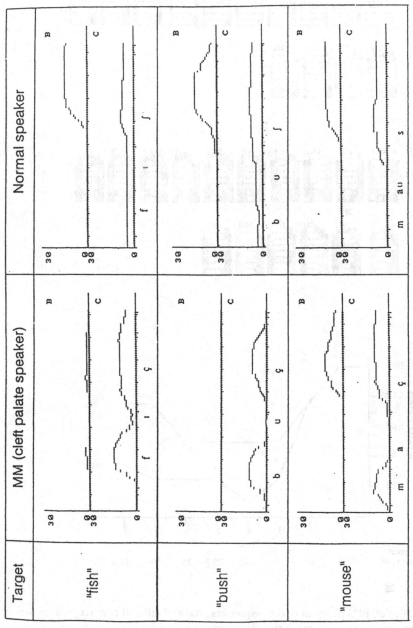

Figure 6.9. Total number of activated electrodes in two regions of the palate: B = rows 3, 4 and 5, the post-alveolar and palatal regions; C = rows 6, 7 and 8, the palatal and velar regions, expressed as a function of time (in frame numbers). This 'totals' graph is for the words 'a fish', 'a bush' and 'a mouse' produced by a cleft palate speaker (on the left) and a normal speaker (on the right). (Individual frames are indicated by the ticks on the x axes.)

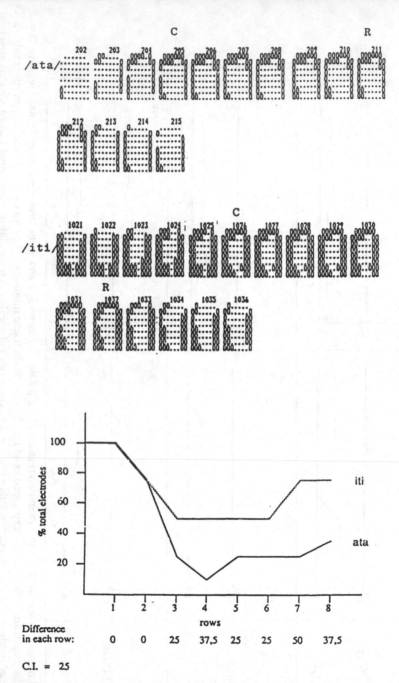

Figure 6.10. Full EPG printout of the sequences /ata/ and /iti/ and contact profiles for the closure point C (= first frame showing complete alveolar closure) for each stop. The contact profiles are calculated by plotting the total number of activated electrodes in each row expressed as a per cent of the total number of contacted electrodes. A coarticulation index (CI) is calculated by averaging the differences between the totals at each row (see numbers below each row).

Table 6.1. Summary of indices developed to quantify different aspects of EPG contact patterns.

Contact Distribution Indices

A. Centre of Gravity (COG)	Expresses the location of the main concentration of activated electrodes across the palate. The calculation assigns progressively higher values towards the more anterior rows. Hardcastle, Gibbon and Nicolaidis (1991b). Gibbon, Hardcastle and Nicolaidis (1993a).
B. Anteriority Index	Expresses the location of the main concentration of activated electrodes across the palate. The calculation gives preference to the concentration of contacts in either the anterior or posterior rows. Faber (1989).
C. Anteriority/posteriority/ centrality contact indices	Expresses the degree and concentration of activated electrodes across the palate. The anteriority and posteriority indices quantify changes along the sagittal axis of the palate and the centrality index along the coronal axis. Fontdevila, Recasens and Pallarès (1994). Recasens, Farnetani, Fontdevila and Pallarès (1993).

Other Indices

D. Articulatory reduction index	Expresses changes in electrode activation during a segment produced with different speech styles. Farnetani and Provaglio (1991).
E. Asymmetry Index	Expresses asymmetry of contact pattern between the left and right sides of the palate. Farnetani (1988). Marchal; A and Espesser (1989).
F. Coarticulation Index	Expresses differences in electrode activation during the production of a segment when uttered in two distinct contextual environments. Farnetani (1990). (See Figure 6.10.)
G. 'Trough' Index	Expresses changes in electrode activation reflecting lingual 'relaxation' during the production of an intervocalic consonant. Engstrand (1989).
H. Variability Index	Expresses inter-utterance and/or contextual variability in electrode activation during the production of a segment. Two different indices have been proposed: Farnetani, Provaglio (1991). Sudo, Kiritani and Sawashima (1983).

into differential diagnosis (Dagenais *et al*, 1994a; Gibbon *et al*, 1993b; Hardcastle and Edwards, 1992; Morgan Barry, 1995a). A corollary of EPG-based descriptions is that these generate aims of therapy that are expressed in similar terms. Interpreting the data in order to define these aims is as important as the use of the technique to provide clients with visual feedback during therapy. In addition, recording EPG data before and after therapy makes it possible to quantify the nature and extent of change in tongue activity brought about as a result of intervention. These central themes will be explored and illustrated in the following sections.

EPG-based Description of Error Patterns

EPG error classifications aim to describe atypical articulatory patterns that occur in specific disorders (see the classification systems of Hardcastle and Edwards (1992) for apraxic errors; Suzuki *et al*. (1980) for errors in Japanese-speaking children with cleft palate and Imai and Michi (1992) for an adaptation of the previous scheme for (Japanese) glossectomized speech). These existing classifications are included here and extended by additional categories to encompass error patterns found in a range of speech disorders. The error patterns are broadly divided into spatial distortions, temporal and serial ordering abnormalities, and errors of substitution and omission.

Spatial distortions occur where the configuration of contacted electrodes in individual palatograms is unlike that seen in normal speakers. For instance, studies have shown that (in English) the central palatal region remains relatively free of contact during normal speech production (Fletcher, 1988). Consequently, if the whole of the palate were contacted during production of /s/ or /t/, this would be considered a spatial distortion.

Temporal and serial ordering difficulties are identified where the spatial configuration of the EPG patterns looks normal, but there is an abnormality (in relation to the target) in the timing or sequencing of the gesture. For instance, if the spatial configuration for a stop such as /t/ was normal, but produced with an abnormally long duration (typical of a stutterer, for example) then this would be considered a temporal abnormality. Serial ordering difficulties may be manifested by problems with transitions between speech gestures (which in normal speakers are executed both smoothly and rapidly) or by incorrect sequencing of such gestures. Examples of these types of error patterns include repetitions of gestures, slow transitions between consonants in cluster sequences and metatheses. Often a particular error pattern can be described as being both a temporal and a serial ordering problem.

Substitutions occur where the EPG patterns are spatially and temporally normal, but are not the expected pattern for a given target, and omissions occur where a particular gesture is apparently absent from the EPG trace. These types of difficulties are considered in greater detail below, with examples drawn from a range of different speech pathologies. Spatial distortions produced by speakers with cleft palate have been found to cluster uniquely together, and for this reason are discussed in a separate section.

Distorted Spatial Patterns

Spatial abnormalities differ qualitatively from the normal (idealized) patterns outlined in Figure 6.7. A general spatial characteristic observed in a number of different pathologies is broader or increased tongue-palate contact. This has been found in speakers with repaired cleft palate (Hardcastle et al, 1989a; Michi et al, 1986; Yamashita et al, 1992), glossectomy (Fletcher, 1988; Imai and Michi, 1992), developmental neurological disorders (Hardcastle et al, 1987), and functional articulation disorders (Dagenais et al, 1994a; Gibbon et al, 1995). Dagenais and Critz-Crosby (1991) noted excessive tongue-palate contact in hearing impaired speakers for a proportion of lingual consonants. Wood (1993) found increased contact in a group of stutterers, and Hamilton (1993) noted that this also occurred in young adults with Down's syndrome. One exception is the speech of those with anterior open-bite, where the EPG data shows reduced amounts of contact (Suzuki et al, 1981a) and also more forward, dental articulations.

Spatial distortions frequently occur during abnormal fricative production, particularly in children with functional articulation disorders (Dagenais et al, 1994a; Gibbon and Hardcastle, 1987; Gibbon et al, 1995). These abnormal EPG patterns have been related to general perceptual categories that are well documented in the literature (Powers, 1971) and include lateralized, palatal and dental articulations. EPG has been found to be particularly valuable in the description of lateralized fricatives. These are a common type of distortion, and may present the clinician with a particular problem because they do not always resolve either spontaneously or as a result of therapy. These distortions may be referred to as lateral /s/, lateral lisp, lateral misarticulation or lateralized articulations.

EPG patterns for sounds heard as lateralized fricatives are surprisingly diverse (Gibbon et al, 1995). Figure 6.11 shows EPG patterns (at the point of maximum constriction) for three children (D1–3), all of whom were perceived by listeners as having lateralized /s/ and /ʃ/. Also included in Figure 6.11 is a normal (N1) child's production of /s/ and /ʃ/. The EPG patterns for the lateralized productions are similar in that they all have complete closure across the palate (note that this is not a universal characteristic of lateralized fricatives, see Gibbon and Hardcastle (1987), but they also vary along the following dimensions:

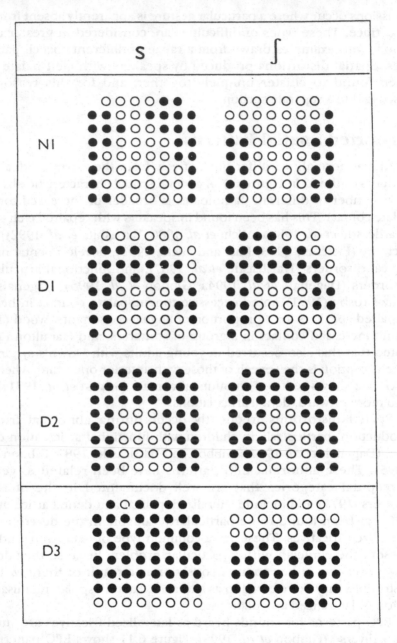

Figure 6.11. EPG frames for /s/ and /ʃ/ targets illustrating the range of EPG patterns for sibilant targets judged auditorily as being lateralized. The data is from three children (D1–3) with functional articulation disorders, all of whom had lateralized productions of /s/ and /ʃ/. EPG frames were taken at the point of maximum contact during the fricative portion of six words containing /s/ (left) and six words containing /ʃ/ (right). Electrodes activated more than 50% of the total possible are indicated as filled circles. EPG patterns from a normal child (N1) for the same words are shown at the top of the diagram.

- location of contact (compare D2's alveolar contact with D3's contact in the alveolar, post-alveolar and palatal regions);
- the extent of contact (note D3's excessive tongue palate contact compared with D1 and D2);
- extent of lateral contact (D1 and D3 show incomplete lateral seal indicating a possible location of friction).

Although speakers with apraxia tend not to produce spatial distortions, one exception is that sibilant sounds are often produced with a characteristically asymmetric 'skewed' configuration (Edwards and Miller, 1989; Hardcastle, 1987; Hardcastle and Edwards, 1992; Hardcastle *et al*, 1985). These distorted spatial patterns have been tentatively interpreted as indicating a slight motoric problem evident only during the production of relatively complex sounds such as fricatives and affricates. Interestingly, these fricatives were generally heard as acceptable productions.

Christensen, Fletcher and McCutcheon (1992) observed a different type of spatial abnormality in oesophageal speakers who produced /s,z/ with a narrower lingual groove than normal speakers. This was interpreted as an articulatory manoeuvre to regulate a limited intraoral air supply so as to produce a more normal fricative duration.

One type of spatial distortion has been termed under- or overshoot of articulatory gestures, and these have been noted to occur in speakers with some forms of acquired dysarthria (Hardcastle *et al*, 1985). Examples of undershoot include incomplete closure for stops and abnormally retracted places of articulation. Examples of overshoot include complete alveolar contact for fricative targets, and abnormally forward or anterior tongue-palate placement.

Spatial distortions in cleft palate speech

A variety of spatial distortions have been identified in speakers with cleft palate. These spatial distortions generally involve both excessive, and more posterior, tongue-palate contact, and can be related broadly to perceptual categories (see Edwards, 1980; Trost, 1981). A classificatory system for Japanese cleft palate speakers was devised by Suzuki *et al*. (1980) based on the Rion palate (see Figure 6.12). This system involves classifying individual EPG frames along several dimensions including: (1) presence/absence of complete constriction; (2) location of contact; and (3) area of contact. This classification has been expanded and related to perceptual categories in a large cohort (53) of cleft palate speakers (Yamashita and Michi, 1991; Yamashita *et al*, 1992). A number of general categories emerge from these and other studies.

Lateralized articulations, particularly of /s, z, ʃ, ʒ, tʃ, dʒ/ are common and have been referred to as Lateral Misarticulation in the Japanese literature (Michi *et al*, 1986; Suzuki *et al*, 1981b). This type of articulation

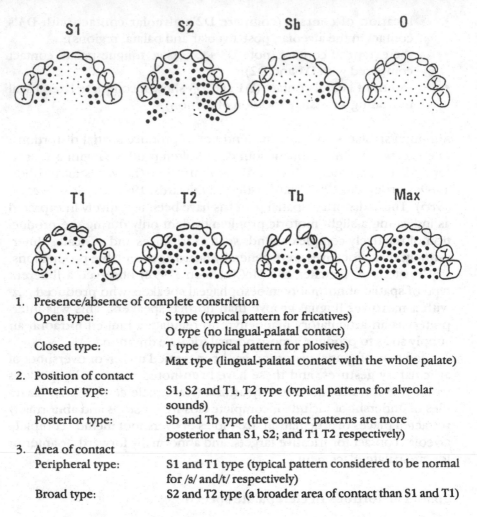

1. Presence/absence of complete constriction
   Open type: S type (typical pattern for fricatives)
                             O type (no lingual-palatal contact)
   Closed type: T type (typical pattern for plosives)
                             Max type (lingual-palatal contact with the whole palate)
2. Position of contact
   Anterior type: S1, S2 and T1, T2 type (typical patterns for alveolar
                             sounds)
   Posterior type: Sb and Tb type (the contact patterns are more
                             posterior than S1, S2; and T1 T2 respectively)
3. Area of contact
   Peripheral type: S1 and T1 type (typical pattern considered to be normal
                             for /s/ and /t/ respectively)
   Broad type: S2 and T2 type (a broader area of contact than S1 and T1)

Figure 6.12. EPG classification system used by Suzuki *et al* (1980) to describe error patterns that occur in Japanese cleft palate speakers. The electrode configuration is that of the Japanese Rion palate.

involves the tongue dorsum making complete contact across the palate (i.e. there is no evidence of tongue grooving), and lateral release of air (i.e. air directed out of the occluded dental arch posterior to the molar teeth). Similar distortions have been found to occur in British children with cleft palate (Hardcastle *et al*, 1989a).

   Palatal/velar place of articulation can occur for alveolar targets (Gibbon and Hardcastle, 1989; Hardcastle *et al*, 1989a). Palatal misarticulations are described as involving the posterior tongue dorsum and mid-dorsum elevated to make a relatively posterior, palatal contact (Okazaki *et al*, 1980). A central groove (located in the palatal/velar region of the palate) is often present during the production of palatal fricatives, with air being directed over the midline of the palate (Michi *et al*, 1986; Yamashita and Michi, 1991).

Nasopharyngeal articulations have been found to involve complete constriction in the velar region of the palate, accompanied by posterior friction (probably in the velopharyngeal region) and simultaneous escape of air through the nose (Abe, 1987; Dent *et al*, 1992; Gibbon and Hardcastle, 1989).

Pharyngeal/glottal articulations have been described using EPG in a small number of children with a history of velopharyngeal incompetence (but not necessarily cleft palate). During the production of these sounds, the EPG patterns show minimal tongue-palate contact (Dent *et al*, 1995).

Double articulations occur where there is closure in two regions of the vocal tract simultaneously, and EPG has revealed two specific types in children with cleft palate (Dent *et al*, 1992; Gibbon and Hardcastle, 1989), both of which involve complete velar constriction.

First, *double labial-velar articulations* (for labial targets) involve labial closure occurring simultaneously with complete velar constriction. This is illustrated in Figure 6.13, which shows the word 'biscuit' produced by a child with a repaired cleft palate. In the display, nasal airflow is shown below the acoustic waveform, and below this is the EPG printout for the initial /bɪs/ sequence. Note that there is some (abnormal) airflow occurring during production of the bilabial stop /b/, the alveolar fricative /s/ and on release of the /t/. While /b/ was judged auditorily to be produced at the lips, the EPG data during this stop (frames 181–215) shows simultaneous velar closure. This type of double articulation is particularly difficult to detect either visually or auditorily, as it occurs during the closure phase of the bilabial stop. In the case described by Gibbon and Hardcastle (1989), oral airflow showed a brief negative pressure during the release phase of the double labial-velar articulation. The articulatory and airflow characteristics of this type of double articulation could be similar to the double closure stops found in many West African and Northern Central African languages, e.g. Yoruba (Ladefoged, 1968), although the relative timing of the two components of the closure may be different.

Second, *double alveolar-velar articulations* (for alveolar targets) involve alveolar closure occurring simultaneously with complete velar constriction (see Dent *et al*, 1992). This configuration resembles that found during the period of overlap seen in normal speakers during a /kt/ sequences (see Figures 6.5 and 6.6) but differs in that the tongue tip and tongue body are both raised simultaneously throughout the duration of the closure.

In a study by Whitehill, Stokes, Hardcastle and Gibbon (1995), simultaneous alveolar/velar lingual contact during production of velar targets was noted in two Cantonese-speaking children with cleft palate. Both

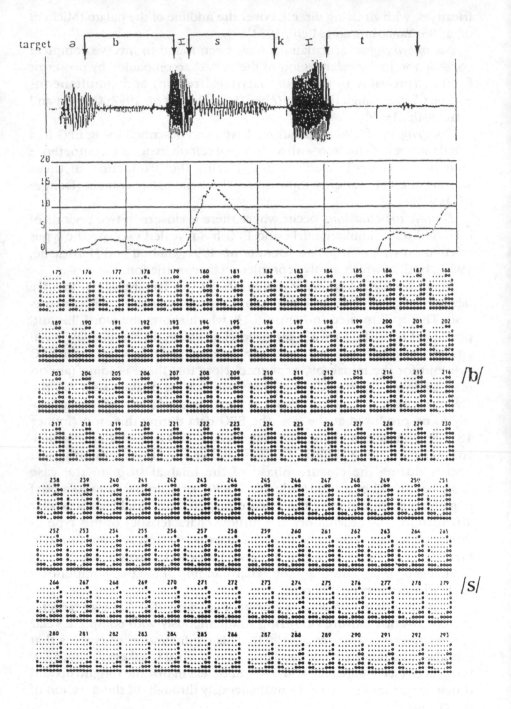

Figure 6.13. Computer display of data recorded from a cleft palate child saying 'a biscuit' (see text for details).

children had residual alveolar clefts, which were unobturated at the time of the EPG recording. It was hypothesized that the tongue tip/blade was being raised in an attempt to 'block' the alveolar cleft.

When interpreting EPG data from speakers with abnormal dento-facial morphology, in particular clefts of the hard palate, several factors should be kept in mind. First, electrode placement according to prescribed anatomical landmarks is not easy where there are hard palate deformities, such as intrusive teeth, shallow and misshapen dental arches and so on. Here the relationship between electrode placement, oral morphology (including the presence of a malocclusion) and the schematic palatograms needs to be considered carefully. Second, it is not simple to define what a 'normal' spatial EPG pattern would be for these speakers, and likewise what would constitute a spatial distortion.

Temporal Abnormalities

Abnormal durations

Some speakers produce obstruent sounds with abnormally long durations. For example, Figure 6.14 shows an EPG printout of the sequence /ɛkstɪ/ from the word 'extinct' produced by a stutterer and a normal subject. Note the prolonged duration of /s/, measured from the acoustic record (not shown here) as 430 ms (frames 170–212). This can be judged as abnormally long compared with the normal speaker's duration of 120 ms (frames 136–147). Prolonged closure phases for stops have been found to be associated with misdirected articulatory gestures (Hardcastle and Edwards, 1992) and complex stop gestures produced by children with functional articulation disorders (Gibbon *et al*, 1993b). Long contact times were also noted by Washino *et al* (1981) in a subject with apraxia of speech, and this was interpreted as at least partially explaining the slow effortful speech often observed in these clients.

Temporal and spatial variability

Variability is a characteristic of disordered speech, but it is a feature that is not easy to quantify using auditory-based analysis. Excessive variability has been linked particularly with apraxia of speech, and this has been corroborated in EPG studies of these speakers (Hardcastle and Edwards, 1992; Washino *et al*, 1981). In the study by Hardcastle and Edwards (1992) the variability was particularly noticeable in the transitions between elements in sequences such as /tk, kt, kl/ etc., and in the occurrence of misdirected articulatory gestures.

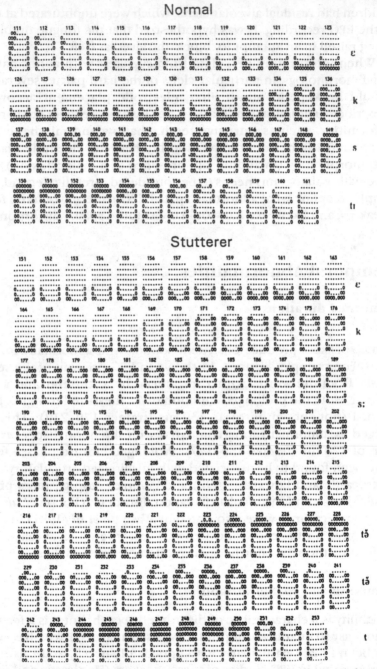

Figure 6.14. EPG patterns for the cluster /ɛksti/ in the word 'extinct' produced by a normal speaker and a stutterer. The stutterer's production was transcribed as [ɛks:tətətɪ]. Several things are noteworthy: (1) an intrusive velar gesture in between the alveolar fricative and the first stop (frames 216–218) which was not detected by listeners; (2) an abnormally long /s/ duration; and (3) the multiple repetitions of the /t/

Spatio-temporal distortions

These are complex articulations involving both the tongue body and tongue tip/blade systems, and are considered complex in relation to the target, which would normally be produced as a single gesture. Gibbon, Dent and Hardcastle (1993b) describe a child who produced complex gestures for alveolar targets. These involved an initial complete velar closure, which was followed (during the closure phase of the stop) by the tongue moving forward to the anterior regions of the palate, so producing secondary and even double velar-alveolar articulations. These gestures were found to be associated with long durations, and were heard variously as velar/palatal substitutions or acceptable alveolar stops. Gibbon (1990) describes a similar case of a child who was identified from an auditory analysis as using the phonological process of alveolar backing. The velar/alveolar contrast was judged auditorily to be neutralized, but the EPG records showed that the alveolar targets involved quite different articulatory manoeuvres from velar targets.

Serial Ordering Abnormalities

Misdirected articulatory gestures

These have been found to be one of the most frequently occurring error patterns in apraxic speech. Misdirected gestures occur where the EPG patterns themselves are spatially normal, in that they can be identified as one of the idealized patterns described in Figure 6.7, but they occur in an inappropriate place. For example, a feature that occurs frequently in the EPG data from apraxic speakers is a velar gesture 'intruding' immediately before or after an alveolar gesture. Figure 6.15 shows the EPG patterns produced by an apraxic and a normal speaker saying 'a deer'. The EPG records from the apraxic speaker show evidence of an abnormal velar gesture (frames 0598–0608) occurring before the alveolar, but note that the two gestures overlap temporarily (frames 0606–0608). This type of gesture can be differentiated from the double alveolar-velar articulation typical of cleft palate speakers, as in the latter case, the two articulations occur more or less simultaneously for the duration of the closure period. However, in the apraxic data, while there may be a brief period of overlap at one point during the closure phase of the two stops, they do not occur simultaneously, and the amount of articulatory overlap is variable.

Misdirected gestures are one of the most interesting atypical EPG patterns, as they are often undetected by an auditory-based analysis. These gestures can occur during the closure phase of a stop where there is little acoustic energy and as a consequence no audible cues present. The production shown in Figure 6.15 was judged to be a normal /d/ by

Normal

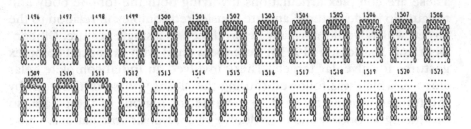

Apraxic

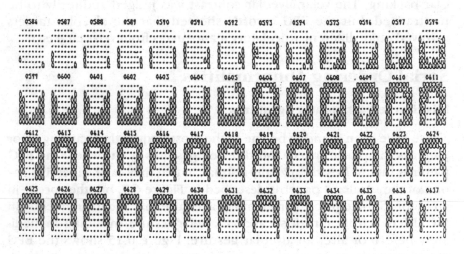

Figure 6.15. EPG patterns of 'a deer' produced by a normal speaker and an apraxic speaker. The EPG records from the apraxic show evidence of an abnormal (intrusive) velar gesture occurring before the alveolar.

listeners, but similar intrusive gestures have been judged variously as substitutions, distortions or acceptable productions. These misdirected gestures have also been observed in the speech of stutterers. An example of an intrusive velar is given in Figure 6.14, which shows EPG patterns extracted from the word 'extinct' produced by a stutterer. Note that there is an intrusive velar gesture in between the long alveolar fricative and the first repetition of the stop (frames 216–218). The brevity of the intrusive gesture coupled with its unexpected location probably contributed to listeners failing to detect its presence.

Transitional difficulties

Abnormal transitional timing for successive articulatory gestures, particularly in consonant sequences, has been noted to be typical of speakers with acquired apraxia and dysarthria. Hardcastle and Edwards (1992) found that for speakers with apraxia, there was often audible release of the first element in clusters, such as the /kl/ sequence in 'clock' or the /tk/ sequence in 'catkin', and this was often accompanied by a relatively long delay between the two elements. Excessively long transition times have been observed in a speaker with a mixed dysarthria following a head injury. Figure 6.16 shows EPG patterns for this speaker's production of the /kt/ sequence in 'tractor'. Note the abnormally long time lag of 100 ms between the release of the /k/ (frame 193), which was produced with

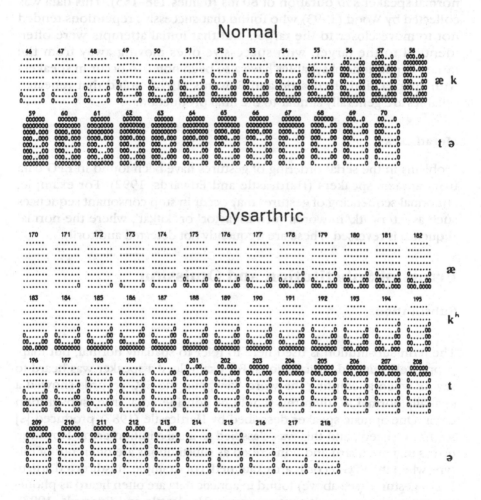

Figure 6.16. EPG patterns for the /kt/ sequence in 'tractor' produced by a normal speaker and a speaker with mixed dysarthria.

audible aspiration, and the closure for the /t/ (frame 203). Compare this with the articulatory overlap of the /k/ and /t/ in the normal speaker.

Repetitions

Gestures that are produced a number of times in succession are called repetitions. This phenomenon is illustrated in Figure 6.14, which shows a stutterer's production of the /ɛkstɪ/ cluster in the word 'extinct' (transcribed as [ɛks:tə̆tə̆tɪ]). The repetitions of the alveolar stop can be observed in considerable detail from the EPG trace. The first repetition occurs between frames 223 and 228 (60 ms), the second between 236 and 238 (30 ms) and the final one between frames 243 and 250 (90 ms). The durations of the first and second repetitions are briefer than the normal speaker's /t/ duration of 80 ms (frames 148–155). This data was collected by Wood (1993) who found that successive repetitions tended not to move closer to the target, and that initial attempts were often identical to the target, with successive ones moving away from the target. Repetitions of syllables have also been noted to occur in speakers with apraxia, and Hardcastle and Edwards (1992) noted that repeated syllables are generally similar to the final production.

Metatheses

Problems in the serial ordering of gestures have been found in EPG data from apraxic speakers (Hardcastle and Edwards, 1992). For example, abnormal sequencing of gestures may occur in stop-consonant sequences such as /kt/ or /tk/ in words such as 'ac_tor' or 'kit_kat', where the normal sequence is reversed. These are frequently not detected auditorily.

Errors of Substitution and Omission

Substitutions

The term substitution is used here to refer to spatially normal, but inappropriately selected, articulations. For example, if a speaker was heard to say /ti/ when attempting the word 'key', and the EPG records showed a spatially normal /t/, then this would be considered a 'true' substitution error. One apraxic speaker described by Hardcastle (1987) produced [s] for /ʃ/ in 'sheep', and this was classified as a substitution error. However, errors that are heard and transcribed as substitutions are often not of this type when the EPG records are examined. For example, misdirected articulatory gestures (see above) found in apraxic data are often heard as phonemic paraphasias, or substitution errors (Hardcastle and Edwards, 1992). Also, it has been found that some children with phonological disorders, who are heard by listeners to be neutralizing sound contrasts, are in fact producing a consistent contrast at the articulatory level (Gibbon, 1990).

Omissions

Omissions occur where an expected gesture is missing from the EPG record. Omissions have been observed in both apraxic speakers (Sugishita *et al*, 1987) and adults with acquired dysarthria (Hardcastle *et al*, 1985). In the study by Hardcastle and Edwards (1992), there were instances where apraxic speakers omitted the second element in clusters and also the fricative phase of affricates. These were often heard as omissions, but the records often showed subtle changes in contact pattern that were not perceived.

Interpretation of EPG Error Patterns

Interpretation of EPG data is a qualitative task, for current knowledge does not allow us to state absolutely the boundaries of 'normality' and 'normal variation' in terms of EPG records. Phonetic context, rate and style of speech all need to be considered, as do physical factors such as palatal morphology and electrode configuration. For example, in order for incomplete alveolar closure for /t/ to be categorized as an error (e.g. as undershoot), both the phonetic and linguistic environment have to be considered (for example, incomplete contact for /t/ occurs in normal speakers, particularly in syllable final position).

With these caveats in mind, classifying EPG errors in the way described above assists the clinician in identifying patterns of abnormal articulatory behaviour, which can be subsequently targeted in therapy. EPG has been found to reveal general tendencies or patterns of articulatory behaviour not detected from an auditory-based analysis. For example, similar EPG error patterns can have varying perceptual consequences, depending on factors such as the exact articulatory timing involved in the production (Gibbon and Hardcastle, 1989; Hardcastle and Edwards, 1992), the phonetic context (Gibbon *et al*, 1993b), and the sound class affected (Dent *et al*, 1992; Gibbon and Hardcastle, 1989).

An EPG classification also provides insight into possible underlying causes. In terms of diagnosis, temporal and serial ordering errors, for example, have been interpreted as being due to higher level motor programming deficits. Spatial distortions, on the other hand, have been attributed to lower level motoric deficits, such as weakness and incoordination in adults with acquired disorders, or faulty motor learning and impaired sensory feedback in children. Such interpretations influence the therapeutic process in terms of selection of strategies and tasks presented to the client.

Using EPG as a Visual Feedback Device in Therapy

The use of biofeedback in therapy derives its effectiveness from making ambiguous internal cues (for example, those associated with tongue position and movement in the case of EPG) explicit, and enabling conscious control of such cues to develop. In relation to the remediation of speech disorders, Shuster, Ruscello and Smith (1992) suggest that biofeedback is particularly effective where details of target sound production are difficult to describe to clients. This applies particularly to the activity of the tongue, which may be too subtle or automatic for the client to be aware of under normal circumstances. A further advantage of computer-mediated procedures is that some clients are more inclined to persist with tasks when performance is measured objectively (i.e. by a computer) rather than when it is judged by another person (i.e. the clinician) (Volin, 1993).

When confronted with the task of learning new motor skills, evidence suggests that feedback in the visual modality can be highly effective (Mulder and Hulstijn, 1985). The more controversial and unresolved issue in our present state of knowledge, is the process by which new articulatory skills acquired using visual feedback are integrated into natural speech. EPG therapy operates essentially within a behavioural framework, and as such is based on principles of learning theory. The problem of carry-over needs careful attention when using EPG, and for this reason, EPG should be viewed as an additional strategy to be used in conjunction with other approaches to improve overall speech intelligibility. The exact and specific contribution that EPG makes within the total learning process is difficult to establish at present, but is an important issue that future work needs to address.

EPG has been used extensively as a therapy tool for a variety of disorders (Dent *et al*, 1995; Hardcastle *et al*, 1991a; Morgan Barry, 1989, 1995b; Shibata *et al*, 1979). The technique has been found to be particularly effective in the treatment of children with cleft palate, who have abnormally broad or posterior tongue placement (Michi *et al*, 1986, 1993) or abnormal double articulations (Dent *et al*, 1992; Gibbon and Hardcastle, 1989). Michi *et al* (1993) combined EPG with a display of friction and treated six children with distorted /s/, and found that those with excessive posterior tongue elevation made faster progress with visual feedback than those who were treated without EPG. Whitehill, Stokes and Man (1996) used EPG to treat an 18-year-old woman who had undergone primary repair of the palate at 13 years of age. The client showed rapid improvement in articulatory placement for /s/ and /t/, which were produced with more anterior placement following therapy, and there was good carry-over to non-target phonemes. Interestingly, this speaker showed a 'spontaneous' reduction in nasal emission and nasal plosion during production of these sounds after treatment, although this aspect of speech was not directly targeted in therapy.

A number of studies have investigated the use of EPG with speakers who are hearing impaired. In a study by Fletcher, Dagenais and Critz-Crosby (1991), five profoundly hearing impaired children were treated using EPG. They showed that there were changes in EPG patterns for a wide range of lingual consonants and listener perceptions indicated significant improvements for all subjects. They concluded that visual articulatory modelling and feedback of EPG contact patterns were effective in improving speech intelligibility. In a more recent paper, Dagenais, Critz-Crosby, Fletcher and McCutcheon (1994b) compared the effectiveness of EPG in teaching profoundly hearing impaired children to produce a range of consonants with traditional aural/oral approaches. This study showed that, immediately post-treatment, the EPG-trained group produced more normal-looking EPG patterns than the group who had received traditional therapy. In addition, the EPG group often showed dramatic progress, for example most learned how to produce velar gestures in one therapy session (see also Crawford, 1995, for a description of using EPG to teach velar stops to profoundly deaf children).

EPG has been successfully used in the treatment of older children with functional articulation disorders who present with persisting difficulties with sounds such as lingual fricatives, affricates and stops (see Dagenais, 1995, for a summary). Dent, Gibbon and Hardcastle (1995) report the results of therapy for a group of children with a variety of distorted /s/ productions. Before therapy, these children showed a wide range of articulatory configurations (described in Gibbon et al, 1995), but one consistent finding was that none had an anterior groove during production of /s/ targets. For those children who completed therapy, all showed evidence of anterior groove configurations and perceptually acceptable sounding /s/ productions after treatment. Figure 6.17 gives examples of EPG patterns for /s/ targets before and after therapy for three of the children. These children presented with different distortions of sibilant sounds prior to treatment: D1 had lateralized productions, D2 palatal fricatives and D3 pharyngeal fricatives for sibilant targets. After therapy, the EPG patterns more closely resembled those of a normal speaker, (see Figure 6.7, alveolar grooved pattern). Dagenais, Critz-Crosby and Adams (1994a) describe two children of a similar age, both of whom had 'lateral lisps'. The EPG patterns for the two children were different, not only for /s/ targets, but also for a range of other sounds. One child's speech was treated successfully using EPG, while the other child had continuing difficulties. They conclude that there may be few commonalties among children with lateralized articulations, and that further research is needed. In addition, changes such as those required during EPG therapy require basic articulatory reorganization, and this can have a wide-ranging effect on the whole sound system (Howard, 1994). This may mean, for example, that the client may enter a period of increased variability before new patterns stabilize.

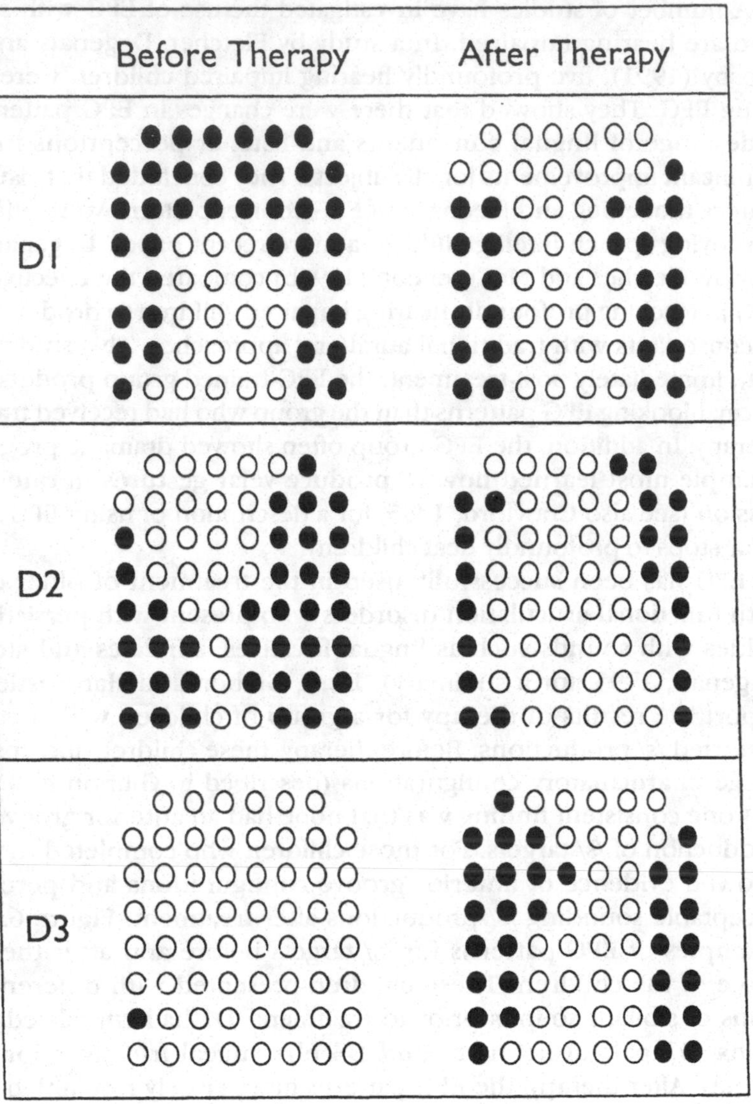

Figure 6.17. EPG patterns of /s/ targets before (left) and after (right) EPG treatment for three children (D1–3) with different types of distortions. D1's /s/ targets were perceived as lateralized fricatives, D2's as palatal fricatives and D3's as pharyngeal fricatives before therapy. EPG frames were taken at the point of maximum contact during the fricative portion of six words containing /s/ and electrodes activated more than 50% are indicated by filled circles. After therapy, all sibilants were heard as acceptable productions.

A number of studies reporting the use of EPG to treat children and adults with motor speech disorders have been published (e.g. Howard and Varley, 1995; Goldstein *et al*, 1994; Morgan Barry, 1995a, b). Howard and Varley (1995) used EPG to treat a patient with severe apraxia of speech, and found that EPG provided the speaker with valuable visual feedback on attempts at speech production and that this information facilitated the gradual modification of abnormal articulatory movements. Goldstein *et al* (1994) combined a palatal lift device with EPG to treat an adult with severe dysarthria. They found that this patient's speech had improved on a number of measures after therapy.

Methodological Issues

Client selection

When considering whether to use EPG in therapy, a number of factors should be investigated. Although an obvious point, the clinician must be of the opinion that overall speech intelligibility/acceptability will be improved by modifying tongue placement and/or dynamics. Possible aetiological or maintaining factors need to have been fully explored. These include sensory loss, particularly hearing and visual; structural and functional abnormalities of the vocal tract (e.g. velopharyngeal insufficiency, muscle weakness etc.); cognitive ability; auditory discrimination or linguistic difficulties; medical factors; psycho-social problems; poor attention; motivation (Morgan Barry and Hardcastle, 1987). These factors do not necessarily preclude clients from being selected for EPG therapy, but they are important in the overall management of individuals, and will affect the ultimate prognosis.

Practical issues relating to the wearing of the palate need to be considered. These include whether the client is currently undergoing orthodontic or dental treatment, is expected to lose teeth imminently, or has special dental requirements such as a denture. It is important that the individual will tolerate wearing the palate, and although this is difficult to determine in advance, full discussions prior to therapy are essential. Recommending EPG therapy for young children has to be considered carefully, as they may still make progress using other forms of therapy. Also, while young children are able to understand what is involved in EPG therapy, they do not always have the determination or motivation to persist with what is recognized as a demanding and exacting form of treatment.

The client and carers need to be engaged in full consultations prior to therapy, particularly regarding the process of making and wearing the artificial palate. Before having an artificial palate made, they should have the opportunity to view EPG in a live demonstration, in order to observe the type of visual feedback EPG provides, and to allow time for discussion.

Assessment protocol

EPG is an additional assessment procedure that supplements information gathered from routine procedures and other instrumental investigations, in particular acoustic analysis and airflow measurements (particularly relevant for speakers with cleft palate). A standard word list (Hardcastle *et al*, 1985), designed to elicit a range of consonants and consonant sequences, is often used when recording EPG data. Additional lists or tasks can be devised to investigate specific difficulties, and could include any of the following:

*   nonsense, or non-speech items, such as diadochokinetic tasks, imitating a rhythm using the tongue, etc. (see Edwards and Miller, 1989);
*   imitation as well as spontaneous production of speech items;
*   lists of potential homonyms in the client's speech production;
*   connected speech. With EPG3, reliable segmentation of long sequences of spontaneous speech is possible;
*   several repetitions of the word lists, or additional items. This is desirable in order to estimate the variability of a client's production, and is particularly valuable for those with neuromotor disorders, such as dyspraxia.

High-quality audio-tape recordings are made routinely for the purpose of carrying out auditory-based transcriptions. Tape recordings are made with and without the palate being worn, so that it is possible to estimate the effect that the palate is having on the client's speech. Detailed assessments are undertaken, as described above, typically on a minimum of three occasions for each client, if a course of treatment is to be carried out. The first recording is made prior to receiving treatment, the second on completion of therapy, and a third follow-up assessment takes place, usually 3 months or more after completion of therapy. Long-term follow-up using EPG is not always possible in children because dento-facial growth means that the artificial palate will not fit comfortably for indefinite periods.

Following the initial recording, EPG data is observed simultaneously with the acoustic signal, and the patterns described according to the error classification scheme outlined above. Diagnosis is considered in the light of the profile of error patterns, bearing in mind other factors such as: the shape of the palate and electrode configuration; the auditory analysis; knowledge of and assumptions about 'normality'; and known organic pathology. For detailed examples that illustrate this process for individual clients, see Gibbon, Dent and Hardcastle (1993b); Dent, Gibbon and Hardcastle (1992); and Hardcastle, Gibbon and Dent (1993).

EPG Therapy

During EPG therapy, the client sits directly in front of the computer screen which contains a real-time display of tongue-palate contact on the left and a static palatogram on the right (see Figure 6.3 and Dent *et al*, 1995, for further details). EPG3 has the facility for two multiplexers to be connected, one for the client and one for the clinician, with a switch that allows the clinician to sit next to the client and toggle between the two. The clinician can demonstrate EPG targets and capture or 'freeze' specific aspects of tongue-palate contact on to the static palatogram. Clients can then compare their own patterns with a permanent target. This simple yet effective display is flexible and provides only the essential information. Incentives and interest may need to be added for some clients, and clinicians can adapt many materials and activities to liven up tasks if necessary. The following provide general guidelines that have been used in treatment using EPG for a variety of disorders (see Hardcastle *et al*, 1989a, 1991a; Morgan Barry, 1989). Therapy typically includes a number of stages:

- *Demonstrations and verbal explanations*. These help the client to develop knowledge about articulation which will assist the therapy process. This stage aims to establish awareness of (1) the relationship between tongue patterns (as displayed on the EPG screen) and the resulting sound heard; (2) linking the visual display to the client's own tongue and hard palate; and (3) the difference between the client's patterns and those of a normal speaker.

- *Learning new motor skills*. In practice, it has been found that, initially, clients need to establish and practise a new articulatory pattern without other speech features present, such as airstream or voicing, and as a static posture. A number of stages have been found to be useful in helping clients to progress from artificial gestures to their use in naturalistic contexts (see Hardcastle *et al*, 1991a, for more details of these stages).

- *Transfer into naturalistic contexts*. At each stage of treatment, time is spent ensuring that skills can be maintained without the presence of visual feedback. A first step might be to remove the visual feedback, but keep the artificial palate *in situ*. This might simply involve covering the computer screen, or unplugging the artificial palate. The next stage could involve short assignments gradually increasing the complexity and naturalness of the tasks. Assignments are better if devised by the client to be implemented in real-life situations and the client should feel ready and responsible for carrying them out.

Conclusions

EPG is a good example of an instrumental technique that was originally designed for phonetic research, but which has subsequently proved to be a useful clinical procedure. In assessment, EPG data allows the clinician access to details of an important aspect of speech production not routinely available. In many instances, however, the interpretation of EPG data needs to be verified by the use of additional procedures. Ultrasound (another non-invasive procedure) can be combined with EPG to determine the proximity of the tongue to the palate as well as its surface shape (Stone *et al*, 1992). Such an analysis, together with accurate three-dimensional measurements of the palate, would make it possible to take into account differences in oral morphology, and would assist in the interpretation of EPG contact patterns. In therapy, EPG can be seen as an effective additional procedure for certain types of speech disorders. However, therapy using EPG has focused almost entirely on remediating abnormal spatial distortions, with the remediation of temporal and serial ordering difficulties receiving comparatively little attention. The use of EPG to improve these aspects of speech motor control promises to be an exciting future direction, but strategies and guidelines to develop these specific aspects of production need to be devised.

Applications of EPG in other fields are now being explored (see Jack and Gibbon, 1995, for the use of EPG in describing aspects of swallowing). Also, EPG may prove to be a useful supplement to traditional methods in second language teaching and learning. A pilot study exploring the use of EPG with Japanese learners of English has been successful in improving their productions of the /r/, /l/ distinction (Gibbon *et al*, 1991). Larger-scale studies focusing on other common sources of difficulty for the foreign language learner are envisaged.

Acknowledgements

Part of the work described in this paper was supported by a project grant from the British Medical Research Council (Project no. G8912970N), from Daiwa Anglo-Japanese Foundation and from the British Council (under the Hong Kong-British Academic Link Scheme). Thanks are due to Hilary Dent who collaborated on the MRC project, to Wilf Jones who designed EPG3 and provided technical support and finally to Katerina Nicolaidis and Sara Wood who made helpful comments on an earlier draft of the chapter.

References

Abe M. Pathophysiology of nasopharyngeal articulation: sound analysis and observation of articulatory movement. The Japan Journal of Logopedics and Phoniatrics (Japanese) 1987; 28: 239–50.

Abercrombie D. Direct palatography. Zeitschrift für Phonetik 1957; 10: 21–25.

Ahmed S. An experimental investigation of 'emphasis' in Sudanese colloquial Arabic.

Unpublished PhD thesis, University of Reading, 1984.

Barry WJ, Timmermann G. Mispronunciations and compensatory movements of tongue operated patients. British Journal of Disorders of Communication 1985; 20: 81–90.

Butcher A. Measuring coarticulation and variability in tongue contact patterns. Clinical Linguistics and Phonetics 1989; 3: 39–47.

Butcher A, Weiher E. An electropalatographic investigation of coarticulation in VCV sequences. Journal of Phonetics 1976; 4: 59–74.

Byrd D. Articulatory timing in English consonant sequences. UCLA Working Papers in Phonetics, 86, May 1994.

Byrd D. Influences on articulatory timing in consonant sequences. Journal of Phonetics 1996; 24: 209–44.

Byrd D, Tan CC. Saying consonant sequences quickly. Journal of Phonetics 1996; 24: 263–82.

Byrd D, Flemming E, Mueller CA, Tan, CC. Using regions and indices in EPG data reduction. Journal of Speech and Hearing Research 1995; 38: 821–27.

Christensen JM, Fletcher SG, McCutcheon MJ. Oesophageal speaker articulation of /s,z/: a dynamic palatometric assessment. Journal of Communication Disorders 1992; 25: 65–76.

Crawford R. Teaching voiced velar stops to profoundly deaf children using EPG, two case studies. Clinical Linguistics and Phonetics 1995; 9: 255–70.

Dagenais PA. Electropalatography in the treatment of articulation/phonological disorders. Journal of Communication Disorders 1995; 28: 303–29.

Dagenais PA, Critz-Crosby P. Consonant lingual-palatal contacts produced by normal-hearing and hearing impaired children. Journal of Speech and Hearing Research 1991; 34: 1423–35.

Dagenais PA, Critz-Crosby P, Adams JB. Defining and remediating persistent lateral lisps in children using electropalatography: preliminary findings. American Journal of Speech-Language Pathology 1994a; September: 67–76.

Dagenais PA, Critz-Crosby P, Fletcher SG, McCutcheon MJ. Comparing abilities of children with profound hearing impairments to learn consonants using electropalatography or traditional aural-oral techniques. Journal of Speech and Hearing Research 1994b; 37: 687–99.

Dagenais PA, Lorendo LC, McCutcheon MJ. A study of voicing and context effects upon consonant linguapalatal contact patterns. Journal of Phonetics 1994c; 22: 225–38.

Dent H, Gibbon F, Hardcastle W. Inhibiting an abnormal lingual pattern in a cleft palate child using electropalatography. In Leahy MM, Kallen JL. (Eds), Interdisciplinary Perspectives in Speech and Language Pathology, pp. 211–21. Dublin: School of Clinical Speech and Language Studies, 1992.

Dent H, Gibbon F, Hardcastle W.The application of electropalatography (EPG) to the remediation of speech disorders in school-aged children and young adults. European Journal of Disorders of Communication 1995; 30: 264–77.

Edwards M. Speech and language disability. In Edwards M, Watson ARH. (Eds), Advances in the Management of Cleft Palate, pp. 83–96. Edinburgh: Churchill Livingstone, 1980.

Edwards S, Miller N. Using EPG to investigate speech errors and motor agility in a dyspraxic patient. Clinical Linguistics and Phonetics 1989; 3: 111–26.

Eek A. Observations on Estonian palatalization: an articulatory study. Estonian Papers in Phonetics, pp. 18–36. Tallinn: Academy of Science of the Estonian S.S.R. Institute for Language and Literature, 1973.

Engstrand O. Towards an electropalatographic specification of consonant articulation in Swedish, pp. 115–56. Stockholm: PERILUS X (Phonetic Experimental Research at the Institute of Linguistics, University of Stockholm), 1989.

Faber A. Studies in Sibilant Articulation. Unpublished manuscript. Haskins Laboratories, 270 Crown Street, New Haven, CT 06511, 1989.

Farnetani E. Asymmetry of lingual movements: EPG data on Italian. Quaderni del Centro di Studio per le Ricerche di Fonetica del CNR 1988; 7: 211–28.

Farnetani E. An articulatory study of 'voicing' in Italian by means of dynamic palatography. Speech Research International Conference, Linguistic Institute of Hungarian Academy of Sciences, pp. 395–98. Budapest: T. Szende, 1989.

Farnetani E. V-C-V lingual coarticulation and its spatiotemporal domain. In Hardcastle WJ, Marchal A. (Eds), Speech Production and Speech Modelling, pp. 93–130. Dordrecht: Kluwer, 1990.

Farnetani E, Provaglio A. Assessing variability of lingual consonants in Italian. Quaderni del Centro di Studio per le Ricerche di Fonetica del CNR 1991; 10: 117–45.

Farnetani E, Vagges K, Magno-Caldognetto E. Coarticulation in Italian /VtV/ sequences: a palatographic study. Phonetica 1985; 42: 78–99.

Fletcher S. New prospects for speech by the hearing impaired. In Lass N. (Ed.), Speech and Language: Advances in Basic Research and Practice, pp. 1–42. New York: Academic Press,1983.

Fletcher S. Speech production and oral motor skill in an adult with an unrepaired palatal cleft. Journal of Speech and Hearing Disorders 1985; 50: 254–61.

Fletcher S. Speech production following partial glossectomy. Journal of Speech and Hearing Disorders 1988; 53: 232–38.

Fletcher SG, McCutcheon MJ, Wolf MB. Dynamic palatometry. Journal of Speech and Hearing Research 1975; 18: 812–19.

Fletcher S, Hasegawa A, McCutcheon M, Gilliom J. Use of linguo-palatal contact patterns to modify articulation in a deaf adult. In McPherson D, Schwab M. (Eds), Advances in Prosthetic Devices for the Deaf: A Technical Workshop, pp. 127–33. Rochester, NY: NTID, 1980.

Fletcher SG, Dagenais PA, Critz-Crosby P. Teaching consonants to profoundly hearing-impaired speakers using palatometry. Journal of Speech and Hearing Research 1991; 34: 929–42.

Fontdevila J, Recasens D, Pallarès MD. The contact index method of electropalatographic data reduction. Journal of Phonetics 1994; 22: 141–54.

Fujimura O, Tatsumi IF, Kagaya R. Computational processing of palatographic patterns. Journal of Phonetics 1973; 1: 47–54.

Gibbon F. Lingual activity in two speech-disordered children's attempts to produce velar and alveolar stop consonants: evidence from electropalatographic (EPG) data. British Journal of Disorders of Communication 1990; 25: 329–40.

Gibbon F, Hardcastle W. Articulatory description and treatment of 'lateral /s/' using electropalatography: a case study. British Journal of Disorders of Communication 1987; 22: 203–17.

Gibbon F, Hardcastle W. Deviant articulation in a cleft palate child following late repair of the hard palate: a description and remediation procedure using electropalatography. Clinical Linguistics and Phonetics 1989; 3: 93–110.

Gibbon FE, Hardcastle WJ, Suzuki H. An electropalatographic study of the /r/, /l/ distinction for Japanese learners of English. Computer Assisted Language Learning 1991; 4: 153–71.

Gibbon F, Hardcastle W, Nicolaidis K. Temporal and spatial aspects of lingual coarticulation in /kl/ clusters: a cross-linguistic investigation. Language and Speech 1993a; 36: 261–78.

Gibbon F, Dent H, Hardcastle W. Diagnosis and therapy of abnormal alveolar stops in a speech-disordered child using EPG. Clinical Linguistics and Phonetics 1993b; 7: 247–68.

Gibbon F, Hardcastle WJ, Dent H. A study of obstruent sounds in school-age children with speech disorders using electropalatography. European Journal of Disorders of Communication 1995; 30: 213–25.

Goldstein P, Zeigler W, Vogel M, Hoole P. Combined palatal lift and EPG feedback therapy in dysarthria: a case study. Clinical Linguistics and Phonetics 1994; 8: 201–18.

Hamilton C. Investigation of articulatory patterns of young adults with Down's syndrome using electropalatography. Down's Syndrome: Research and Practice 1993; 1: 15–28.

Hamlet SL, Bunnell HT, Struntz B. Articulatory asymmetries. Journal of the Acoustical Society of America 1986; 79: 1164–69.

Hardcastle WJ. Some phonetic and syntactic constraints on lingual co-articulation during /kl/ sequences. Speech Communication 1985; 4: 247–63.

Hardcastle WJ. Electropalatographic study of articulation disorders in verbal dyspraxia. In Ryalls J. (Ed.), Phonetic Approaches to Speech Production in Aphasia and Related Disorders, pp. 113–36. San Diego: College Hill Press, 1987.

Hardcastle WJ. EPG and acoustic study of some connected speech processes. Proceedings of the 1994 International Conference on Spoken Language Processing (ICSLP 94) Yokohama, Japan, 1994; 2: 515–18.

Hardcastle WJ. Assimilation of alveolar stops and nasals in connected speech. In Lewis J, Windsor L. (Eds.), Studies in General and English Phonetics, pp. 49–67. London: Routledge, 1995.

Hardcastle WJ, Roach PJ. An instrumental investigation of coarticulation in stop consonant sequences. In Hollien P, Hollien H. (Eds), Current Issues in the Phonetic Sciences, pp. 531–40. Amsterdam: John Benjamins, 1977.

Hardcastle WJ, Brasington RWP. Experimental study of implosive and voiced egressive stops in Shona: an interim report. Speech Research Laboratory Work in Progress, University of Reading 1978; 2: 66–97.

Hardcastle WJ, Clark JE. Articulatory, aerodynamic and acoustic properties of lingual fricatives in English. Speech Research Laboratory Work in Progress, University of Reading 1981; 3: 51–78.

Hardcastle WJ, Morgan R. An instrumental analysis of articulation disorders in children. British Journal of Disorders of Communication 1982; 6: 47–65.

Hardcastle WJ, Barry W. Articulatory and perceptual factors in /l/ vocalisations in English. Speech Research Laboratory Work in Progress, University of Reading 1985; 5: 31–44.

Hardcastle WJ, Marchal A. EUR-ACCOR: a multi-lingual articulatory and acoustic database. ICSLP 90, Proceedings of the International Conference on Spoken Language Processing, The Acoustical Society of Japan. Kobe, Japan, 1990; 2: 1293–96.

Hardcastle WJ, Edwards S. EPG-based descriptions of apraxic speech errors. In Kent R. (Ed.), Intelligibility in Speech Disorders: Theory, Measurement and Management, pp. 287–328. Philadelphia: John Benjamins, 1992.

Hardcastle WJ, Morgan Barry R, Clark C. Articulatory and voicing characteristics of adult dysarthric and verbal dyspraxic speakers: an instrumental study. British Journal of Disorders of Communication 1985; 20: 249–70.

Hardcastle W, Morgan Barry R, Clark C. An instrumental phonetic study of lingual activity in articulation disordered children. Journal of Speech and Hearing Research 1987; 30: 171–84.

Hardcastle W, Morgan Barry R, Nunn M. Instrumental articulatory phonetics in assessment and remediation: case studies with the electropalatograph. In Stengelhofen J. (Ed.), Cleft Palate: The Nature and Remediation of Communicative Problems, pp. 136–64. Edinburgh: Churchill Livingstone, 1989a.

Hardcastle WJ, Jones W, Knight C, Trudgeon A, Calder G. New developments in electropalatography: a state-of-the-art report. Clinical Linguistics and Phonetics 1989b; 3: 1–38.

Hardcastle WJ, Gibbon FE, Jones W. Visual display of tongue-palate contact: electropalatography in the assessment and remediation of speech disorders. British Journal of Disorders of Communication 1991a; 26: 41–74.

Hardcastle W, Gibbon F, Nicolaidis K. EPG data reduction methods and their implications for studies of lingual coarticulation. Journal of Phonetics 1991b; 19: 251–66.

Hardcastle W, Gibbon F, Dent H. Assessment and remediation of intractable articulation disorders using EPG. Research Institute of Logopedics and Phoniatrics Annual Bulletin, University of Tokyo 1993; 27: 159–70.

Hardcastle WJ, Gibbon F, Scobbie J. Phonetic and phonological aspects of English affricate production in children with speech disorders. Phonetica 1995; 52: 242–50.

Harrington J. Coarticulation and stuttering: an acoustic and electropalatographic study. In Peters H, Hulstijn W. (Eds), Speech Motor Dynamics in Stuttering, pp. 381–92. New York: Springer-Verlag, 1987.

Hayward KM, Omar YA, Goesche M. Dental and alveolar stops in Kimvita Swahili: an electropalatographic study. African Languages and Cultures 1989; 2: 51–72.

Hiki S, Imaizumi S. Observation of symmetry of tongue movement by use of dynamic palatography. Annual Bulletin, Research Institute of Logopedics and Phoniatrics, University of Tokyo 1974; 8: 69–74.

Hoole P, Ziegler W, Hartmann E, Hardcastle W. Parallel electropalatographic and acoustic measures of fricatives. Clinical Linguistics and Phonetics 1989; 3: 59–69.

Hoole P, Nguyen-Trong N, Hardcastle WJ. A comparative investigation of coarticulation in fricatives: electropalatographic, electromagnetic and acoustic data. Language and Speech 1993; 36: 235–60.

Howard S. Spontaneous phonetic reorganisation following articulation therapy: an electropalatographic study. In Aulanko R, Korpijaako-Huuhka AM. (Eds), Proceedings of the 3rd Congress of the International Clinical Phonetics and Linguistics Association, 1993, Helsinki, Finland, Hakapaino Oy 1994, pp. 67–74.

Howard S, Varley R. Using electropalatography to treat severe acquired apraxia of speech. European Journal of Disorders of Communication 1995; 30: 246–55.

Imai S, Michi K. Articulatory function after resection of the tongue and floor of the mouth: palatometric and perceptual evaluation. Journal of Speech and Hearing Research 1992; 35: 68–78.

Itoh H, Matsuda Y, Sugawara J, Fujita Y, Kanuma A, Yamashita S. Relationship between oral cavity shape and articulation of post-operative cleft palate subjects – observation by use of electropalatography, 3, pp.1149–53. Medinfo 1980. IFIP World Conference Series on Medical Informatics, Tokyo, Japan: North Holland Publishing Company 1980, pp. 1149–53.

Jack F, Gibbon F. EPG in the study of tongue movement during eating and swallowing (a novel procedure for measuring texture-related behaviour). International Journal of Food Science and Technology 1995; 30: 415–23.

Jones WJ, Hardcastle WJ. New developments in EPG3 software. European Journal of

Disorders of Communication 1995; 30: 183–92.

Kohler K. The instability of word-final alveolar plosives in German: an electropalatographic investigation. Phonetica 1976; 33: 1–30.

Ladefoged P. A Phonetic Study of West African Languages (2nd edn). Cambridge: Cambridge University Press, 1968.

Marchal A. Coproduction: evidence from EPG data. Speech Communication 1988; 7: 287–95.

Marchal A, Espesser R. L'asymetrie des appuis linguo-palatins. Journal d'Acoustique 1989; 2: 53–57.

Marchal A, Courville L, Belanger D. La palatographie dynamique. Revue de Phonétique Appliquée 1980; 53: 49–72.

Matsuno K. An electropalatographic study of Japanese palatal sounds. Bulletin, The Phonetic Society of Japan 1989; 190: 8–17.

Michi K, Suzuki N, Yamashita Y, Imai S. Visual training and correction of articulation disorders by use of dynamic palatography: serial observation in a case of cleft palate. Journal of Speech and Hearing Disorders 1986; 51: 226–38.

Michi K-I, Yamashita Y, Imai S, Suzuki N, Yoshida H. Role of visual feedback in the treatment for defective /s/ sounds in patients with cleft palate. Journal of Speech and Hearing Research 1993; 36: 277–85.

Miyawaki K, Kiritani S, Tatsumi IF, Fujimura O. Palatographic observation of VCV articulations in Japanese. Annual Bulletin, Research Institute of Logopedics and Phoniatrics, University of Tokyo 1974; 8: 51–57.

Morgan Barry RA. Lingual patterns in a child with severe oral sensory impairment. College of Speech Therapists' Bulletin 1984; December: 4–5.

Morgan Barry RA. EPG from square one: an overview of electropalatography as an aid to therapy. Clinical Linguistics and Phonetics 1989; 3: 81–91.

Morgan Barry RA. Phonetic and phonological aspects of neurological speech disorders. PhD thesis, Department of Linguistic Science, University of Reading, 1990.

Morgan Barry R. The relationship between dysarthria and verbal dyspraxia in children: a comparative study using profiling and instrumental analyses. Clinical Linguistics and Phonetics 1995a; 9: 277–309.

Morgan Barry R. EPG treatment of a child with Worcester-Drought syndrome. European Journal of Disorders of Communication 1995b; 30: 256–63.

Morgan Barry R, Hardcastle W. Some observation on the use of electropalatography as a clinical tool in the diagnosis and treatment of articulation disorders in children. Proceedings of the First International Symposium on Specific Speech and Language Disorders in Children, 29th March – 3rd April, 208–22. Reading: AFASIC, 1987.

Mulder T, Hulstijn W. Sensory feedback in the learning of a novel motor task. Journal of Motor Behaviour 1985; 17: 110–28.

Nicolaidis K. Aspects of lingual articulation in Greek: an electropalatographic study. In Philippaki-Warburton I, Nicolaidis K, Sifianou M. (Eds), Themes in Greek Linguistics, pp. 225–32. Amsterdam: John Benjamins, 1994.

Nicolaidis K, Hardcastle W, Gibbon F. Bibliography of electropalatographic studies in English (1957–1992) – parts I, II and III. Speech Research Laboratory, University of Reading, Work in Progress 1993; 7: 26–106.

Okazaki K, Onizuka T, Abe M, Sawashima M. Palatalised articulation as a type of cleft palate speech: observation by dynamic palatograph and cineradiograph. The Japan Journal of Logopedics and Phoniatrics (Japanese) 1980; 22: 109–20.

Palmer JM. Dynamic palatography: general implications of locus and sequencing patterns. Phonetica 1973; 28: 76–85.

Powers MH. Functional disorders of articulation: symptomatology and etiology. In

Travis LE. (Ed.), Handbook of Speech Pathology and Audiology. Englewood Cliffs, NJ: Prentice Hall, 1971.

Recasens D. Timing constraints and coarticulation: alveolo-palatals and sequences of alveolar + [j] in Catalan. Phonetica 1984a; 41: 125–39.

Recasens D. V-to-C coarticulation in Catalan VCV sequences: an articulatory and acoustical study. Journal of Phonetics 1984b; 12: 61–73.

Recasens, D. Vowel-to-Vowel coarticulation in Catalan VCV sequences. Journal of the Acoustical Society of America 1984c; 76: 1624–35.

Recasens, D. Long range coarticulation effects for tongue dorsum contact in VCVCV sequences. Speech Communication 1989; 8: 293–307.

Recasens D, Farnetani E, Fontdevila J, Pallares MD. An electropalatographic study of alveolar and palatal consonants in Catalan and Italian. Language and Speech 1993; 36: 213–34.

Recasens D, Pallarès MD, Fontdevila J. Co-articulatory variability and articulatory-acoustic correlations for consonants. European Journal of Disorders of Communication 1995; 30: 203-12.

Schönle PW, Muller C, Wenig P. Echtzeitanalyze von orofacialen Bewegungen mit Hilfe der elektromagnetische Articulographie. Biomedizinische Technik 1989; 34: 126–30.

Shibata S, Ino A, Yamashita S. Teaching Articulation By Use Of Electro-palatograph. Tokyo, Japan: Rion Co Ltd, 1979. (English version, translated by K Kakita, H Kawasaki and J Wright, edited by S Hiki, 1982).

Shuster L, Ruscello DM, Smith KD. Evoking [r] using visual feedback. American Journal of Speech-Language Pathology 1992; 1: 29–34.

Speculand B, Butcher GW, Stephens CD. Three-dimensional measurement: the accuracy and precision of the Reflex Microscope. British Journal of Oral and Maxillofacial Surgery 1988; 21: 276–83.

Stone M, Faber A, Raphael LJ, Shawker TH. Cross-sectional tongue and linguapalatal contact patterns in [s], [ʃ], and [l]. Journal of Phonetics 1992; 20: 253–70.

Sudo MM, Kiritani S, Sawashima M. The articulation of Japanese intervocalic /d/ and /r/: an electropalatographic study. Annual Bulletin, Research Institute of Logopedics and Phoniatrics, University of Tokyo 1983; 17: 55–59.

Sugishita M, Konno K, Kabe S, Yunoki K, Togashi O, Kawamura M. Electropalatographic analysis of apraxia of speech in a left-hander and in a right-hander. Brain 1987; 110: 1393–417.

Suzuki N. Clinical applications of EPG to Japanese cleft palate and glossectomy patients. Clinical Linguistics and Phonetics 1989; 3: 127–36.

Suzuki N, Michi K, Takahashi M, Katayose K, Yamashita Y, Ueno T. Study of the articulatory movement of the cleft palate subjects by use of dynamic palatography: an attempt to classify the palatogram pattern. Journal of the Japanese Cleft Palate Association (Japanese) 1980; 5: 162–79.

Suzuki N, Sakuma T, Michi KT, Ueno T. The articulatory characteristics of the tongue in anterior open-bite: observation by use of dynamic palatography. International Journal of Oral Surgery 1981a; 10: 299–303.

Suzuki N, Yamashita Y, Michi K, Ueno T. Changes of the palatolingual contact during articulation therapy in the cleft palate patients: observation by use of dynamic palatography. 4th International Congress of Cleft Palate and Related Craniofacial Anomalies, Acapulco, Mexico, May 1981b.

Trost JE. Articulatory additions to the classical description of the speech of persons with cleft palate. Cleft Palate Journal 1981; 18: 193–203

Volin RA. Clinical applications of biofeedback. American Speech-Language-Hearing

Association (ASHA) 1993; 35(8): 43–44.

Washino K, Kasai Y, Uchida Y, Takeda K. Tongue movement during speech in a patient with apraxia of speech: a case study. In Peng FC. (Ed.), Current Issues in Neurolinguistics. A Japanese Contribution: Language Function and its Neural Mechanisms. Advances in Neurolinguistics, Proceedings of the 2nd ICU Conference of Neurolinguistics, vol 6, Mitaka, Japan: International Christian University, pp. 125–59, 1981.

Whitehill T, Stokes S, Hardcastle WJ, Gibbon F. Electropalatographic and perceptual analysis of the speech of Cantonese children with cleft palate. European Journal of Disorders of Communication 1995; 30: 193–202.

Whitehill TL, Stokes SF, Man YHY. Electropalatography treatment with an adult with late repair of cleft palate. Cleft Palate-Craniofacial Journal 1996; 33: 160–68.

Wolf MB, Fletcher SG, McCutcheon MJ, Hasegawa A. Medial groove width during /s/ sound production. Biocommunication Research Reports, Department of Biocommunication, University of Alabama at Birmingham, USA, 1976.

Wood S. An EPG study of stuttering. Speech Research Laboratory Work in Progress, University of Reading 1993; 7: 107–34.

Wood S. An electropalatographic analysis of stutterers' speech. European Journal of Disorders of Communication 1995; 30: 226–36.

Wright S, Kerswill P. Electropalatography in the study of connected speech processes. Clinical Linguistics and Phonetics 1989; 3: 49–57.

Yamashita Y, Michi K. Misarticulation caused by abnormal lingual-palatal contact in patients with cleft palate with adequate velopharyngeal function. Cleft Palate-Craniofacial Journal 1991; 28: 360–66.

Yamashita Y, Michi K, Imai S, Suzuki N, Yoshida H. Electropalatographic investigation of abnormal lingual-palatal contact patterns in cleft palate patients. Clinical Linguistics and Phonetics 1992; 6: 201–17.

Chapter 7
Imaging Techniques

MARTIN J. BALL AND BERTHOLD GRÖNE

Introduction

The aim of this chapter is to examine a set of different techniques all attempting to image the movement of the organs of speech with the minimum of invasive interruption to normal articulation. Traditionally, imaging in phonetics has involved a variety of X-ray techniques, and this approach is described in some detail in the first part of the chapter. More recently, researchers have favoured methods that do not involve the inherent dangers of X-radiography, and newer developments covered in later parts of the chapter include electromagnetic articulography, ultrasound and magnetic resonance imaging. (Stroboscopic endoscopy, although invasive, might also be included under a general heading of imaging techniques. This approach is not covered in this chapter, but is dealt with in Chapter 5.)

X-ray Techniques

Introduction

Unlike many of the other techniques described in this book, X-ray-related investigations will not normally be readily available to the speech scientist or speech pathologist. There are, of course, straightforward reasons for this: in the wrong hands X-rays can be extremely dangerous; considerable training is necessary to learn how to operate the equipment, which, in turn, is itself very complex and expensive. Therefore, anyone wishing to use an X-ray technique will probably only be able to do so indirectly – through the co-operation of the X-ray department of a hospital or similar research institution. This is not always an easy arrangement to make of course, although permission to use radiography with subjects suffering from a speech disorder is more readily given than to phoneticians pursuing purely theoretical problems.

The purpose of this section of the chapter, therefore, is not to show the reader how to undertake an X-ray study personally, but rather to discuss the various X-ray techniques that are available and to help the reader decide which of these techniques would be most useful for any particular problem. It should also be noted at this stage that in the field of speech pathology, the major use of X-ray techniques is as an assessment and diagnostic tool, rather than as an aid to remediation.

X-rays and their properties

X-rays were discovered in 1895 by Professor W.K. Röntgen, and for this reason they are sometimes referred to as Röntgen-rays. X-rays are in principle similar to rays of light or heat and radio waves, they are all classed as belonging to the electromagnetic spectrum (Van der Plaats, 1969). The difference between the various rays in the spectrum is found in differences of frequency (the number of vibrations per second), although this can also be expressed as differences in the length of the wave — wavelengths being measured in divisions of a metre. For example, the wavelength of a radio transmission may be about 1 km, whereas visible light lies within a range of 760–400 nm (100 nm = 0.001 mm), and X-rays have wavelengths below 0.5 nm (Ridgway and Thumm, 1968; Van der Plaats, 1969), although 0.1 nm is often considered the upper limit for X-rays in medical usage.

X-rays are produced when electrons strike any solid body, and special *electron tubes* are used to achieve this. Design of the tubes differs according to whether a diagnostic or therapeutic (i.e. radiation therapy) function is required. The tube voltage will further decide whether the resultant rays will have a short wavelength, high X-ray energy and great penetration power (the so-called *hard X-rays*), or a longer wavelength, less X-ray energy and smaller penetration power (*soft X-rays*).

The major properties of X-rays of interest to the speech pathologist can be listed as follows (see Ridgway and Thumm, 1968; Van der Plaats, 1969). First, X-rays are able to penetrate materials that would absorb and reflect visible light. This is, of course, their most useful property, and is reinforced by the fact that absorption does take place to some extent. This absorption (and in fact the scattering of the X-ray beam) is differential, by which it is meant that while all material is susceptible to penetration by X-rays, usually the more dense the material, the greater will be the absorption of the X-rays by that material. In this way it is possible to gauge density from X-rays films. A third important property showing the usefulness of X-rays is the fact that they travel in straight lines and are not easily refracted or reflected.

It is often necessary to have permanent records of X-ray information, and the following two properties are of importance here: X-rays affect photographic film in a similar way to visible light; and X-rays produce fluorescence (visible radiation) in certain materials. These aspects are further discussed below.

X-rays also have the property of producing ionization in gases and this feature can be used to measure the amounts of radiation. Radiation meters are, of course, important in ensuring that patients do not receive too great a degree of exposure to X-radiation. This leads to the last property of X-rays: they are able to damage or kill living cells. In radiation therapy this is, of course, a benefit, but in diagnostic work as in speech pathology, this is a danger to be avoided and is the reason why access to X-ray equipment is so strictly vetted.

Although the general principles discussed above are common to all X-ray techniques, there are several different ways in which studies have been undertaken in the field of speech research, and it is the purpose of this section to outline the most important of these different techniques.

Perhaps the major choice facing the speech scientist in terms of X-ray techniques is that between still or cine film. (The distinction between direct and indirect radiography to be discussed below is to be found whether still or cine apparatus is used.) In terms of speech research, as speech is a serial activity it has always been considered more appropriate to use X-ray cinematography (see Bladon and Nolan, 1977), although previous researchers have used still photography, often due to the dictates of circumstance; though it does have a value when non-dynamic aspects of the speech mechanism are under consideration. Taking X-ray cinematography as a general term covering all methods of moving X-ray film, we can follow Ridgway and Thumm (1968) in their first major division between direct and indirect methods:

1.   **Direct**. This area is also termed *radiography*. It is direct in the sense that the X-rays are recorded directly on to a photographic film or plate. For recording dynamic events *serial radiography* may be used. This involves the taking of a series of radiographs of the area concerned. Serial radiography can be as fast as 12 exposures per second. If the radiographs are reproduced on cinefilm the technique is termed *cineradiography*.

2.   **Indirect**. This area is generally termed *fluorography*, because it involves the photography of a fluoroscopic screen. X-radiation falls on to the screen where it is converted into light energy. This light energy is proportional to the rate of absorption of the X-rays, so the various densities shown by the X-ray image, and the movements of the image in time are all reproduced on the screen. Still, serial and cine film may be used to record the screen of course, but the main drawback of fluorography is the low intensity of the image on the screen. This can be overcome by the use of an *image intensifier*. The most common type of image intensifier is a vacuum tube which

converts the light image from the fluoroscopic screen into an electron image. The electrons are accelerated and reconverted into a smaller, brighter light image (see Figure 7.1). Using an image intensifier the resultant image may be recorded on to cine film, or more popularly these days, videotape. As Bladon and Nolan (1977) point out, video has the added advantages of live monitoring, instant playback and low X-ray dosage compared with other methods.

There are many specialist techniques using X-rays, and brief mention may be made of those relevant to speech science.

1. **Panoramic Radiography**. This is often used for dental purposes as it gives a complete picture of the upper and lower jaw in one picture, by employing a special X-ray tube, which produces a wide beam.

2. **Kymography**. A technique used to show broad movements of internal organs (such as the heart). The method is explained more fully in Van der Plaats (1969: p. 112), but normally will not give quite the amount of detail required by the speech scientist.

3. **Tomography (or Laminography, Planigraphy or Stratigraphy)**. This technique provides a cross-section of structures instead of a view of all planes. The X-ray source and the film are rotated in an arc in relation to the subject, and only the anatomic plane that has maintained the same distance from the source and the film will remain in focus. This method has been used extensively in speech research (particularly in larynx studies) but has the drawbacks of requiring a lot of film and a relatively high radiation dose. However, more recently, *computerized tomography* has overcome these drawbacks to some extent.

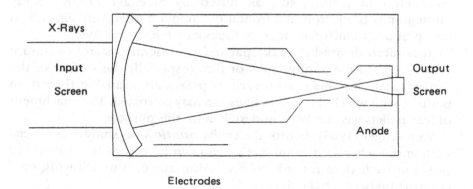

Figure 7.1. The image intensifier.

4.   **Xeroradiography**. This method uses a special plate, which avoids the necessity of using a photographic chemical plate. Pictures may be obtained immediately, and the plate used again. This is particularly useful when ongoing monitoring of pictures is needed, although it does usually require a high radiation dosage. (Polaroid cameras are of course another way of accomplishing speed in obtaining pictures.) As Dicenta and Oliveras (1976) commented, xeroradiography is especially good at showing the relative densities of tissues.

5.   **Tracking and X-ray microbeams**. Techniques under this heading involve the tracking via X-ray film of objects attached to the vocal organs of the subject. From this information the movements of the organs of speech may be followed. Tracking has been combined with the use of X-ray microbeams, which is a comparatively recent development involving computer-controlled low dosages of X-radiation. Perhaps the best descriptions of this are provided by Kiritani, Itoh and Fujimura (1975) and Kiritani (1986). The system involves tracking tongue movements by following small lead pellets affixed to its surface. The X-ray microbeams involved ensure a very low dosage of radiation. This technique has already been used in speech pathology, and this work will be discussed below.

It must be remembered that this section has only dealt with techniques likely to be of use to speech pathology and the speech sciences in general. Other techniques exist outside the scope of this chapter.

Radiographic methods in phonetics

Most X-ray studies conducted into speech have concentrated on the supra-glottal vocal tract. It is also the case that most studies have been conducted in profile, for, as noted by Strenger (1968), X-ray photographs taken from the frontal position are often very difficult to interpret due to the dense mass of the bone of the lower jaw.

It is often desired to make particular structures stand out more clearly in the final photographs or film (especially the surface of the tongue), and for this reason various pastes are available (based on barium) with which the area in question may be coated. The attachment of lead pellets has also been undertaken for this purpose.

As Strenger (1968) reports, the *cephalostatic* X-ray study uses special equipment whereby the subject's head can be placed in an identical position each time recordings are being made; thus allowing easy comparison between the developed films.

A series of anatomical reference points, and lines derived from these (see Figure 7.2) are used where precise measurements are required;

these measurements should be made from a single frame in the case of cine or video films. Strenger (1968) notes four areas where reasonably precise measurements may be obtained: (1) the angle between the jaws; (2) the movement of the upper and lower lips on the horizontal axis; (3) the gap between the surfaces of the incisors; and (4) the position and type of stricture between the tongue and the palate. Moll (1965) also notes that measurements can be made of velar height, tongue pharynx distance and vocal fold opening; and Painter (1979) mentions larynx height. A review of radiographic studies in the phonetics of normal speech is given in MacMillan and Keleman (1952) and Ball (1984).

X-rays in speech pathology

Some of the more important and more recent research in the various areas of speech pathology that have used X-ray techniques will be reviewed in this section. Those areas of research which have used X-rays

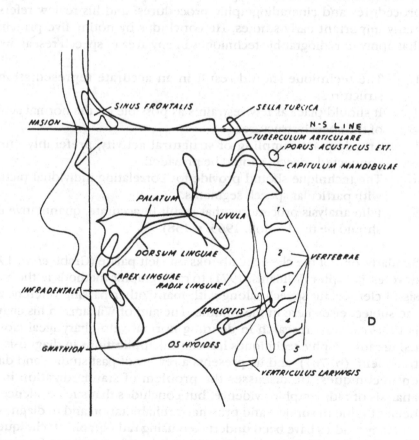

Figure 7.2. A view of the reference points and lines necessary for a phonetic analysis of articulation. (Source: Malmberg, 1968.)

a great deal are reviewed before those that have used them less although this does not necessarily imply that the techniques are best suited to any particular area.

Cranio-facial disorders

The term *cranio-facial disorder* is used here to cover the conditions *cleft palate* and *velopharyngeal insufficiency/inadequacy*. It is perhaps not surprising that these areas of speech pathology have seen the greatest use of X-rays in research due to the fact that treatment often involves medical attention, which in turn will usually necessitate the taking of X-rays. This section will review some of the studies undertaken with these disorders.

Moll (1965), in a contribution to the 1963 conference on cleft palate, discusses the use of radiographic techniques in speech research with special emphasis on its role in cleft palate research. He divides X-ray techniques into three main types: still X-ray procedures, laminographic procedures and cineradiographic procedures; and his review refers to many important early studies. He concludes by noting five principles that apply to radiographic techniques in any area of speech research:

1.   The technique should result in an accurate representation of structures.
2.   It should place as few restraints as possible on the normal activity of the speech structures.
3.   An adequate sampling of structural activity, preferably during connected speech, should be provided.
4.   The technique should provide for correlating individual pictures with particular speech segments.
5.   Film analysis procedures that result in accurate, quantitative data should be used. (Moll, 1965: p.138)

Similarly, one of the classic textbooks on cleft palate (Grabb *et al*, 1971) devotes a chapter (Williams, 1971) to radiographic methods in the analysis of cleft palate speech, along with many other passing references to the subject elsewhere in the volume. The aim of Williams in his chapter is to 'show how research in defining normal velo-pharyngeal closure using radiographic techniques has clinical applications in diagnosis and treatment' (p. 767), and he presents a review of past studies and different techniques. He discusses the problem of standardization in the analysis of radiographic evidence, but concludes that such evidence has been of value in surgical and prosthetic rehabilitation and in diagnosis.

Many studies have been undertaken using radiographic techniques in the field of cranio-facial disorders and, of course, it will not be possible to review all of them. However, a study of the literature reveals various areas of specific interest. First, there is the use of X-ray techniques as a straightforward description of a particular disorder, or as a diagnostic tool. An example of the former is found in Shprintzen, Croft, Berkman and Rakoff (1980) who used videofluoroscopy and endoscopy to study patients suffering from the facio-auriculo-vertebral malformation complex. They discovered that while over half of the patients suffered from velopharyngeal insufficiency, only two out of the 12 actually had cleft palate.

In terms of a diagnostic study, Bowman and Shanks (1978) used cephalometry to study a group of patients with suspected velopharyngeal insufficiency. Looking at radiographs of the /i/ and /s/ phonemes they concluded that the former gave a better indication of the presence of insufficiency.

Certain recent studies have been concerned with comparing perceived aspects of cleft palate speech (such as nasalization) with data from X-ray studies of speech movements. For example, Karnell *et al* (1985) used cinefluorography to examine this area, whereas Hardin *et al* (1986) found that lateral X-rays taken on /s/ did not consistently match the other criteria (including perceptual) that were used to group subjects into those showing minimal but consistent nasalization. It seems, therefore, that touch closure or minimal velopharyngeal opening is not always found with speakers exhibiting excessive nasal resonance, or such minimal opening is highly variable and not always clearly seen in X-ray studies.

A second group of studies is concerned with comparisons between disordered subjects and normals. This is usually in terms of the description of a particular physiological feature, for example Glaser, Skolnick, McWilliams and Shprintzen (1979) compared the dynamics of Passavant's ridge in normal subjects and those with velopharyngeal insufficiency using videofluoroscopy; whereas Zwitman, Gyepes and Ward (1976) examined velar and lateral wall movements.

A third important area is the assessment of subjects post-operatively. Kuehn and Van Demark (1978) assessed velopharyngeal competency following a Teflon pharyngoplasty. Pre- and post-operative X-ray information suggested considerable improvement in competency during the first 3 months following the operation. Lewis and Pashayan (1980) examined the effects of pharyngeal flap surgery on 20 patients and found that lateral pharyngeal wall movement had not improved in these cases. Finally, in a slightly different area, Enany (1981) examined the effects of primary osteoplasty in unilateral cleft lip and palate subjects.

The fourth area which has attracted much work is that of longitudinal studies of child development. The use of metal implants trackable by X-rays is often found to provide detailed information on growth patterns in subjects suffering from a variety of cranio-facial disorders. However, these studies rarely include direct reference to speech disorders.

Lastly, there are those studies concerned with evaluating different investigative techniques in the context of cranio-facial disorders. For example, Williams and Eisenbach (1981) compare still X-radiography with cinefluorography in a study of velopharyngeal insufficiency. The authors conclude that 'one is apt to misdiagnose the presence or absence of velopharyngeal insufficiency on the order of 30% of the time when relying on the lateral still X-ray technique alone' (p. 45). This is attributed to the limited speech sample that can be used in still filming as opposed to cine.

Zwitman *et al* (1976) compared cineradiography with endoscopy. In this particular instance the radiographic technique was used to assess the accuracy of endoscopy in the examination of velar and lateral wall movement. The authors found that cineradiography confirmed endoscopic observation in a larger percentage of patients.

Shelton and Trier (1976) discuss the use of cinefluorography in the measurement of velopharyngeal closure, and conclude that measures in addition to fluorography are needed, and a comparison of various measure types is provided. Later, Zimmerman *et al* (1987) compared cineradiography and photodetection techniques for assessing velopharyngeal function.

We can also note a study by Spolyar *et al* (1993) where the authors describe a procedure for correcting image parallax errors that can detract from the reliability of studies using cephalometric analyses of cleft palate speakers.

Laryngeal disorders

This section will review some of the work done on disorders of the larynx resulting in voice disorders, including such areas as vocal fold tension, laryngeal disease and laryngectomy.

From quite early on the advantages of X-ray techniques in the study of laryngeal disorders have been recognized. In one of the major textbooks on voice (Luchsinger and Arnold, 1965), a whole section is included on the use of radiographic methods in voice analysis. The section reviews various suitable techniques (e.g. kymography, fluoroscopy, tomography and cineradiography), and references to many of the pioneering studies in the application of X-ray techniques to voice may be found, particularly the use of tomography. Many of these studies were concerned with normal voice characteristics, but Van den Berg (1955) is mentioned for his cineradiographic study of the production of oesophageal pseudovoice.

Another study concerned with oesophageal voice was conducted by De Santis *et al* (1979). They noted that sometimes the attempt to introduce oesophageal voice to laryngectomy patients fails, and state that other research has shown the importance of the cervical portion of the oesophagus in the production of oesophageal voice. Their investigation concerns the advantages and disadvantages of various radiographic techniques in the study of this area.

Ward *et al* (1979) compare various techniques in the study of laryngeal disease. Computerized tomography appeared to the authors to be the clearest technique for showing tumours, cystic lesions and traumatic lesions. There were reduced radiation doses, and the technique was cheaper to use, also eliminating the need for conventional tomography or laryngography. (See also Pahn, 1981, for an X-ray diagnosis method for superior laryngeal nerve palsy.)

Pruszewicz, Obrebowski and Gradzki (1976) used both tomography and lateral radiography to examine the larynxes of several groups of patients undergoing different drug treatments. Voice quality in the patients had been affected, with a generally lowered pitch, smaller pitch range, shortened phonation time and a tendency to tire easily. The study showed an increase of calcification of the larynx cartilages and an asymmetry of the vocal folds and related structures.

Ardran and Kemp (1967) used tomography and radiography in a study of the function of the larynx following the King-Kelly operation involving the lateral fixation of a vocal cord in patients suffering from bilateral vocal cord palsy. The X-ray pictures clearly show pre- and postoperative conditions, and are compared with previous work undertaken by the same authors on normal vocal cord activity.

These studies are representative of the sort of work done in the general area of laryngeal disorders, but more recently a new technique based on xeroradiography has been developed, and this has been applied to many types of voice disorder (Berry *et al.*, 1982a; MacCurtain, 1981). The full name of this new development is *Xeroradiography-Electro-Laryngography* (XEL), and it encompasses a joint use of xeroradiography with the electrolaryngograph (see Chapter 5). This produces simultaneous information on soft tissue changes in the vocal tract in terms of a visual display of the Lx and Fx waves on the electrolaryngograph, and the xeroradiographic picture. One of the advantages claimed for the technique is that in most cases the need for direct laryngography is eliminated.

This particular technique has been developed to be used easily in the clinic, and for this purpose the reading of the xeroradiograms is facilitated through the drawing up of a set of 17 voice quality parameters, easily located on the xeroradiograph (see Figure 7.3). This technique is concerned with both diagnosis and treatment, although it should be noted that the xeroradiographic aspect is mostly helpful for diagnosis.

A representative study using XEL is found in Ranford (1982). Evidence is presented from XEL to show the nature of a voice disorder in a patient who had previously been undiagnosed. The xeroradiograms seemed to show a loss of smoothness in the vocal fold vibration and some tilting of the laryngeal assembly in phonation due to an imbalance

1. vocal folds
2. laryngeal airway
3. ventricular folds
4. laryngopharynx
5. vestibule of the larynx
6. epiglottis
7. vallecula
8. oropharynx

9. hyoid bone
10. hypopharynx
11. thyroid cartilage
12. length of vocal tract
13. cricothyroid vizor
14. nasopharynx
15. retropharyngeal soft tissue
16. tongue gesture

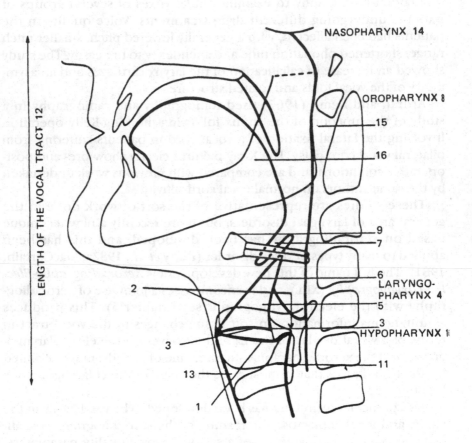

Figure 7.3. Anatomical parameters used in XEL listed in order of frequency of use in analysing voice disorders. (Source: Reprinted with permission from Berry *et al*, 1982a, b. Courtesy of F. MacCurtain.)

of muscle activity. (See also Berry *et al*, 1982a, b for investigations of normal and disordered voice.)

The development of XEL, bringing together two of the techniques described in this book, is a very interesting step forward for speech pathologists, for it brings a very sophisticated diagnostic ability within the reach of the clinic. Examples of the clarity obtained in xeroradiograms are shown in Figure 7.4a and 7.4b, which illustrate the supraglottal vocal organs at rest, and producing the vowel [i] respectively.

Stuttering

A series of publications will be examined which show the value that X-ray techniques could have in the area of stuttering. Zimmerman (1980a, b, c) used high-speed cinefluorography to examine articulation in stutterers. In the first of the three studies, he examined the speech of six stutterers in comparison with seven normal speakers. The passages that were recorded from all the speakers on this occasion contained only speech

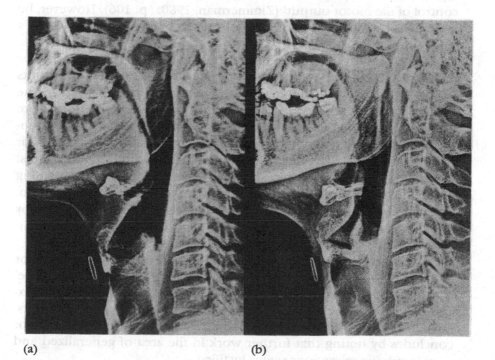

(a)   (b)

Figure 7.4a. Xeroradiograph taken at rest. (Courtesy Evelyn Abberton and Frances MacCurtain.)

Figure 7.4b. Xeroradiograph taken of the vowel [i]. (Courtesy Evelyn Abberton and Frances MacCurtain.)

that was perceptually fluent. The aim was to describe the movement of the articulators in terms of space and time, and to see what differences there were, if any, between stutterers and normals during what appeared to be fluent speech. The second investigation used the same technique to look at a group of stutterers, comparing their fluent and non-fluent utterances. The third study sought to combine information gained from the previous two to propose a model of disfluency.

The results obtained in the first study suggested that stutterers and normal speakers differ in how speech production is organized even in speech that appears fluent perceptually. These differences manifested themselves in consistently longer durations between movement onsets, achievements of peak velocity, and voice onsets for the stutterers in comparison with the normals. Zimmerman (1980a) also reported that the stutterers showed 'longer steady state positioning for the lip and jaw during vowel production and a greater asynchrony between lip and jaw movement' (p.95). The stutterers' utterances were also of longer duration than the normals. Zimmerman feels that an explanation for these findings could be found in terms of compensatory behaviour. He notes that 'reducing the amount of movement (displacement) and/or increasing the duration of a production might allow the stutterer to gain better control of the motor output' (Zimmerman, 1980a: p. 106). However, he concludes by warning about generalizations being made from such a small subject population.

The second investigation utilized the same X-ray technique on four male stutterers in comparison with one female non-stutterer. The results of this study showed that articulator relationships occurred in the speech of stutterers (both in fluent and disfluent utterances) that were not usually found in normal speakers, and that 'a systematic repositioning [of articulators] occurs preceding the release from oscillatory or tonic (posturing) behaviors' (p. 117). Zimmerman notes that the most frequent of these relationships involved lowering of the jaw, reshaping of the tongue towards the rest position, and lowering of the lower lip. Zimmerman suggests that some of these effects can be accounted for by reflex interactions among the muscles of articulation: 'imbalances in afferent-efferent interactions among brainstem structures' (p. 119).

The author feels that these conclusions have direct implications for therapy, 'therapy might be geared to putting the system back in balance' (p. 119), and he quotes as an example, 'instead of dealing with relaxation of the lip muscles when they are involved in oscillatory behaviors, jaw closers might advantageously be relaxed' (p. 119). The author concludes by noting that further work in the area of generalized and muscle specific relaxations seems justified.

Zimmerman (1980c) proposes a model of stuttering as a disorder of movement, drawing on information from the first two studies. He suggests that the movement of articulators in time and space (and the interactions between articulators) operate within a permissible range of variability. When this range is exceeded for whatever reason, the articulatory system is thrown out of balance, resulting in oscillatory behaviour or static positioning (stuttering and blocking). Further research is suggested, as only the movement patterns of the upper articulators have been studied.

Zimmerman's work has shown how X-ray techniques can add much to our knowledge of articulatory behaviour in stuttering and in the theoretical consideration of this problem. One other study can be briefly mentioned here: Fujita (1966) who, as part of an examination into the role of phonation in stuttering, took posterior-anterior X-rays of one Japanese stutterer. He reported irregular or inconsistent opening and closing of the pharyngolaryngeal cavity and asymmetric tight closure of the pharyngeal cavity. Again, there are obvious drawbacks in this study from the small subject population.

Aphasia, apraxia, dysarthria

Some X-ray studies have been undertaken in this area of speech pathology, though it has not proved as popular a technique as in the field of cranio-facial disorders for instance.

In the case of dysarthria, Kent and Netsell (1975) conducted cineradiographic and spectrographic investigations into the speech of an ataxic dysarthric. They found abnormalities in speaking rate, stress patterns, articulatory placements, velocities of articulator movements and fundamental frequency contours; and they conclude, 'perhaps . . . ataxic dysarthria is characterized by a generalized hypotonia . . .' (p. 129), this hypotonia resulting in the slowness of movement that was observed.

Hirose, Kiritani, Ushijima and Sawashima (1978) used the X-ray microbeam system to analyse abnormal articulatory movements in two dysarthric patients: the first an ataxic dysarthric of cerebellar origin, the second a case of amyotrophic lateral sclerosis. Different patterns of articulator movement were recorded, with additional evidence provided by electromyography. The authors feel that this sort of study is a 'promising approach for elucidating the nature of central problems of speech production and for a differential diagnosis of various types of dysarthrias' (p. 96). The same technique is employed by Hirose et al (1981) in a study of dysarthric movements in patients with Parkinsonism.

An X-ray microbeam investigation was also employed in a study of apraxia (Itoh et al, 1980). The authors found that temporal organization among the articulators was disturbed, and also that the 'pattern and velocity of the articulator movements of the patient . . . were different from those of typical dysarthric patients' (p. 66).

In the field of aphasia, X-rays in the form of tomography have been used as a diagnostic tool to locate the position of lesions in the brain.

However, this use of X-rays is more properly described as medical than as part of speech pathology, and is therefore not within the scope of this chapter.

Articulation disorders

X-ray techniques have also been used in other areas of speech pathology, although to a lesser extent. Various studies have been undertaken in the area of articulation and articulation disorders. To understand better the role of proprioceptive feedback, Putnam and Ringel (1976) investigated articulation in subjects with temporarily induced oral-sensory deprivation, finding a loss of precision in lip, tongue and jaw movements. Kuehn and Tomblin (1977) looked at child speech in the specific area of /w/ - /r/ substitutions. Their findings suggested that while the subjects were 'possibly differentiating between /w/ and intended /r/, . . . the articulatory target configurations appeared to be nondiscriminatory' (p. 462), and that systematic lip, jaw and tongue differences were required successfully to discriminate the two sounds.

Also in the field of articulation, studies have been carried out on articulation problems involving dental and oral surgery. Zimmerman, Kelso and Lander (1980) and Shelton, Furr, Johnson and Arndt (1975) discussed two such cases.

Studies of articulation have also been a focus of X-ray microbeam studies in recent times. Westbury (1994) gives a good account of the Microbeam project at the University of Wisconsin, and the large-scale database of normal speech that was one of the aims of that work. Some of the normative data from this work is found, for example, in Adams *et al* (1993), and other studies cited in Westbury (1994). Westbury *et al* (1995) used microbeams to study tongue shape of /r/ in American speakers. This concluded that a variety of tongue shapes were used (rather than the simple dichotomy between retroflex and bunched), and this could clearly have implications for speech pathology where /r/ problems occur frequently in English-speaking subjects.

Clearly, if adequate funding is forthcoming to continue work like this, X-ray microbeam would be a valuable tool to investigate articulation disorders. Like other tracking systems (e.g. EMA described later in this chapter), X-ray microbeam studies provide traces of the movement of the set of pellets (affixed, for example, to the tongue) in relation to landmarks such as the palate and pharyngeal wall, during speech. Figure 7.5 shows the trace patterns of the four tongue pellets (T1–4), upper lip and lower lip pellets (UL, LL), mandibular molar pellet (MNm), and mandibular incisor pellet (MNi) for a subject (JW27) for a stretch of speech. The y-axis in the figure represents position with regard to maximillary occlusal plane, and the x-axis represents position with regard to central maxillary incisors.

Hearing impairment

X-ray studies have also been undertaken in the field of hearing problems. For example, Seaver, Andrews and Granata (1980) discussed velar positioning in hearing-impaired adults and concluded that the hypernasality found in the hearing impaired is of a different character to that found in cleft-palate patients. Lock and Seaver (1984) examined nasality and velopharyngeal function in hearing-impaired adults, and note that cineradiography showed that only two of their five subjects had velopharyngeal opening, despite perceived nasality in all the subjects. Still in the area of resonance, Subtelny *et al* (1989) used cineradiography to investigate aspects of deviant resonance in hearing-impaired subjects. They looked at oral-pharyngeal relationships in vowels between normal and hearing-impaired subjects, and concluded that the latter showed variability in tongue root retraction and tongue height.

Bergstrom (1978) discusses the differences between congenital and acquired deafness in cleft-palate patients.

Clinical applications

The above review has shown the versatility of radiographic techniques in

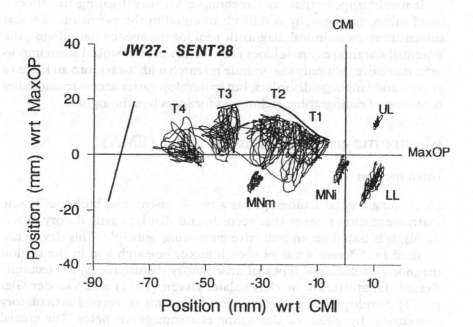

Figure 7.5. Mid-sagittal plane trajectories with both palate and pharyngeal outlines from X-ray microbeam data. (Courtesy John Westbury.)

speech pathology, both as a general research tool to aid our understanding of different disorders, but also as a method of diagnosis. In terms of its clinical applications, the diagnostic ability of each technique is of primary importance. X-ray techniques as they have been defined here play no direct role in treatment (radiotherapy is outside the scope of this chapter), though of course accurate diagnosis is in itself a pre-requisite to effective treatment.

As the review has shown, radiography can play an important role in the diagnosis of various cranio-facial disorders, voice disorders, dysarthrias and so on, and that different techniques are suitable for different areas. However, the major problem of accessibility remains. Comparatively few speech pathologists have ready access to these techniques, although the XEL project in Britain promises well for the assessment of laryngeal disorders.

Other problems remain in assessing the usefulness of radiography to the clinician. Returning to Moll's (1965) five principles, it might be argued that in many cases accurate film analysis is not made, and that the technique can become too invasive through the introduction of barium paste on the tongue, lead pellets or other marking devices, thereby going against Moll's principle of placing as few restraints as possible on normal speech activity. There are also, of course, the dangers from radiation to consider, even though recent developments do seem to have minimized these.

It would appear that, as a technique for investigating the speech mechanism, radiography is difficult to equal in the provision of visual information. As a clinical diagnostic tool for the speech pathologist, the potential advantages are seldom realised however. It would seem important, therefore, not only to continue research with X-rays into all kinds of speech and language disorders, but to develop easier access to and fuller provision of radiographic techniques for speech pathologists.

Electromagnetic Articulography (EMA)

Introduction

Electromagnetic articulography is a non-invasive, and biologically safe instrumentation system that records and displays articulatory movements. It is based on an inductive measuring principle. This device can be used in different areas of speech motor research and in the clinical diagnosis of different types of articulatory disturbances, for example dysarthria, stuttering or cleft palate. Hixon (1971) and Van der Giet (1977) developed early articulograph-systems to record articulatory movements by means of alternating electromagnetic fields. The crucial problem with these devices was the lack of any correcting mechanism for misalignment between the transmitter coils and the receiver coils, which could lead to measurement errors. At present, there are three different commercially available systems that differ in technical details. The Carstens Electromagnetic Articulograph AG 100 (Schönle *et al*, 1987; Tuller *et al*, 1990), the Electromagnetic Midsagittal Articulometer EMMA (Perkell *et al*, 1992), and the Movetrack from Sweden (Branderud, 1985), which has, in contrast to the others, no automatic tilt correction.

Measuring principle

A transmitter coil generates an alternating magnetic field; the strength of the field decreases with the distance from the transmitter. A receiving coil positioned with its axis in parallel to the transmitter induces an alternating low voltage, which changes with the distance of the receiver from the transmitter. By using two transmitter coils with different frequencies the distance between the receiver and the transmitter can be calculated from the strength of the voltages induced in the receiver. But when the detector is tilted, distances appear to be too large, and the position of the detector cannot be determined. Therefore, a third signal from a third transmitter has been added, which allows an iterative correction of the tilt angle. The three signals from the transmitters can be interpreted as radii of three circles around the transmitters. If the receiver coil is tilted, these three circles do not intersect at one point as all three radii are too great. In a step-by-step algorithm the radii are then reduced by the same factor until intersection occurs at a single point. This point represents the actual coil position.

Technical realization

The technical realization of the three articulograph systems differs in details. Different computer systems or different software for data analysis are used. Therefore full details of the extended calibrating procedures (e.g. Hoole, 1993), or of reference systems (Schönle, 1988) are excluded from this chapter. This description is based on the Schönle-articulograph, a non-commercial device for clinical research, that is close to Carstens AG 100, but provides some extra features for data recording (e.g. A/D-converter) and analysis (SIEMA-software package).The transmitter coils are aligned in parallel and perpendicular to the mid-sagittal plane on a light-weight helmet, worn around a speaker's head. The positions of the coils are in front of the forehead, the mandible, and the neck. In this manner, the speaker's head is just inside the alternating electromagnetic field. Up to five detector coils can be fixed on the articulators for simultaneous recording (about 800 Hz), e.g. the upper and lower lips, the mandible, the tongue tip and the tongue dorsum. The speech signal is also recorded as an acoustical reference (about 16 kHz). Detector coils, which are 2–4 mm in size, are fixed with surgical glue (Hystoacryl). From these coils a very small wire, about 0.4 mm in diameter, leads out of the corner of the mouth (for coils that are fixed on the tongue surface) to the pre-amplifier of the recording unit of the device. The hardware requirements are an 80386 IBM-compatible Personal Computer with 80387 math-coprocessor (or an 80486 PC) and a DAP AD/DA-converter (not in AG 100). For auditory control of the displayed data, a second low cost D/A-converter is used to replay the recorded utterances acoustically.

EMA-data

Electromagnetic articulography provides a two-dimensional mid-sagittal display of articulatory movements. As a constant reference structure, the shape of the palate can be recorded. Therefore, the investigator fixes one receiver coil on top of his forefinger and moves it along the palate. The recorded mid-sagittal outline of the palate can be displayed in the online mode and for offline analysis of the data (see Figure 7.6). As an example of data recording and analysis, Figures 7.7 and 7.8 demonstrate the functional bicompartmentalization of the tongue, its selective innervation in a normal speaker and the loss of selective innervability in a patient with spastic dysathria during the production of the utterance [kata] in the context 'ich habe Kater gehört' (literally: 'I have heard cat'). Figure 7.7a shows the movement of the tongue blade in the y-direction (solid line) together with the velocity in this direction (dashed line); Figure 7.7b shows the movement of the tongue tip correspondingly. Comparison of Figures 7.7a and 7.7b indicates a reciprocal behaviour of the tongue blade and tip during [k] versus [t] production. While the blade reaches its highest position during [k] the tip is lowered, and subsequently the tip moves up for [t] while the blade reaches its lowest point. The same reciprocal behaviour can be seen with their respective velocities. At point 1 velocity is at the maximum value for the blade and at a relative minimum for the tip, while at point 3 the tongue tip peaks in its maximum velocity and the blade is at its minimum. In other words, during the [kata]-production we find a distinct two-component activity pattern of the tongue: tongue blade raising/tongue tip lowering versus tongue blade lowering/tongue tip raising. This flip-flop movement pattern is grossly disturbed in the dysarthric speaker (Figure 7.8). Tongue tip and tongue dorsum work as one unit without selective innervation.

Conclusions

As the example shows, EMA can be a useful tool in investigating articulatory movements in both normal and dysarthric speech. The accuracy within the major working space is satisfactory. Honda and Kaburagi (1993) made a comparison of EMA and ultrasonic measurement of tongue movements under realistic conditions. Their results demonstrated that the measured positions of both systems differed only by 0.43 mm, if the coils were fixed in optimal positions. The resolution in time is extremely high. This allows a precise calculation of velocity and acceleration, and an accurate measurement of the temporal structure of movement co-ordination in coarticulatory tasks of different articulators.

Software is used for sophisticated data analysis. Further, the online mode provides the opportunity for biofeedback training with patients. However, there are still some unresolved problems. EMA provides only a two-dimensional diagram, omitting lateral movements, but in dysarthric speech lateral movements are often of great interest, because they can

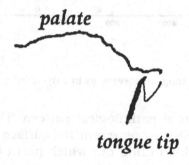

Figure 7.6. EMA data for tongue tip movements compared with mid-sagittal outline of the palate.

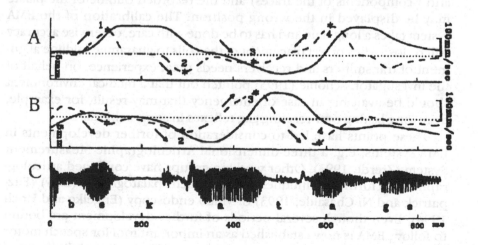

Figure 7.7. EMA data for tongue movements in a normal speaker.

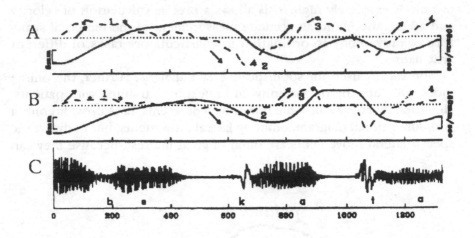

Figure 7.8. EMA data for tongue movements in a dysarthric speaker.

demonstrate the crucial pathological pattern. The measurement of single points is not able to represent the surface of the tongue. The investigator is not able to find out which part of the tongue makes palatal contact, for example in oral stop-consonants. This may lead to palatal contact being missed because the coil has been placed on different tongue position than that used in the contact.

Uncontrolled movements of the helmet may cause a misalignment of the coordinate system. The orientation of the movement changes (the x- and y-components of the traces) and the recorded outline of the palate may be displayed in the wrong position. The calibration of the EMA system takes a long time and has to be done with care, otherwise accuracy will be lost. The correct placement of the coils to guarantee midline alignment of transmitters and receivers needs great experience, on behalf of the investigator. Schönle (1993) pointed out that a medical environment should be available in case of emergency that may result, for example, from long-lasting over-reacting gag reflexes in some subjects.

These points have led to consideration of further developments in EMA systems, e.g. a three-dimensional Articulographic Measurement System (Zierdt, 1993). Other working groups have combined articulography with further techniques such as electropalatography (EPG) (Fitzpatrick and Ní Chasaide, 1993) or video endoscopy (Engelke and Hoch 1994). Even though several periods of further development are bound to follow, EMA is now established as an important tool for speech motor research, and is going to be more widely available in clinical diagnosis of articulatory disturbances.

Ultrasonic Measurements of Articulatory Movements

Introduction

Ultrasonic measurements provide kinematic information about the tongue or the larynx during speech production. Ultrasound techniques are non-invasive and do not cause any ionization hazard in the patient. They use the reflection of ultrasonic sound beams at the marginal surface of different acoustic resistances, such as the tongue-air boundary within the oral cavity.

Measuring principle and technical realization

The measuring principle is based on analysing the resulting echo of a given pulse ((im)pulse-echo-method). This may be illustrated by the following example with 'normal' sound. A sound moves through the air with a velocity of 331 metres per second, e.g. the crack of a gun shot. If the sound reaches a place with a different acoustic resistance, for example a rock, the sound wave will be partly reflected back to the signal source.

This typical echo is characterized by two important attributes.

1.   The running time from sending the pulse to receiving the echo is determined by the equation:

$$2s = v \cdot t$$

where s represents the distance from the source of the sound to the reflecting marginal surface, v the velocity of sound spread, and t is the running time.

2.   The intensity of the echo depends on the size of the resistance differences of two different tissues. A great difference causes an intense echo, a small difference a less intense echo. The acoustic resistance r is a product of the density of the tissue d and the sound velocity v:

$$r = d \cdot v$$

There is an echo if the sound beam passes tissues with different acoustic resistance and there is no echo within a homogeneous medium, such as water or air. In a biological system the sound will be reflected at the boundary of soft parts with air or with bone, because of the different acoustic resistance. One example is the tongue-air boundary inside the oral cavity.

For medical diagnosis audible sound cannot be used, because it does not possess a sufficient resolution (about 0.75 m). For this reason a sound with higher frequencies is used (2–20 Mhz). This non-audible sound is named ultrasound. Using a frequency of 2.5 MHz, the spatial resolution is about 0.6 mm within the mean direction of the sound beam. The lateral resolution at the same frequency is only about 4 mm. The ultrasound is generated by a piezoelectrical crystal, which effects high-frequency vibrations: the ultrasound.

When striking the transducer, reflected beams cause deformations of the crystal, which result in a change of voltage. The voltage can be displayed on the monitor of an oscillograph monitor or on a computer screen. The amplitude of the displayed voltage rises corresponding to the intensity of the echo. This property of the crystal allows the use of the same crystal as a sound source and as a receiver. The transducer generates at first a short ultrasonic pulse of about two oscillations. Then it is switched into receiver mode to register the reflected sound. A working system is in receiving mode 99.7% of the time, and only about 0.3% of the time is used to send ultrasonic waveforms.

The time delay between the burst emission and the reception of the echo is measured. Knowing the speed of sound and the acoustic resistance of the sound-conducting material, e.g. the tongue, it is possible to calculate the distance from the sound source to the marginal surface of different acoustic resistances. This surface may represent the surface contour of the tongue or any other anatomical structures. If the tongue is moved, for example while speaking, the pulse-echo time delay alters. From examining different time delays, different tongue positions can be calculated. At each millisecond interval, a measurement corresponding to the distance between the transducer and the tongue dorsum is obtained (Keller and Ostry, 1983).

The necessary equipment for an ultrasonic measuring device consists of an ultrasound generator, an amplifier, an A/D-converter, and an oscillograph/computer. The transducer is placed in a vertical position beneath the chin along the inferior midline of the mandible, although a different placement is used for recording vocal fold vibrations. For this purpose, Kaneko et al (1981) placed the transducer on the thyroid lamina.

Ultrasonic data

Basically we have to distinguish two different ultrasound display methods. The first is the 'A-scan mode' or 'amplitude modulating mode'. The horizontal axis of display represents the running time of the echo, that means the distance from the reflecting marginal surface to the transducer. The intensity of the echo is displayed by proportional modulating of the amplitude in a vertical direction.

A schematic display of the A-scan is given in Figure 7.9.

Kaneko *et al* (1981), for example, used the A-scan mode to investigate the vibration echo from the margin of the vocal fold during phonation. They were able to register and analyse vocal cord activity period by period directly.

The second mode is the 'B-scan' or 'brightness-scan'. In contrast to the A-scan mode, the intensity of the echo is represented by the brightness of a corresponding light spot on the monitor. A higher echo intensity evokes a brighter light spot, and a less intense echo is represented by a less bright spot. There are brightness scales of 8, 16, or more grades for the different sound intensities. A schematic illustration of the B-scan is given in Figure 7.10.

Kaneko and his co-workers (1981) gave examples of different B-scan investigations of the larynx, representing the vocal folds together with a sketch of anatomical structures, and their pathological deformation, e.g. by tumour. Furthermore, this work group provided kinematic data of the larynx for different vowels and different voice characteristics.

A central goal of applying ultrasonic methods in clinical phonetics is the investigation of articulatory movements of the tongue. Watkin and

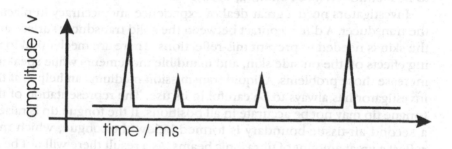

Figure 7.9. A-scan display (ultrasound).

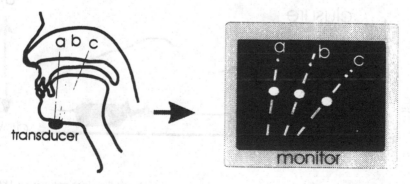

Figure 7.10. B-scan display (ultrasound).

Zagzebski began this work in 1973. Keller and Ostry (1983) recorded the kinematic signal of tongue movements while speaking, and worked out further analysis through the use of computer software. The configuration of the midline contour of the tongue for different articulatory gestures is displayed as a chain of bright light spots on the monitor.

Also, the main direction of the tongue movement can be investigated in a time-related display of selected points on the tongue surface. These traces allow us to calculate velocity and acceleration of the movement. Simultaneously the speech signal is recorded, and can be displayed as a reference to the movement tracks. A schematic illustration of this kind of data is given in Figure 7.11.

Keller and Ostry (1983) revealed a set of articulatory data for tongue movements for normal speakers, for different dysarthrias, and for stuttering.

Conclusion

Ultrasonic investigations of laryngeal and tongue movements provide very interesting data on speech kinematics. It is, and will be, an important tool in clinical phonetics. But there are also limitations, which have to be mentioned (see Fujimura, 1990).

Investigators need a great deal of experience and accuracy in placing the transducer. A direct contact between the solid transducer surface and the skin is needed to prevent mis-reflections. There are mechanical loading effects on the outside skin, and mandible movements while speaking increase those problems. A liquid transmission medium can help, but the investigator has always to be careful in its use. The representation of the tongue tip may not be accurate in all positions. If the tongue tip is raised, a second air-tissue-boundary is formed below the tongue, which may reflect a great amount of ultrasonic beams. As a result there will not be an accurate representation of the anterior part of the tongue.

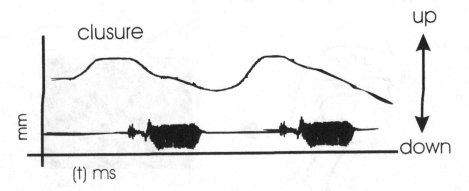

Figure 7.11. Trajectory of tongue movement (selected point) repetitive [kɑ] — schematic illustration.

Even though there are some limitations, there is no doubt about the importance of ultrasound measurements in the investigation of articulation. One great advantage is the representation of the whole tongue, as opposed to selected single points (as in, for example, articulography and X-ray microbeam systems).

Magnetic Resonance Imaging (MRI)

Introduction

Magnetic resonance imaging (or nuclear magnetic resonance imaging) is a non-invasive imaging technique giving three-dimensional views of biological tissue with good resolution compared with many other approaches (particularly of the soft tissue of the vocal tract). Its main drawback currently is temporal, in that, due to the time required to obtain a magnetic resonance image, static images only are possible although recent developments towards a more dynamic system can produce images very frequently: Westbrook (1994) quotes every 6 seconds, whereas Foldvik *et al* (1995) note 1 second or less is now possible; still too slow for speech of course. It is only recently that MRI has been applied to speech (see below), but is seems likely that combinations of different imaging techniques — some with good resolution, and others with dynamic temporal abilities — may well provide information of great interest to speech scientists in the future.

Nuclear magnetic resonance was first seen in 1945 by groups of scientists at Stanford and at MIT (Morris, 1986). However, it was only in the early 1970s that magnetic resonance imaging was developed, and early studies in the analysis of (among other areas) biological tissue were published. Since then, there has been a dramatic increase in the application of MRI to medical diagnosis and, as just noted, more recently to speech. Rokkaku *et al* (1986) and Baer *et al* (1987) were some of the earliest publications to apply MRI to speech analysis, but the continual improvement of MRI equipment means that more recent publications show clearer images than those in this early work.

Measuring principle and technical realization

MRI works by taking advantage of the magnetic properties of hydrogen nuclei, protons, which occur abundantly in biological tissue (Moore, 1992). If a large and constant magnetic field is applied to the biological tissue (for example, the vocal tract), then the protons in the area concerned will align parallel to that field. The next step in the imaging procedure requires the application of a radio frequency orthogonal to the magnetic field. This results in the dipoles tipping away from their primary axis and precessing in a cone-shaped spinning path. During the free induction decay of the precession of the dipole, a small electromotive force is emitted. This force can be detected by a receiver, which is tuned to the radio frequency used, and in the final stage of imaging, the electromotive force is converted via a processor unit to an image (see, for example, Morris, 1986, for fuller information).

Due to the range of equipment available for MRI, it is not feasible to provide detailed technical specifications of MRI equipment. A recent publication, such as Westbrook and Kaut (1993), can be consulted if more information is required.

MRI Data

The majority of MRI studies on speech have concentrated on examining the vocal tract, and comparing MRI results with those obtained from other methods (such as the acoustic record or X-radiography). Rokkaku *et al* (1986) were interested in vocal tract measurement, and Baer *et al* (1987) looked at pharynx shape during the production of the vowels /i/ and /ɑ/ in two subjects. The results of this latter study were checked with X-ray data from the same subject, and it appeared that the dimensions obtained from the two methods did not fully agree: the MRI results were significantly larger than those from the X-ray study. Various sources were suggested to account for this discrepancy (including body posture), but it did not prove possible to explain them unambiguously.

Baer *et al*. (1991) built on this first study, by adding data for the vowels /æ/ and /u/, together with axial pharyngeal images of the vowels /ɪ, ɛ, ɔ, ʊ, ʌ/. In this study also, the authors used the MRI images to build models of the vocal tract, which they then used to resynthesize the four vowels /i, æ, ɑ, u/. The real and synthesized versions were played to a panel of naive listeners who had to identify which vowel they heard. While the real data was recognized correctly more often than the synthesized data, the differences were slight. Other recent MRI studies of vowel production can be found in Lakshminarayanan *et al* (1991), and Greenwood *et al* (1992).

Investigation of errors in MRI data was one of the main aspects of the study by Moore (1992). The author used various analysis procedures to calculate vocal tract volumes from the magnetic resonance images, and to see how these fitted in with well-established acoustic transmission theory. Five subjects were used in the investigation, which looked at a limited set of both vowel and consonant articulations. Interestingly, one of the subjects had a slight articulatory disorder in that sibilants were produced with noticeable lateral distortion; this appears to be one of the first MRI studies to include any account of disordered speech.

Moore's results clearly demonstrate the lateral articulation of /s/ with the subject noted above. However, more interestingly, the article describes sources of error in analysing images and ways of correcting these. Finally, the resulting vocal tract volumes obtained from the study, when applied to acoustic resonance theory, accurately predict the acoustic make-up of the vowels studied. Moore believes, therefore, that MRI can be used effectively in studies of speech production. Figure 7.12 illustrates some of the images obtained during this study, and demonstrates tongue position for a variety of vowels and consonants.

Other studies mainly concerned with modelling the vocal tract, or aspects of it, include Foldvik *et al* (1993) and Yang and Kasuya (1994); while Foldvik *et al* (1995) compares MRI with ultrasound. Studies are also beginning to appear that examine specific classes of speech sounds. We have noted above various vowel studies; there have now been studies on nasals (Dang *et al* 1993) and fricatives (Narayanan *et al* 1995).

Clearly, we are only at the beginning of research using MRI. We can confidently predict that studies of disordered speech using this approach will be reported in the literature with increasing frequency. It may well be that MRI will continue to be used with other dynamic systems for the time being, but if image acquisition times can be improved still further, it could become one of the dominant techniques in speech imaging.

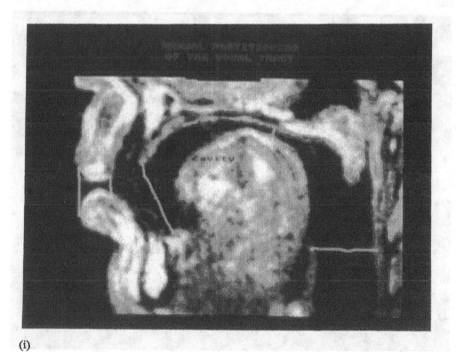

(i)

Figure 7.12. Magnetic resonance images: manual partitioning of the vocal tract; mid-sagittal images of tongue positions for the sounds /i/, /a/, /u/, /s/, /r/; serial sagittal images of /s/: 3 mm slices, 1 mm separation. (Courtesy Christopher Moore.)

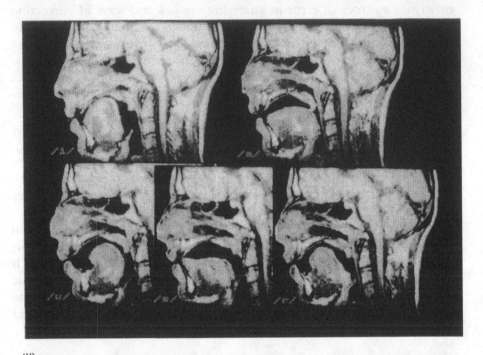

(ii)

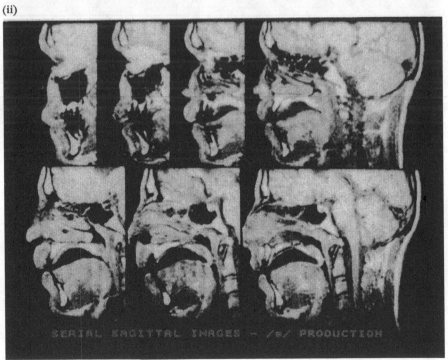

(iii)

Figure 7.12. Contd.

References

Adams S, Weismer G, Kent R. Speaking rate and speech movement velocity profiles. Journal of Speech and Hearing Research 1993; 36: 41–54.

Ardran GM, Kemp FH. Laryngeal function following lateral fixation of the vocal cord. British Journal of Disorders of Communication 1967; 2: 15–22.

Baer T, Gore J, Boyce S, Nye P. Application of MRI to the analysis of speech production. Magnetic Resonance Imaging 1987; 5: 1–7.

Baer T, Gore J, Gracco V, Nye P. Analysis of vocal tract shape and dimensions using magnetic resonance imaging: vowels. Journal of the Acoustical Society of America 1991; 90: 799–828.

Ball MJ. X-ray techniques. In Code C, Ball MJ. (Eds), Experimental Clinical Phonetics, pp. 107–28. London: Croom Helm, 1984.

Bergstrom LV. Congenital and acquired deafness in clefting and craniofacial syndromes. Cleft Palate Journal 1978; 15: 254–61.

Berry RJ, Epstein R, Fourcin AJ, Freeman M, MacCurtain F, Noscoe N. An objective analysis of voice disorder: Part one. British Journal of Disorders of Communication 1982a; 17: 67–76.

Berry RJ, Epstein R, Freeman M, MacCurtain F, Noscoe N. An objective analysis of voice disorder: Part two. British Journal of Disorders of Communication 1982b; 17: 77–85.

Bladon RAW, Nolan FJ. A video-fluorographic investigation of tip and blade alveolars in English. Journal of Phonetics 1977; 5: 185–93.

Bowman SA, Shanks JC. Velopharyngeal relationships of /i/ and /s/ as seen cephalometrically for persons with suspected incompetence. Journal of Speech and Hearing Disorders 1978; 43: 185–91.

Branderud P. Movetrack — a movement tracking system. Proceedings of the French-Swedish Symposium on Speech, 22-24 April 1985. Grenoble: GALF, pp. 113–22.

Dang J, Honda K, Suzuki H. MRI measurement and acoustic investigation of the nasal and paranasal cavities. Journal of the Acoustical Society of America 1993; 94: 1765 (A).

De Santis M, Cellini N, Minuto I, Modica V, Ciarniello V. Xeroradiography, teleradiography at high voltage, opaque contrastography in the dynamic study of the cervical portion of esophagus in patients who are [sic] undergone laryngectomy and radiotherapy. Acta Medica Romana 1979; 17: 255–59.

Dicenta M, Oliveras J. La Xerorradiología Laríngea. Acta Otorrinolaringologica Española 1976; 27: 99–106.

Engelke W, Hoch G. Simultane elektromagnetische Artikulographie und Videoendoskopie. Ein Kasuistische Beitrag zur objektiven Diagnostik des velopharyngealen Sphinkters. 55; 297–303.

Enany NM. A cephalometric study of the effects of primary osteoplasty in unilateral cleft lip and palate individuals. Cleft Palate Journal 1981; 18: 286–92.

Fitzpatrick L, Ní Chasaide A. Using EMA, EPG and acoustic data to look at quantal theory: an account of work in progress. Forschungsberichte der Institut für Phonetik und Sprachliche Kommunikation der Universität München (FIPKM) 1993; 31: 229–38.

Foldvik A, Kristiansen U, Kværness J, Bonnaventure H. A time-evolving three-dimensional vocal tract model by means of magnetic resonance imaging (MRI) Proceedings Eurospeech 1993; 1: 557–58.

Foldvik A, Kristiansen U, Kværness J, Torp A, Torp H. Three-dimensional ultrasound and magnetic resonance imaging: a new dimension in phonetic research. In

Elenius K, Branderud P. (Eds), Proceedings of the XIIIth International Congress of Phonetic Sciences, Vol. 4, pp. 46–49. Stockholm: KTH and Stockholm University, 1995.

Fujimura O. Methods and goals of speech production research. Language and Speech 1990; 33: 195–258.

Fujita K. Pathophysiology of the larynx from the viewpoint of phonation. Journal of the Japanese Society of Otorhinolaryngology 1966; 69: 459.

Glaser ER, Skolnick ML, McWilliams BJ, Shprintzen RJ. The dynamics of Passavant's Ridge in subjects with and without velopharyngeal insufficiency: a multiview video-fluoroscopic study. Cleft Palate Journal 1979; 16: 24–33.

Grabb WC, Rosenstein SW, Bzoch KR. (Eds), Cleft Lip and Palate. Little, Brown and Co., Boston, 1971.

Greenwood A, Goodyear C, Martin P. Measurement of vocal tract shapes using magnetic resonance imaging. IEEE Proceedings I (Communication, Speech, Vision) (UK) 1992; 139: 553–60.

Hardin M, Morris H, Van Demark D. A study of cleft palate speakers with marginal velopharyngeal competence. Journal of Communication Disorders 1986; 19: 461–73.

Hirose H, Kiritani S, Ushijima T, Sawashima M. Analysis of abnormal articulatory dynamics in two dysarthric patients. Journal of Speech and Hearing Disorders 1978; 43: 96–105.

Hirose H, Kiritani S, Ushijima T, Yoshioka H, Sawashima M. Patterns of dysarthric movements in patients with Parkinsonism. Folia Phoniatrica 1981; 33: 204–15.

Hixon THJ. An electromagnetic method for transducing jaw movements during speech. Journal of the Acoustical Society of America 1971; 49: 603–6.

Honda M, Kaburagi T. Comparison of electromagnetic and ultrasonic techniques for monitoring tongue motion. Forschungsberichte der Institut für Phonetik und Sprachliche Kommunikation der Universität München (FIPKM) 1993; 31: 121–36.

Hoole P. Methodological considerations in the use of electromagnetic articulography in phonetic research. Forschungsberichte der Institut für Phonetik und Sprachliche Kommunikation der Universität München (FIPKM) 1993; 31: 43–64.

Itoh M, Sasanuma S, Hirose H, Yoshioka H, Ushijima T. Abnormal articulatory dynamics in a patient with apraxia of speech: X-ray microbeam observation. Brain and Language 1980; 11: 66–75.

Kaneko T, Uchida K, Suzuki H, Komatsu K, Kanesaka T, Kobayashi N, Naito J. Ultrasonic observations of vocal fold vibrations. In Stevens KN, Hirano M. (Eds), Vocal Fold Physiology, pp. 107–18. Tokyo: University of Tokyo Press, 1981.

Karnell M, Folkins J, Morris H. Relationships between the perception of nasalization and speech movements in speakers with cleft palate. Journal of Speech and Hearing Research 1985; 28: 63–72.

Keller E, Ostry DJ. Computerized measurement of tongue dorsum movements with pulsed-echo ultrasound. Journal of the Acoustical Society of America 1983; 73: 1309–15.

Kent R, Netsell R. A case study of an ataxic dysarthric: cineradiographic and spectrographic observations. Journal of Speech and Hearing Disorders 1975; 40: 115–34.

Kiritani S. X-ray microbeam method for measurement of articulatory dynamics: techniques and results. Speech Communication 1986; 5: 119–40.

Kiritani S, Itoh K, Fujimura O. Tongue-pellet tracking by a computer-controlled X-ray microbeam system. Journal of the Acoustical Society of America 1975; 57: 1516–20.

Kuehn DP, Tomblin JB. A cineradiographic investigation of children's w/r substitutions. Journal of Speech and Hearing Disorders 1977; 42: 462–73.

Kuehn DP, Van Demark DR. Assessment of velopharyngeal competency following Teflon pharyngoplasty. Cleft Palate Journal 1978; 15: 145–49.

Lakshminarayanan A, Lee S, McCutcheon M. MR imaging of the vocal tract during vowel production. Journal of Magnetic Resonance Imaging 1991; 1: 71–76.

Lewis MB, Pashayan HM. The effects of pharyngeal flap surgery on lateral wall motion: a videoradiographic evaluation. Cleft Palate Journal 1980; 17: 301–4.

Lock R, Seaver III E. Nasality and velopharyngeal function in five hearing-impaired adults. Journal of Communication Disorders 1984; 17: 47–64.

Luchsinger R, Arnold GE. Voice — Speech — Language. London: Constable, 1965.

MacCurtain F. Pharyngeal factors influencing voice quality. PhD thesis, University of London, 1981.

MacMillan AS, Keleman G. Radiography of the supraglottal speech organs. A survey. AMA Archives of Otolaryngology 1952; 55: 671–88.

Malmberg B. (Ed.), Manual of Phonetics. Amsterdam: North Holland, 1968.

Moll KL. Photographic and radiographic procedures in speech research. ASHA Reports 1965; 1: 129–39.

Moore C. The correspondence of vocal tract resonance with volumes obtained from magnetic resonance images. Journal of Speech and Hearing Research 1992; 35: 1009–23.

Morris P. Nuclear Magnetic Resonance Imaging in Medicine and Biology. Oxford: Oxford University Press, 1986.

Narayanan S, Alwan A, Haker K. An articulatory study of fricative consonants using magnetic resonance imaging. Journal of the Acoustical Society of America 1995; 98: 1325–47.

Pahn J. Röntgenologische Untersuchungsmethode der Nervuslaryngeus-superior-Parese. Folia Phoniatrica 1981; 33: 15–22.

Painter C. An Introduction to Instrumental Phonetics. Baltimore: University Park Press, 1979.

Perkell JS, Cohen MH, Svirsky MA, Matthies ML, Garabieta I, Jackson MTT. Electromagnetic midsagittal articulometer system for transducing speech articulatory movements. Journal of the Acoustical Society of America 1992; 92: 3078–96.

Pruszewicz A, Obrebowski A, Gradzki J. Postmedicamentous voice virilisation. X-ray examination of the larynx. In Loebell E. (Ed.), Proceedings XVlth International Congress of Logopedics and Phoniatrics. Interlaken 1974. Basel: S. Karger, 1976.

Putnam AHB, Ringel RL. A cineradiographic study of articulation in two talkers with temporarily induced oral sensory deprivation. Journal of Speech and Hearing Research 1976; 19: 247–66.

Ranford HJ. 'Larynx-NAD'? CST Bulletin 1982; 359: 5.

Ridgway A, Thumm W. The Physics of Medical Radiography. Reading, MA: Addison-Wesley, 1968.

Rokkaku M, Hashimoto K, Imaizumi S, Niimi S, Kiritani S. Measurements of the three-dimensional shape of the vocal tract based on the magnetic resonance imaging technique. Annual Bulletin Research Institute of Logopedics and Phoniatrics 1986; 20: 47–54.

Schönle PW. Elektromagnetische Artikulographie — Ein neues Verfahren zur klinischen Untersuchung der Sprechmotorik. Berlin: Springer, 1988.

Schönle PW. The developmental geneology of Electromagnetic Articulography (EMA). Forschungsberichte der Institut für Phonetik und Sprachliche Kommunikation der Universität München (FIPKM) 1993; 31: 83–89.

Schönle PW, Wenig P, Schrader J, Höhne J, Bröckmann E, Conrad B. Electromagnetic articulography — use of alternating magnetic fields for tracking movements of multiple points inside and outside the vocal tract. Brain and Language 1987; 31: 26–35.

Seaver EJ, Andrews JR, Granata JJ. A radiographic investigation of velar positioning in hearing impaired young adults. Journal of Communication Disorders 1980;13: 239–47.

Shelton RL, Furr ML, Johnson A, Arndt WB. Cephalometric and intra-oral variables as they relate to articulation improvement with training. American Journal of Orthodontics 1975; 67: 423–31.

Shelton RL, Trier WC. Issues involved in the evaluation of velopharyngeal closure. Cleft Palate Journal 1976; 13: 127–37.

Shprintzen RJ, Croft CB, Berkman MD, Rakoff SJ. Velopharyngeal insufficiency in the facio-auriculo-vertebral malformation complex. Cleft Palate Journal 1980; 17: 132–37.

Spolyar J, Vasileff W, MacIntosh R. Image corrected cephalometric analysis (ICCA): design and evaluation. Cleft Palate Craniofacial Journal 1993; 30: 528–41.

Strenger F. Radiographic, palatographic, and labiographic methods in phonetics. In Malmberg B. (Ed.), Manual of Phonetics, pp. 334–64. Amsterdam: North Holland, 1968.

Subtelny J, Li W, Whitehead R, Subtelny JD. Cephalometric and cineradiographic study of deviant resonance in hearing-impaired speakers. Journal of Speech and Hearing Disorders 1989; 54: 249–63.

Tuller B, Shao S, Kelso JAS. An evaluation of an alternating megnetic field device for monitoring tongue movements. Journal of the Acoustical Society of America 1990; 88: 674–79.

Van den Berg J. On the role of the laryngeal ventricle in voice production. Folia Phoniatrica 1955; 7: 57–69.

Van der Giet G. Computer-controlled method for measuring articulatory activities. Journal of the Acoustical Society of America 1977; 61: 1072–76.

Van der Plaats GJ. Medical X-ray technique. Eindhoven: Centrex, 1969.

Ward PH, Hanafee W, Shallit J, Mancuso A, Berci G. Evaluation of computerized tomography, cinelaryngoscopy, and laryngography in determining the extent of laryngeal disease. Annals of Otology, Rhinology and Laryngology 1979; 88: 454–62.

Watkin KL, Zagzebski JA. On-line ultrasonic technique for monitoring tongue displacements. Journal of the Acoustical Society of America 1973; 54: 544–47.

Westbrook C. Handbook of MRI Technique. Oxford: Blackwell, 1994.

Westbrook C, Kaut C. MRI in Practice. Oxford: Blackwell, 1993.

Westbury J. X-Ray Microbeam Speech Production Database. User's Handbook. Version 1.0. Madison, WI: University of Wisconsin, 1994.

Westbury J, Hashi M, Lindstrom M. Differences among speakers in articulation of American English /r/: an X-ray microbeam study. In Elenius K, Branderud P. (Eds), Proceedings of the XIIIth International Congress of Phonetic Sciences, vol 4, pp. 50–57. Stockholm: KTH and Stockholm University, 1995.

Williams WN. Applications of radiological measures. In Grabb WC, Rosenstein SW, Bzoch KR. (Eds), Cleft Lip and Palate, pp. 767–75. Boston: Little, Brown and Co, 1971.

Williams WN, Eisenbach CR. Assessing VP function: the lateral still technique vs cinefluorography. Cleft Palate Journal 1981; 18: 45–50.

Yang C-S, Kasuya H. Accurate measurement of vocal tract shapes from magnetic resonance images of child, female and male subjects. Proceedings of the International

Congress of Speech and Language Processing, pp. 623–26. Yokohama: ICSLP, 1994.

Zierdt A. Problems of electromagnetic position transduction for a three-dimensional articulographic measurement system. Forschungsberichte der Institut für Phonetik und Sprachliche Kommunikation der Universität München (FIPKM) 1993; 31: 137–42.

Zimmerman G. Articulatory dynamics of fluent utterances of stutterers and non-stutterers. Journal of Speech and Hearing Research 1980a; 23: 95–107.

Zimmerman G. Articulatory behaviors associated with stuttering: a cinefluorographic analysis. Journal of Speech and Hearing Research 1980b; 23: 108–21.

Zimmerman G. Stuttering: a disorder of movement. Journal of Speech and Hearing Research 1980c; 23: 122–36.

Zimmerman G, Dalston R, Brown O, Folkins J, Linville R, Seaver E. Comparison of cineradiographic and photodetection techniques for assessing velopharyngeal function during speech. Journal of Speech and Hearing Research 1987; 30: 564–69.

Zimmerman G, Kelso JAS, Lander L. Articulatory behavior pre and post full-mouth tooth extraction and alveoplasty: a cinefluorographic study. Journal of Speech and Hearing Research 1980; 23: 630–45.

Zwitman DH, Gyepes MT, Ward PH. Assessment of velar and lateral wall movement by oral telescope and radiographic investigation in patients with velopharyngeal inadequacy and in normal subjects. Journal of Speech and Hearing Disorders 1976; 41: 381–89.

Chapter 8
Experimental
Audioperceptual
Techniques

CHRIS CODE

In this chapter, I examine two important auditory techniques which have been widely applied in research and treatment in communication disorders. These are delayed auditory feedback and dichotic listening. I look at the role and impact of each technique in speech science and its application in research and treatment in speech pathology.

Delayed Auditory Feedback

In the normal individual, speech sounds are fed back to the inner ear via air (air-conducted feedback) and bone (bone-conducted feedback) with a delay of about 0.001 seconds (Yates, 1963). Delayed auditory feedback (DAF), sometimes called delayed sidetone, involves extending the time between the utterance of a speech sound and its auditory perception.

The DAF effect on a normal speaker, first described by Lee (1950), can be quite dramatic and is characterized by a number of alterations to normal speech described by Fairbanks (1955) as the *indirect* and the *direct* effects of DAF. The indirect effects are reduction in rate of speech, increase in intensity and increase in fundamental frequency. According to Fairbanks, these indirect effects are due to the subject's efforts to overcome the influence of the DAF. The direct articulatory effects that are observed include repetition of syllables and continuants, mispronunciations, omissions, substitutions, additions and omitted word endings. Lee (1950) referred to the DAF effect as 'artificial stuttering'.

Achieving delays in auditory feedback is not difficult and can be accomplished with a good standard reel-to-reel tape recorder with separate record and playback heads, although such machines are becoming rarer in academic departments and clinics. This is a shame because a good reel-to-reel tape recorder permits flexible, high-quality if low-tech access to DAF and dichotic listening, which is discussed later. The subject's speech is recorded on the tape via the record head, the tape passes to the playback head and the speech is fed back to the subject

228

through headphones. The delay in auditory feedback is determined by a combination of the distance between the heads and the speed of the tape. For example, an inter-head gap of 1.25 inches over a tape speed of 7.5 in/s will give a delay of about 160 ms. Four delay times (80, 160, 330 and 660 ms) are therefore available from such a tape recorder with the four tape speeds, 1.875, 3.75, 7.5 and 15 in/s.

More delay times are available with a tape recorder that has either a moveable record or playback head, and Tiffany, Hanley and Sutherland (1954) and Huggins (1967) describe different devices for converting tape recorders in such a way that a large variety of accurate delay times can be achieved. The device described by Huggins utilizes a micrometer bolted to the surface of a tape recorder, which can be adjusted to vary the length of the tape path between the heads. The device has the advantage that it does not involve moving heads and the tape recorder can still be used in the normal way when not required for DAF. An even simpler method is described by Code (1979) for varying the length of the tape path. All that is required is a tape pulley, a length of wire about 1 mm thick and a clamping screw that can hold the wire and allow adjustment. The clamping screw can be bolted to the upper surface of the tape recorder and the length of wire can be calibrated.

Siegel, Fehst, Garber and Pick (1980) describe a versatile method for obtaining a range of delay times employing two tape recorders arranged in series. The subject's speech is delayed on one recorder and then fed to the other where the delay produced by the first recorder is combined with the delay chosen on the second. This method can provide a range of delay times depending on the tape speeds and inter-head gaps available on the machines.

Apart from using standard tape recorders there are a number of commercially produced DAF machines available. The 'Phonic Mirror' is a multiplehead tape machine (one record and five playback heads), which employs a tape loop. This machine gives a range of five delay times (50, 100, 150, 200 and 250 ms). A number of tapeless, solid-state devices, which achieve delays electronically, have become available with developments in silicon chip technology. The Aberdeen Speech Aid (Low and Lindsay, 1979) is a device developed in Britain which comes in two models. The larger desk model is for clinical and laboratory use and the pocket size model (10 × 5 × 2.5 cm) is for personal use and includes a lapel microphone and earphones. The device provides continuous delay from 30 to 300 ms, and is capable of binaural and mononaural presentation of DAF. It gets over the problem of delaying the voices of others close to the user by employing a switch that is activated by the higher intensity of the user's voice but not of others close by. In this way only the user's voice is delayed.

The Danish Phonic Mirror PM 505 is a similar device slightly larger than the Aberdeen Speech Aid (11 × 6.4 × 3.8 cm), and provides continuous delays from 25 to 220 ms. It also employs a lapel microphone and earphones. The Dystech 1000 is a body-worn DAF device, developed in the United States and briefly described by Muellerleile (1981). Using microcomputers to alter auditory feedback is discussed in Chapter 9 by Zeigler *et al.*

There is variability in the degree of disruption experienced by different groups of normal speakers under DAF. Chase, Sutton, First and Zubin (1961) found that children between 4 and 6 years show less disturbance of speech than older children between 7 and 9 years under a delay of 200 ms. Mackay (1968) tested the same age groups as Chase *et al* (1961) with a variety of delay times. He found that the delay required to produce disruption in speech decreases with age. Children in the younger group (4–6 years) showed maximum disturbance under a delay of 500 ms, whereas children in the older group (7–9 years) experienced peak disruption at 400 ms delay. In addition, Mackay reports that the disturbances of the younger group were more severe than those of the older group, which were in turn more severe than the disruptions observed in an adult group (20–26 years). In agreement with most other studies, Mackay also reports that 200 ms is the delay that produces maximum disruption in adults.

Work by Buxton (1969) and Siegel *et al* (1980) tends to confirm Mackay's findings. Moreover, Buxton found that the most disruptive delay-time for older adults between 60 and 81 years was 400 ms. It therefore appears that the maximumly disruptive delay time decreases with age from 500 ms in early childhood, to 400 ms in later childhood, and to 200 ms in adults where some kind of peak is reached. It then increases with old age to 400 ms. It also appears that the disruption caused by DAF becomes more pronounced with age, which suggests that there is a reduction in reliance on auditory feedback with increasing age (Siegel *et al*, 1980).

The relationship between gender and DAF is less clear. Timmons and Boudreau (1972) report that when delays of 0–500 ms were presented in random order to male and female subjects no differences in reactions were observed, but differences do emerge when the delay times are compared in order of their presentation. However, Buxton (1969), in his study, found no differences at all between sexes. Those studies that have found differences tend to indicate that males are more vulnerable to DAF than females.

It seems to be generally established that more fluent and rapid speakers show less disruption under DAF (Beaumont and Foss, 1957; Buxton, 1969; Mackay, 1968). Mackay found that the slower a subject's speech was without DAF the more disruption of speech occurred under DAF. This correlation was observed in all the age groups that Mackay investigated — young children, older children and adults. Conversely, Buxton found that naturally rapid speakers show less disturbance in their speech under delays ranging from 100 to 600 ms. Furthermore, evidence indicates that a rapid speaker requires a shorter delay time to produce maximum instability, whereas naturally slow speakers show maximum disruption under longer delay times.

In summary, there are individual differences in reactions to DAF by normal speakers. Some speakers are comparatively unaffected while others show severe distortions of fluency, vocal pitch and intensity. Disturbances in speech appear to decrease with age with adults being less affected than children. However, older adults are more affected than younger adults. There is some evidence that male subjects show more disturbance than female subjects, and more rapid fluent speakers are less affected than less rapid and less fluent speakers.

The role of delayed auditory feedback in speech science

The main thrust of research into the DAF effect with normal speakers has been the examination of the role of auditory feedback in speech production. Explanations for the DAF phenomenon abound (see Code, 1980 for some discussion). Lee (1950) was among the first to propose a model of speech production that took account of the effect. The model is made up of feedback loops, which are approximately proportional in length to the time necessary to perform the speech activity associated with the particular loop. Four hierarchically arranged loops make up the model: an articulatory loop (phonemes), a voice loop (syllables), a word loop and a thought loop. It is the shorter loops — articulatory and voice — that are affected by DAF. An important property of the model is that any unit may be repeated if monitoring is dissatisfied with the first performance, and there is a common junction for all the loops that represents a cortical speech centre. Lee suggested, therefore, that stuttering and 'artificial' stuttering result from a dysfunction or instability of closed-loop feedback at the phonemic and/or syllabic level.

Since Lombard (1911) first described the effect that bears his name, it has been known that the presentation of masking noise causes the speaker to increase vocal intensity (*the Lombard effect*). Cherry and Sayer (1956) conducted a classic series of experiments using white masking noise with 54 severe stutterers and were able to show that intense auditory feedback masking resulted in almost complete fluency. They found, however, that band-pass filtering of the white noise to allow only high frequencies above 500 Hz through to the speaker, reduced stuttering; whereas filtering to allow only low frequencies below 500 Hz did not reduce dysfluency. The authors concluded that stuttering must be related to an individual's perception of their own low-frequency, bone-conducted feedback that produces instability in a closed-loop feedback system.

The model of speech production proposed by Fairbanks (1954), which accounts for the DAF effect, includes a comparator to which auditory, tactile and proprioceptive information is fed back via a sensor unit. These signals are compared with output and a calculation is performed by the comparator to determine discrepancies between the two signals.

This model, like Lee's, is dominated by auditory feedback and assumes closed-loop control. Contemporary wisdom considers that an entirely automatic closed-loop model or an entirely open-loop model, with no feedback control, cannot explain all that is now known about speech production. It is also established that auditory feedback is far too slow to achieve *ongoing* monitoring and correction of articulatory events. Auditory feedback can only be post-event in its influence on the control of speech production. For ongoing closed-loop control, proprioceptive feedback via the gammaloop system of the muscle spindles appears to hold the best promise, and some theoretical predictive *feedforward* capabilities of the central nervous system have been proposed (see Borden, 1979, for review).

Borden, Dorman, Freeman and Niimi (1976) examined the electromyographic (EMG) performance of normal speakers under DAF and found EMG activity associated not only with the dysfluent speech produced, but also with aborted articulatory attempts. The study concludes that the DAF effect is due to a conflict between proprioceptive feedback providing information to proceed and auditory feedback providing information to wait. Borden (1979) also points out that EMG data taken while subjects are under DAF is characteristically inconsistent, indicating an intermittent attentiveness to the auditory signal on the part of the speaker rather than true closed-loop error correction.

Applications in speech pathology and therapeutics

There have been a number of applications of DAF in speech pathology and therapeutics. Most research, predictably, has been into stuttering, although there have been studies employing DAF with aphasic, apraxic and dysarthric subjects.

Stuttering

While the DAF effect on normal speakers is generally a negative disruption of the normal speech pattern, interference with auditory feedback in stutterers can have surprisingly positive effects upon fluency (Van Riper, 1973). But where it is the more fluent normal speaker who reacts less to DAF, in the case of stutterers it has been shown that it is the more severe who respond most positively (Soderberg, 1969; Van Riper, 1971). Harrington (1988) has more recently reviewed the application of DAF in stuttering.

While the critical delay time for producing maximum disruption in normal speakers is fairly well established, there appear to be more individual differences among stutterers with regard to critical delay times for producing improvements in fluency. For an individual stutterer who benefits from DAF there is probably a critical delay time that produces maximum fluency, probably a relatively short delay time; and a separate critical delay time, which produces maximum dysfluency, probably a longer delay time. Sark, Kalinowski, Armson and Stuart (1993) recently compared the DAF delay times of 0 ms (no delay), 25 ms, 50 ms and 75 ms in 14 adult (12 male, 2 female) stutterers under a fast and a normal speech rate while reading. Although they found significant reductions in dysfluency under all delay times, there was a gradual and significant decrease in dysfluency as delays increased from 25 ms and 50 ms with a smaller decrease in stuttering between 50 ms and 75 ms. However, these effects were observed in both fast and normal speech rates.

The relationship between genuine and artificial stuttering

It is a common observation that stuttering is often at its worst in the initiation of utterances where auditory feedback does not come into play. This observation is not consistent with a perceptual theory of stuttering, although this is not to say that auditory feedback does not play some part in stuttering. It is clear, for instance, that DAF and, perhaps to a greater extent, auditory feedback masking can have a beneficial effect upon the speech of stutterers, which is more than mere 'distraction'. If DAF was simply acting as a distraction, then *any* delay-time would produce fluency. The same goes for auditory masking. For masking to eliminate dysfluency, it must be the low bone-conducted frequencies that are masked.

It is also clear that DAF causes a sort of 'artificial' stuttering in normal speakers. However, there is evidence to suggest that the two phenomena are mediated by separate mechanisms. Neely (1961) found that the characteristics were different and amount of adaption to DAF was different between stutterers and normal speakers, and in a perceptual study listeners were able to distinguish successfully between the speech of stutterers and normal speakers under DAF. Code (1979) was able to provide some support for Neely's view that stuttering and artificial stuttering are separate phenomena in a study that compared the EMG signals taken from the upper lip of a severe stutterer without DAF and a normal speaker made dysfluent by DAF. An analysis of the amplitudes and durations of the EMG signals revealed that there were significant differences in the muscular activity of the two subjects. However, EMG data taken while the stutterer was reading fluently under low frequency (below 500Hz) masking, and while the non-stutterer was reading normally without DAF showed that there were no significant differences in muscular activity, indicating that muscular activity in masking-induced fluency in stutterers cannot be differentiated from muscular activity in normal fluency using EMG. This last finding supports a similar one by Dewar, Dewar and Anthony (1976). This 'normal' muscular activity observed in fluent stutterers under masking would again not support a simple 'distraction' explanation.

However, Venkatagiri (1980) has suggested that genuine and artificial stuttering may share some important features. He examined the recorded DAF-induced dysfluencies of 24 non-stutterers and found that like stutterers, their dysfluency under DAF is characterized by part-word repetitions, high frequency of dysfluency on polysyllabic words, high frequency of dysfluency on initial syllables and adaptation in repeated readings. However, the degree of consistency of stuttering between initial and subsequent oral readings in DAF-induced dysfluency was found to be considerably less. In contrast, Neelly (1961) found that adaptation to repeated oral readings was significantly different in the two groups.

Aphasia, apraxia and dysarthria

There has been interesting research into the effect of DAF on the speech of aphasic individuals. In an early study, Stanton (1958) tested 13 aphasic patients and found that three responded similarly to normal subjects, two were unaffected by the DAF and five benefited. For three other patients, Stanton described responses as 'atypical'. Singh and Schlanger (1969) compared the effects of a DAF delay-time of 180 ms on 10 aphasic, 10 dysarthric and 10 intellectually impaired subjects. The aphasic group were described as having mild or moderate 'expressive' aphasia. The aim of the study was to compare sentence duration, vocal intensity and speech errors in the three groups during the production of read or repeated sentences of three levels of meaningfulness. Sentence durations were distorted in seven aphasic patients, and the level of vocal intensity also increased in the groups as a whole under DAF. Phone production errors for all groups increased also as a function of the meaningfulness of the sentences, with the aphasic group making most errors, followed by the dysarthric group, and then the mentally impaired group. Moreover, sentence durations were longest, for all three groups taken together, for the least meaningful sentences. Among the aphasic subjects, two produced longer sentence durations under the no-delay condition than under DAF and one appeared to be unaffected by DAF.

The remaining seven aphasic subjects all experienced some kind of unspecified disruption under DAF. It appears that vocal intensity also increased under DAF for all groups taken together. The study appears to support Stanton's (1958) finding that there is variability in the reaction of aphasic patients to DAF.

A series of interesting studies during the 1970s extended knowledge of the effects of DAF on aphasic subjects (Boller and Marcie, 1978; Boller *et al*, 1978; Chapin *et al*, 1981; Vrtunski *et al*, 1976). Vrtunski *et al* (1976) compared left-hemisphere damaged individuals, right-hemisphere damaged individuals and a control group under DAF (360 ms) involving an easy and a difficult verbal task (counting and reporting sentences) and an easy and difficult non-verbal task (tapping at a steady rate and tapping a simple Morse Code pattern). The auditory feedback in this non-verbal condition was a 600 Hz tone produced by the tapping pressure. The dependent variables examined were vocal intensity and duration of speech and intensity and duration of tapping.

All subjects across all groups showed the expected DAF effect on most tasks to some degree. Whereas controls showed increased DAF effect on both verbal and non-verbal tasks as the task became more difficult, for the left-hemisphere damaged group the DAF effect reduced as the verbal (but not the non-verbal) task became more difficult. For the right-hemisphere damaged group, however, the DAF effect reduced as the non-verbal (but not the verbal) task became more difficult. The finding that the left-hemisphere group all experienced disruption in duration and intensity is in contrast to the findings of Stanton (1958) and Singh and Schlanger (1969) indicating variability.

Boller *et al* (1978) explored the effects of DAF at 180 and 360 ms on 10 fluent and 10 non-fluent aphasic subjects and 10 controls. All subjects across all groups showed some DAF effect and the 180 ms delay was the most effective in causing disturbance on the variables measured. Fluent subjects produced a significantly smaller DAF effect than non-fluent subjects and a non-significantly smaller effect than the normal control group. The study failed to find any aphasic subject whose speech improved under DAF, except in reading by the fluent group where speech quality was actually better under DAF than under the no-DAF condition. Even so, duration and intensity were increased for this group and it was articulatory speech quality alone that showed improvements.

The smallest DAF effects were produced by three conduction aphasic subjects and one 'recovered' Broca's subject. There was considerable variability in DAF effect relative to speech task used and 'quality of speech' discriminated best between groups. Correlation analysis suggested that duration and quality of speech are closely related variables whereas vocal intensity appears to be independent of the other two. This echos Fairbanks's (1955) earlier distinction between 'direct' and 'indirect' effects. The study concludes that an independent monitoring system controls intensity (indirect), which is affected similarly in aphasic and normal subjects, but a second system responsible for duration and articulatory quality (direct) is affected differently in different aphasic types. Chapin *et al* (1981) examined further the 'speech quality' data from Boller *et al* (1978). A further aim was to determine which speech quality errors could be considered phonological and which phonetic in nature. Phonological errors were processes such as phone or syllabic substitutions, simplifications and additions, and examples of phonetic errors were increases in length of vowels, fricatives and sonorants. The original aphasic subjects (Boller *et al*, 1978) were further subdivided into Broca's, Wernicke's, conduction and posterior (two word-deaf and one transcortical sensory).

The phonetic feature of vowel length was the only speech quality error that was significantly affected and none of the phonological measures contributed significantly to errors in speech quality. Furthermore, the only significant difference between the groups occurred between conduction subjects who were the least affected, and Broca's subjects who were the most affected. The authors conclude that DAF affects ongoing phonetic planning and implementation and not phonological processes, and that the observation that conduction aphasic patients are relatively unaffected by DAF supports the *disconnection* explanation of conduction aphasia, which holds that a disconnection between the sensory and motor images of words underlies this type of aphasia, possibly due to a lesion in the *arcuate fasciculus*, the bundle of interconnecting fibres which joins Wernicke's area and Broca's area. Finally, they interpret the Broca patients' poor performance under DAF to indicate a highly fragile articulatory system, supporting the view (Code, in press; Darley *et al*, 1975; Johns and LaPointe, 1976) that an apraxia of speech is a significant component of the disorder we call Broca's aphasia. The findings of a study by Lozano and Dreyer (1978), who investigated the effects of DAF (180 ms) on the speech of five subjects with fairly 'pure' apraxia of speech, supports this general finding.

The experimental task involved reading single monosyllabic and polysyllabic words and the number of speech production errors was calculated. No significant differences were detected by judges in the number of errors in the DAF and no-DAF conditions suggested by the researchers to support the view that apraxia of speech is primarily a motor speech disorder without auditory system involvement. The problem in interpreting the result of this study is that the use of a single-word reading task rather than longer utterances might have produced the smaller DAF effect. Also, indirect effects were not measured.

Boller and Marcie (1978) compared a single conduction subject with a group of normal subjects who repeated words and a short sentence under no-DAF and DAF (200 ms). The repetitions of the conduction patient improved under DAF on all measures whereas the normal subjects showed the expected negative effects of DAF. The authors suggest that this confirms the view that conduction aphasia entails a delay in what they call 'external phonemic' feedback (at the phonetic actualization level) as well as a delay in 'internal phonemic' feedback (at the phonological selection level). For normal subjects, DAF interferes only with internal feedback.

In summary, the indicators are that when sufficiently sensitive measures are employed most aphasic subjects show some disturbance in speech production as a result of DAF. It would appear that conduction patients are affected the least (less than normal subjects) and Broca's patients the most. It seems that it is the phonetic aspects of speech quality (mainly vowel length) and duration that are most affected. These variables constitute Fairbanks's indirect effects.

Clinical applications of DAF

Stuttering

Clinical application of DAF has been mainly as a means of training stutterers to reduce their dysfluency by learning a slower-paced method of speech often referred to as *prolonged speech*. A therapeutic approach, which employs DAF as part of an operant treatment programme designed to train prolonged speech, began with work by Goldiamond (1965) and has been developed and described in a number of subsequent studies (Curlee and Perkins, 1969; Ryan, 1971; Ryan and Van Kirk, 1974). The method involves systematic 'step-by-step procedures which include prescribed reinforcement schedules and criterion levels' (Ryan and Van Kirk, 1974: p. 3). The procedures described by Ryan and Van Kirk illustrate well how DAF is used as part of a behavioural programme. The aim of the programme is to establish fluent conversational speech in the clinical setting, to transfer fluency to a variety of settings outside the clinic and finally to maintain fluency over a long period of time. Each of these three phases of the programme (establishment, transfer, maintenance) is made up of a number of steps (in the case of the establishment phase, 27 steps). During the establishment phase the stutterer is taught first to read, then speak in monologue and finally to engage in conversation, in a slow, prolonged speech with the aid of DAF. The delay time starts at 250 ms and is gradually reduced in 50 ms steps to a no-delay condition until the patient is using fluent prolonged speech without the aid of DAF. The criterion set for progression to a following step is 5 minutes of fluency at each step. Ryan and Van Kirk report that the programme, which lasts approximately 20 hours, was effective in establishing and maintaining fluency in a large population of stutterers of both sexes with a wide range of ages and varying degrees of severity.

Kalinowski, Armson, Stuart, Mieszkowski and Gracco (1993) report that a slow speech rate is not necessarily required to enhance fluency, as has been thought for so long. They asked stutterers to speak at normal and fast rates under a range of altered feedback conditions, including DAF (50 ms). They found that the stutterers could maintain fluency under altered feedback at fast as well as at normal rates.

Van Riper (1973) proposed a number of therapeutic applications of DAF with stutterers based on clinical observation. At an early stage of therapy, the clinician can demonstrate the effects of DAF on his or her own speech and thereby show the patient that normal speakers can be made to stutter. DAF can also be used to show the patient that stuttered speech is modifiable. Van Riper also advocates a procedure that trains the patient to ignore auditory feedback and rely instead on proprioceptive and tactile feedback. Through a systematic behavioural approach the stutterer learns to 'beat the machine', as Van Riper puts it, and becomes more fluent through reliance on forms of feedback other than auditory.

With the recent silicone chip revolution, body-worn DAF devices, like those described in an earlier section, will perhaps become cheaper and more accessible and be used to a much greater extent in the stutterer's everyday life. This should improve control over the transfer and maintenance stages of a therapeutic programme.

Applications with other communication disorders

There are indications (Adams and Lang, 1992; Downie *et al* , 1981) that DAF and auditory feedback masking may have a therapeutic application in the management of Parkinson's disease. Downie *et al.* examined the responses of 11 hyperkinetic dysarthria patients suffering from Parkinson's disease to the body-worn Aberdeen Speech Aid. Of the 11 patients who tried the device, two showed dramatic improvements in their speech, one showed slight improvement, and the rest did not benefit. Of the two patients who benefited from DAF, one whose speech without DAF was characterized by hesitations, repetitions, excessive rate and short rushes of words, showed dramatic improvement under a delay time of 50 ms (but not 200 ms). The DAF was of great benefit for 3 months, but original speech patterns began to return after this and after 12 months the DAF was discontinued. The other patient who benefited had speech that was low in intensity and excessive in rate, a classical Parkinsonian dysarthria. The patient had had some kind of stutter in early life which he felt had returned since the development of Parkinson's disease. After 2 years using DAF, his speech remains totally fluent with a reduced rate and an improvement in intensity.

Those patients who did not benefit had either mild speech problems or showed marked akinetic features and slow, faint speech. The authors conclude that Parkinson's patients with festinant speech may benefit from permanently available DAF. Recently, Adams and Lang (1992) examined the therapeutic effects of auditory feedback masking at 90 dB, without delay, in 10 Parkinson's patients. All patients were judged to have low vocal intensity and were at various stages of onset from 1 to 26 years and at various levels of severity. These patients, in contrast to Downie *et al*'s subjects, had no prominent orofacial dyskinesia. All subjects showed a significant increase in vocal intensity in the masking condition compared with the no masking condition (a mean group increase of 4.7 dB) although there was individual variability. Adams and Lang also compared speech rate and intelligibility under masking and no masking. No significant effects on rate and intelligibility were found.

There would appear to be some useful therapeutic applications of DAF and masking for people with Parkinson's disease. Properly organized therapy programmes, supervised by speech pathologists, may hold promise for such patients and trials might also examine the therapeutic applications of DAF for other types of dysarthria.

From the above review of DAF investigation in aphasia, it seems that there are indications that DAF can have a beneficial effect on the speech quality of conduction aphasic patients and Wernicke's patients while reading, although no major therapeutic application of DAF with such patients has been exploited. It would appear that Broca's patients, and others with apraxia of speech, do not benefit from DAF. There may, however, be a clinical contribution of DAF to be exploited, in aiding diagnosis and prognosis. It may be, for instance, that DAF could be used to help determine the integrity of the auditory-motor speech system in fluent patients and the fragility of articulatory planning in non-fluent patients (Chapin *et al*, 1981). DAF might also prove useful as part of a therapeutic programme to improve the self-monitoring abilities of various types of aphasic patients.

DAF: Summary

DAF has had wide application in speech science since its effects were first described more than 40 years ago. It has contributed to knowledge concerning the role of auditory feedback in the control of ongoing speech production in normal subjects and has shed light on the development of auditory feedback from childhood to adulthood. It has also had a significant impact on theoretical explanations of stuttering, and has been successfully applied to therapeutic management. Research indicates that carefully designed studies, employing a range of tasks and clearly identified measures of change, can contribute to our understanding of neurological and neuropsychological disorders of communication, which may provide future help in clinical management, and the development of a number of body-worn DAF devices is enabling the application of DAF beyond the clinic.

Dichotic Listening

Introduction

Dichotic listening was developed primarily from pioneering work by Broadbent (1954) who was among the first to discover that normal subjects tended to show a right-ear preference, advantage or superiority for verbal material (Broadbent used digits) to the detriment of simultaneously presented, but different, verbal material at the left ear. The dichotic paradigm was further developed and extended to research on cerebral hemisphere asymmetries by Kimura (1961, 1967).

The dichotic method involves the simultaneous auditory presentation of different material to the separate ears of a subject via stereophonic headphones, usually from pre-recorded tape or computer storage. While one item or segment occurs at the left ear, a different item occurs at the right ear (see Hugdahl, 1988, for a recent collection). The materials used have been typically verbal (CVC words, CV syllables, digits, etc.) or non-verbal (tonal contours, music, environmental sounds, etc.), and the general and more or less consistent finding has been that normal right-handed subjects show a right-ear advantage (REA) for verbal material (Kimura, 1961, 1967; Shankweiler and Studdert-Kennedy, 1967; Studdert-Kennedy and Shankweiler, 1970) and a left-ear advantage (LEA) for non-verbal material (Bryden et al , 1982; Gregory, 1982; Gordon, 1970; Haggard and Parkinson, 1971; Kimura, 1964; Knox and Kimura, 1970).

The dominant model invoked to explain the effect is that first proposed by Kimura (1967) and illustrated in Figure 8.1. Two auditory pathways leave the inner ear: the *contralateral pathway*, which travels to the auditory area (Heschl's gyrus) in the temporal lobe of the cortical hemisphere opposite the ear, and the *ipsilateral pathway*, which runs to the auditory area in the temporal lobe of the cortical hemisphere on the same side as the ear. The contralateral pathway contains more fibres, is considered to be stronger and more efficient and is seen as inhibiting or blocking the signal travelling via the weaker ipsilateral pathway (Hall and Goldstein, 1968). On this model, the observed REA for verbal material is explained as a function of the relative superiority of the left hemisphere for verbal processing and the LEA for non-verbal material as a reflection of the relative superiority of the right hemisphere for non-verbal processing.

Consequently, dichotic listening has been widely used as a comparatively simple, cheap, non-invasive technique for inferring *hemispheric* advantage or preference for various materials in a variety of populations. Studies have been carried out with subjects suffering from a variety of communication disorders, including aphasia, apraxia, dysarthria, stuttering, dyslexia, delayed and disordered language and articulation, autism and Down's syndrome, among others.

In normal populations, dichotic listening has been used to examine the relationships between ear advantages (and by implication hemispheric advantages) and such variables as age, gender and handedness. Bryden and Allard (1978) concluded in their review of dichotic studies and language development that there is a 'gradual development of cerebral lateralization which approximates the adult state by the eighth grade' (puberty) (p. 398), although there are indicators to suggest that

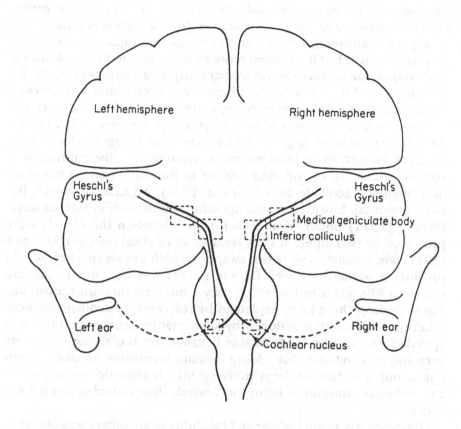

Figure 8.1. The contralateral and ipsilateral auditory pathways. See text for explanation.

the left hemisphere has become superior for speech perception by 5 years of age. These observations become important to questions concerned with whether left hemisphere specialization exists at birth and does not *develop* during childhood — the 'developmental invariance' hypothesis (Kinsbourne, 1975) — or whether there is bilateral hemispheric representation at birth, with both hemispheres being equipotential for language, with subsequent development of unilateral hemispheric specialization (Lenneberg, 1967). The ear advantages observed appear to be dependent upon the different phonetic characteristics of the competing stimuli (Berlin and Cullen, 1977; Darwin, 1974; Speaks *et al*, 1981; Studdert-Kennedy and Shankweiler, 1970). Normal subjects tend to report a preference for voiceless over voiced stops, for velar place of articulation over alveolar place, and for alveolar over bilabial place of articulation. These phonetic effects are so strong that if a

dichotic tape is not properly balanced with regard to phonetic preferences, a consistent *LEA* could be obtained from a normal population.

Right-ear advantages have been demonstrated again and again for
stop consonants but it has been more difficult to obtain significant ear
advantages for vowels (Studdert-Kennedy and Shankweiler, 1970).
This may be due to consonants being more 'encoded' than vowels
(Liberman *et al*, 1967) where consonants are seen as being perceived
'categorically' and vowels as being perceived 'continuously'. Consonant discrimination appears to be based on categorical phonetic
features held in short-term memory, whereas the discrimination of
vowels, which are considerably longer in duration, may be based on
non-linguistic acoustic cues (Darwin, 1974). An REA for vowels has
been obtained, however, by manipulating the stimuli in various ways.
Darwin (1971) obtained an REA for vowels when the vowels were
produced by two different sizes (synthetic) of vocal tract and Haggard
(1971) when subjects were not aware of which of two speakers would
produce a particular vowel. Darwin (1971) was also able to demonstrate an REA for fricatives when they contained formant transitions.
These findings have been explained by reference to acoustic memory
where intelligibility is reduced by such manipulations, and decay is
speeded up. An REA is obtainable because, on the acoustic memory
account, it is thought that adding formant transitions causes the left-
ear stimulus to fade or decay more rapidly in acoustic memory while
the right-ear stimulus is being processed, thus reducing the left-ear
score.

Problems exist with the size and reliability of ear differences observed
in dichotic studies. Despite large *group* differences being obtained, it is
often observed that the ear differences produced by *individuals* sometimes fail to reach statistical significance with the advantage to one ear
over the other usually falling between 2% and 6% (Schulhoff and Goodglass, 1969).

The test–retest reliability of dichotic ear preferences is reported to be
poor, with one study (Blumstein *et al*, 1975) showing that nearly 30% of
normal subjects reversed ear preference on retest. From the clinical
standpoint, it is interesting to note that brain-damaged subjects produce
good test–retest reliability figures (Niccum *et al*, 1981), and the simpler
single-report rhyming CVC word tests also report good test–retest
figures (Code, 1981; Johnson *et al*, 1977) with normal as well as brain-
damaged subjects.

Making a Dichotic Tape

Various methods are described in the literature for preparing dichotic
tapes (Code, 1981; Shankweiler and Studdert-Kennedy, 1967; Vincent
and Bradshaw, 1975). The method chosen will depend on the particular

experimental or clinical requirements of the test as well as the level of sophistication of the equipment available. Recent developments in microcomputing also allow a large variety of manipulations and controls of natural and synthetic speech, and these are discussed in Chapter 9 by Ziegler *et al.*

The method described here uses natural speech, as not only is this the simplest way, but it may be the safest procedure for determining gross preferences for 'speech'. Both natural and synthetic speech are used in dichotic tapes, with the advantage that synthetic speech segments can be stringently controlled for duration, onset, frequency and intensity, as well as selectively manipulated for various experimental motives. Manipulations may involve staggering presentation of items, specifying degree of friction in fricatives, duration of vowels and varying the transitions of formants in stops.

The equipment required includes a stereophonic reel-to-reel tape recorder, two mono reel-to-reel recorders, a sound-level meter, a dual-beam storage oscilloscope, a good-quality unidirectional microphone and a tape-editing kit. All tape-recorder heads must be cleaned and the two channels of the stereo machine must be checked for between-channel asymmetries before commencing. (For detailed discussion on the relative merits of different kinds of recording equipment and methods, see Chapter 1 of this book.)

It will first be necessary to decide on the type of stimulus material to be used (words, syllables, digits, etc.). For various reasons to be discussed below, a number of investigators who have completed dichotic studies with the communicatively impaired have preferred to use high frequency, CVC, simple, concrete words.

The next step is to decide on a mode of presentation. Stimuli can be presented in single pairs (one to the left and one to the right ear) with a pause between pairs to allow the subject to respond, or several pairs (typically three) can be presented in rapid succession followed by a pause for response.

Different patterns of response may be obtained depending on whether a *forced-choice* method is employed, where the subject is required to choose between one of the pairs of items presented, or *free-recall*, where subjects report as many items as they can remember. *Precued partial report* is also used where the subject is required to report the item or items at the ear specified by the examiner for a given trial. Typically, the subject is tapped on the left shoulder if the left-ear item is required or the right shoulder for the right-ear item. The mode of response must also be considered, especially with clinical populations who may have severe expressive difficulties, auditory retention or attentional impairments. The mode can be oral, written or gestural, where the subject points to written word or digit or a picture from a multiple-choice array.

There are a number of problems with the method of presentation that requires the subject to respond to several pairs of items presented in rapid succession, especially with clinical populations where patients may have auditory retention or attention difficulties. There is evidence to suggest that an increased memory load increases the right-ear score (Yeni-Komshian and Gordon, 1974) thereby giving an artificially enhanced laterality score (Bryden and Allard, 1978). One way to eliminate possible memory effects is to require subjects to report only a single stimulus item (Studdert-Kennedy and Shankweiler, 1970). The majority of studies with aphasic subjects have used single pairs for this reason. Shanks and Ryan (1976) in their study suggest that 'an ear advantage cannot be detected on trials where both stimulus items are correctly or incorrectly perceived' (p. 102). However, other studies have shown that ear differences are enhanced when both stimulus items are reported and it is the item reported second which is compared across ears rather than the one reported first (Goodglass and Peck, 1972; Satz *et al*, 1965).

Once the stimulus material has been chosen, a complete list of pairs should be written out, ensuring that each pair occurs an equivalent number of times for each ear. For instance, if the pair 'gun bun' is to be used six times on the tape, then the other pairs must occur six times, with one word of the pair occurring three times at each ear. The pairs must also be arranged on the tape in a quasi-random sequence and in such a way that half-way through the test (after 18 presentations for a 36-item test) the headphones can be reversed to control for any between-channel asymmetries in the playback equipment during testing.

The following method (after the test described by Starkey, 1974) uses six pairs of natural rhyming CVC words, all beginning with a stop consonant. Because the method uses only six pairs of words it is relatively simple, requires less time and produces a high-quality, second-generation tape. The stimulus word pairs first have to be recorded on one of the mono machines on fresh tape and the resulting tape spliced into loops, each loop bearing one pair (see Chapter 1 for advice on optimum recording conditions). Using a tape speed of 7.5 in/s, it is advisable to record the pairs about 10 s apart with a gap of about 3 s between each member of the pair. In this way, one word of the pair will be recorded, followed by a pause of 3 s, followed by the other member of the pair. This in turn is followed by about a 10 s pause before the next pair. Care must be taken at this stage to record words at similar levels by reference to the VU meter of the recorder. The resulting mono tape is then spliced into the separate loops, each loop containing a single word pair.

If a tape speed of 7.5 in/s has been used during recording, each loop will be about 75 in long with an inter-word gap of about 22.5 in. The time gaps allowed during recording between words and between word pairs must be doubled if a tape speed of 3.75 in/s is used. Whichever is used, the resulting loops can be shortened or lengthened by splicing in leader tape. Loops may need to be shorter or longer depending on the sizes of the mono machines used. The two mono tape recorders are then placed side-by-side on a bench and a chosen loop is threaded in such a way that the tape passes through the heads of both machines. The two machines are then connected to the two separate channels of the storage oscilloscope to check for simultaneity and amplitude. The recorders are switched to playback, and gradually moved closer to each other or further apart until the onsets of the two words are seen to be within +2 ms simultaneity on the screen of the oscilloscope. Once this has been achieved, the pairs can then be recorded on a master tape. To do this, the stereo machine is loaded with a fresh tape and the outputs of the two mono machines are connected to the two separate channels of the stereo recorder.

At this stage it is again advisable to check the equivalence of the amplitudes of the two words by playing the loop through the stereo machine without recording. The amplitudes can be checked on the VU meters of the stereo machine and the gain controls on the tape recorders adjusted until the results are satisfactory. A maximum of 4 dB discrepancy between words is recommended.

Once satisfied with simultaneity of onset and equivalence of amplitude, two words can be recorded on fresh tape on the separate channels of the stereo machine. Once this has been done, the master tape can be moved on to the next spot where it has been decided that the same pair will occur again (use a stopwatch to ensure equal distance on the master tape between pairs; 10 s between pairs is usual). For a 36-item test, the pair on the loop is recorded three times on the master tape so that one word of the pair occurs at the left ear during testing. The connecting leads from the two mono machines to the stereo recorder are then switched and the pair is then recorded three times so that the *other* word of the pair occurs at the left ear during testing.

Once this simple but laborious process is complete for all pairs, a master tape of high quality is available, which is only a second-generation tape. This dichotic tape can be preceded by a non-dichotic (binaural) trial tape where the individual words used in the test are presented several times in quasi-random sequence at 10 s intervals. Any number of reel-to-reel or cassette copies can be made from this master tape.

Using a computer with speech recording and storage capability can speed up this process and ensure more reliably controlled manipulation of the stimuli (see Chapter 9). The audio tapes with the stimulus items recorded on them can be recorded on the computer and manipulated using a speech analysis system. The resulting dichotic material can then either remain on the hard disk of the computer (taking care to make backup copies on diskette, of course) or transferred back to audio tape for experimental use.

Applications of dichotic listening in speech pathology and therapeutics

Dichotic listening studies have been conducted with most groups of communication disorders as the following review shows. The approach has been most widely utilized in aphasic and stuttering populations, and these studies are examined in detail.

Aphasia

A variety of response methods, stimulus materials and test lengths and diffi-culties have been employed in dichotic investigations with aphasic patients.

In an early study, Moore and Weidner (1975) found that their control group obtained significantly higher right-ear scores (RES) than either of three aphasic subgroups classified according to months post-onset (MPO). Furthermore, the left-ear score (LES) for the controls was signifi-cantly lower than for the aphasic group. No significant difference between the mean dichotic performance was obtained for the three onset groups, although Group 1(1–6 MPO) showed a small non-signifi-cant LEA, and Groups 2 (7–12 MPO) and 3 (+ 12 MPO) obtained signifi-cantly more mean correct LESs than RESs. Moore and Weidner suggest that there is a shift to the right undamaged cerebral hemisphere for language processing that increases as a function of time post-onset and this is reflected in ear advantages.

Johnson et al (1977) examined the relationship between the dichotic scores of aphasic subjects and initial severity of aphasia as determined by assessment within 4 weeks of onset of aphasia. Subjects were also grouped into less than 6 MPO and more than 6 MPO. All 20 controls produced the expected REA and 18 of the aphasic subjects (N = 20) an LEA. The factor of time since onset did not reach significance, but subjects more than 6 MPO did demonstrate a greater LEA than subjects of less than 6 MPO. Initial severity did significantly influence the results, however. The LEA scores of the initially mild-to-moderate group were significantly smaller than the LEA scores of the initially moderate-to-marked group. The authors interpreted these results to mean that there was a shift to the right hemisphere for linguistic processing, which was greater in the more severely aphasic subjects.

A longitudinal study (Pettit and Noll, 1979) measured dichotic perfor-mance and recovery in a group of subjects on two occasions separated by 2 months. Retest scores on aphasia tests indicated a significant improve-ment although there was much variability in individual performance. There was a significant improvement in LESs on retest, but no significant change in RESs. This result also was interpreted as strong support for the view that a lateral shift takes place as the patient improves in language ability.

Crosson and Warren (1981) compared Broca's and Wernicke's

patients and found no significant difference between the two groups with both groups producing a significant LEA as compared with the REA of the control group. The Wernicke's group producing the larger, but non-significant, LEA and the Broca's subjects produced the greatest variability in responses.

Dominance and lesion effects

Inferring hemispheric advantages from dichotic advantages assumes the integrity of the subject's entire auditory system, including the primary auditory cortices of both left and right hemispheres and the interconnecting commissural pathways. A number of studies have identified and examined a *lesion effect* in the dichotic performance of brain-damaged subjects (Kimura, 1961; Milner *et al*, 1968; Schulhoff and Goodglass, 1969; Sparks *et al*, 1970; Damasio and Damasio, 1979; Hugdahl *et al*, 1991) which should be separated from the *dominance effect*. The lesion effect tends to result in an impairment, suppression or total extinction of stimuli presented to the ear contralateral to the lesion, whereas the dominance effect produces the expected higher scores for material presented to the ear contralateral to the hemisphere specialized for processing that material (Schulhoff and Goodglass, 1969).

Schulhoff and Goodglass (1969) compared left-brain damaged and right-brain damaged subjects on a dichotic digit (verbal) and a dichotic musical (non-verbal) test and a 'neutral' dichotic click-counting task. On the basis of group analysis they found a bilateral decrement for material for which the damaged hemisphere is specialized. The left-brain damaged group showed a non-significant REA for digits, although six of the 10 subjects actually produced an LEA. These subjects produced a near-normal performance (LEA) for music and a reduction in the RES for neutral clicks. The results for the right-brain damaged group paralleled the findings for the left-brain damaged group. There was a bilateral decrement for digits, but a clear REA. A lesion effect was not observed for music however, but click-counting showed a lesion effect with a larger deficit for the left ear.

Sparks *et al* (1970) provide further confirmatory evidence that verbal dichotic information travels from left ear to right temporal lobe and thence to left temporal lobe via the corpus callosum and from right ear to left temporal lobe via the auditory pathways. On this interpretation, a left-hemisphere lesion can impede stimuli from the left ear via the corpus callosum, whereas a right hemisphere lesion can affect only a stimulus that has arrived directly from the left ear to the right temporal lobe via the auditory pathway. A diagrammatical representation of this model is shown in Figure 8.2.

Damasio and Damasio (1979) extended the dichotic paradigm to map the probable interhemispheric auditory pathway via the corpus

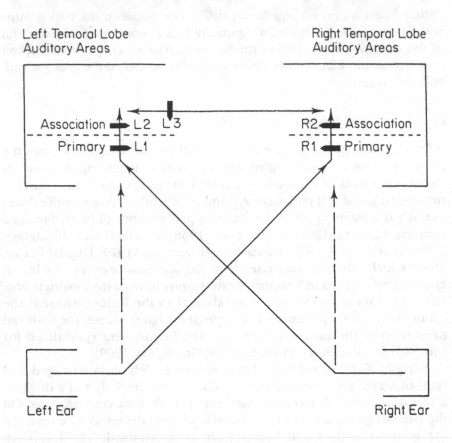

Figure 8.2. Model proposed by Sparks, Goodglass and Nickel (1970) to explain extinction of dichotic stimuli in brain damaged patients. The broken lines represent the ipsilateral pathways and the areas L1, L2, L3, R1, R2 represent the sites of lesions which can produce extinction.

callosum. They did this by comparing dichotic performance with actual lesion sites detected by computerized axial tomography (CAT) scans. Left ear extinction was found to be associated with lesions in the left and right posterior parieto-occipital and right mid-temporal region; and right ear extinction was related to lesions in the left temporal and right parieto-occipital regions. Subjects who obtained 'normal' ear preferences had lesions in the right frontal, left frontal and left posterior occipital region. The authors conclude that left-ear extinction in brain damaged subjects is associated with a lesion at any point along the course of the interhemispheric auditory pathway, irrespective of hemisphere, which runs from the geniculocortical pathways posteriorly and upwards to arch around the lateral ventricles joining the posterior region of the corpus callosum.

The question is how much credibility can be given to dichotic investigations with aphasic patients that have interpreted ear preference scores as indicative of a shift in hemispheric preference, as a function of time since onset, severity, or type of aphasia? Probably ear preferences produced by aphasic patients are determined by a combination of site of lesion (lesion effect) *and* hemispheric advantage (dominance effect). However, it may be possible to separate these effects in dichotic listening. The most consistent and robust result obtained is the increase in LESs scores over RESs as a function of time since onset. Studies that have examined other variables such as severity and type of aphasia have produced inconsistent results, which can unfortunately be explained just as well in terms of lesion effects. The lesion effect cannot explain the increase in LEA scores as a function of time since onset, however, nor does it explain why patients with anterior lesions (non-fluent aphasia), presumably with intact auditory cortex, should show an LEA. This is not to ignore the probable intimate relationship between the anterior (Broca's) and posterior (Wernicke's) areas. As Crosson and Warren (1981) have also pointed out, a lesion in the anterior area might interfere with the processing capabilities of the posterior area such that dichotic performance could be affected. Even so, current knowledge might indicate that non-fluent patients showing an LEA are demonstrating a genuine shift in hemispheric preference for verbal material, especially if this LEA can be shown to increase with time since onset.

The discussion of lesion effects has recently centred on a distinction between a perceptual effect and a cognitive one (Hugdahl and Wester, 1994) where a lesion outside the auditory pathways may still cause a lesion effect, but the underlying cause is due to a cognitive impairment with attention or orientation. Code (1983) attempted to examine whether it was possible to distinguish between aphasic subjects producing a lesion effect and those producing a dominance effect. The ear advantages of 27 aphasic subjects grouped into fluent (posterior) and non-fluent (anterior) were compared on a simple CVC word test. Results revealed highly significant increases in LESs and decreases in RESs in non-fluent subjects who were more than 12 MPO compared with non-fluent subjects who were less than 12 MPO. Significant differences were not found, however, in fluent subjects who were less than and more than 12 MPO. Such results may suggest that for non-fluent subjects with anterior damage and intact posterior mechanisms, superior LESs may reflect an increased involvement of the right hemisphere in verbal processing (dominance effect), but for fluent subjects with damage to posterior auditory processing mechanisms, dichotic responses reflect a lesion effect and cannot be reliably interpreted in terms of hemispheric shift. It could be that a lesion effect may mask any dominance effect in posteriorly damaged patients. However, this interpretation assumes that posterior mechanisms are unaffected by anterior damage, and this may be too simplistic and unrealistic a characterization of the relationship between anterior and posterior mechanisms.

The results are in general agreement with those reported by Castro-Caldas and Botelho (1980) who tested 117 aphasic subjects on three dichotic tests. In both a retrospective and longitudinal analysis, non-fluent patients showed a tendency towards an LEA with time since onset and fluent subjects a tendency towards REA with time since onset.

Stuttering

Dichotic listening has been used to examine the hypothesis first advanced by Orton (1928) and Travis (1931) that cerebral organization in stutterers is in some way different from that of non-stutterers. Curry and Gregory (1969) compared 20 adult stutterers and 20 adult non-stutterers on a dichotic CVC word test, a dichotic environmental sound test and a dichotic pitch test. Both groups showed the expected REA for the word test, although the REA was statistically significant only for the non-stutterers. No differences were obtained between the two groups on either the environmental sound or pitch tests. However, when the size of the absolute between-ears difference scores were compared, a highly significant superiority was observed for the control group. Moreover, 11 (55%) of the stutterers actually showed an LEA on the word test which was masked by the group analysis. It was also reported that a number of those stutterers (73%) producing an LEA showed an REA for one or other of the non-verbal tests.

Brady and Berson (1975) examined 35 severe adult stutterers and a matched group of controls, all right-handed. The CVC test developed by Shankweiler and Studdert-Kennedy (1967) was used where subjects responded by circling one of the two written nonsense syllables. All controls produced the expected REA, with six (17%) of the stutterers producing an LEA that failed to reach significance. No differences in severity or gender were apparent between the LEA and REA subgroups of stutterers. Stutterers also showed smaller between ear differences than non-stutterers. The study concludes that there may be a subset of stutterers whose hemispheric organization is different.

Dorman and Porter (1975) compared 16 right-handed moderate/severe adult stutterers and 20 controls. The test used 120 single-pair presentations of synthetic CV syllables and subjects responded by writing both syllables down. Male stutterers and male and female non-stutterers produced a significant REA on the test, but female stutterers as a group (N = 4) did not, although three of these subjects did produce large REA scores. No significant differences between groups emerged and the authors suggest that there is no support for the Orton-Travis theory.

Rosenfield and Goodglass (1980) conducted a study that attempted to avoid some of the methodological shortcomings of earlier studies in the hope of producing more unequivocal results. They restricted the study to well-matched male stutterers and controls and examined non-verbal ear preferences with Kimura's (1964) dichotic melodies test. The verbal test was a natural CV syllable single-pair test which required written report of both syllables. Order of report was also controlled for by the examiner tapping subjects on either right or left shoulder before each pair. Each subject was required to write down first the CV syllable corresponding to the side which had been tapped.

As mentioned earlier, some studies have shown that ear differences are enhanced when the stimulus which is reported *second* is compared across ears rather than the first stimulus (Satz *et al*, 1965; Goodglass and Peck, 1972). The investigators also conducted a retest for all subjects one week after the first testing to compare stability of preferences in the groups. Group analysis of the degree of REA showed no differences between the two groups on the CV test. Controls produced a greater difference between ears on the stimuli reported second than on those reported first, in agreement with previous studies. However, the stuttering groups produced the opposite result — ear differences on the stimuli reported first were greater than those reported second. This pattern for stutterers and non-stutterers was repeated on retest. On examining the consistency of *individual* subjects between tests and retests it was found that subjects in both groups changed ear preference on retest on the verbal task, but the proportion of control subjects who showed consistent REA was greater than stutterers. Over 25% of stutterers produced a consistent LEA. Group analysis showed that non-stutterers and stutterers showed an LEA for the musical test. Individual results on test and retest revealed that consistency between the two tests for both groups was poor, but worse for the stutterers.

These results suggest 'abnormal' lateralization for verbal and non-verbal material for a subgroup of stutterers which would support the Orton-Travis theory, as although group analysis revealed no differences, the individual performances of some stutterers showed marked deviations.

It was indicated earlier that the dichotic listening paradigm constitutes a *perceptual* task. Consequently, direct inferences about hemispheric processing of speech *production* or expression cannot legitimately be made. In conventional dichotic studies, the most that can be claimed is that ear advantages may reflect a hemispheric perceptual preference, even in those studies using oral report. Sussman and MacNeilage (1975) developed a method, which they considered measured hemispheric perceptual and production processes. They combined a dichotic listening task with a paradigm they called *pursuit auditory tracking* to compare language lateralization in adult stutterers and non-stutterers. The procedure required the subject to match a tone in one ear with a tone in the second ear. The tone in the second ear varied randomly in frequency and amplitude under computer control.

The subject could manipulate the tone in the first ear by movement of the jaw or tongue. This movement was transformed into signals that varied the tone in the first ear so that the subject could attempt to match up the tones. Sussman and MacNeilage argue that pursuit auditory tracking is capable of measuring hemispheric involvement in speech production. A comparison of stutterers and non-stutterers on this combined paradigm showed that non-stutterers as a group were more adept at the articulatory task (i.e. non-stutterers were better at manipulating the right ear tone to match the randomly varied tone in the left ear). This was interpreted as an REA (left-hemisphere preference) for speech production in non-stutterers. Stutterers did not show such a preference, which suggests that, as a group, the stutterers demonstrated less left-hemisphere superiority for perception and production than the normal group. However, a subgroup again emerged whose hemispheric superiority matched that of the non-stutterers, confirming a consistently observed finding that some stutterers do perform as if they were less lateralized for language processing.

Some studies have examined dichotic advantages in stuttering children. Gruber and Powell (1974) found no significant differences between 28 stuttering and 28 non-stuttering children using a test employing the presentation of digits in sets of three. However, the ages ranged from 8 years 5 months to 18 years 8 months.

In contrast, Sommers, Brady and Moore (1975) in their comparison of right-handed stuttering and non-stuttering children and adults obtained different results. This study examined dichotic word and digit performance of 78 subjects, between the ages of 41 and 48 years and classified into three age groups, with 13 stutterers in each group. The dichotic word test consisted of four pairs of CVC rhyming words and the digit test of four pairs of digits. A single-pair presentation oral-report method was used with all subjects. Results on the word test showed that non-stutterers produced larger ear-preference scores. A larger proportion of stutterers failed to show an REA and only 16 of the 39 stutterers across all three age groups produced an REA. On the digit test, 9 non-stutterers and 17 stutterers failed to produce an REA, and 9 stutterers across all age groups produced an LEA score. Excluding the effect of age, no differences were found for non-stutterers, but stuttering children produced significantly lower REA scores than stuttering adults.

These results again support the finding that separate subgroups of stutterers exist, some of whom may have a lack of lateralization for linguistic processing or bilateral representation. The authors also speculate that the spontaneous remission of stuttering in older children may have something to do with the development of speech perception or the establishment of hemispheric dominance, and that these functions may be slower to develop in stutterers.

Some consistent trends appear to emerge from an inspection of the research on dichotic listening in stutterers. Studies that have examined individual scores more closely have found that there are grounds for believing in the existence of two distinct subgroups: one which shows ear advantages similar to non-stutterers and one which does not. There are some indications that severity of stuttering and age may be related to this finding. It would appear that the variables of sex and handedness (particularly familiar left-handedness) need to be examined in future studies.

Dichotic studies have been completed with a range of other speech, language and learning disordered groups relevant to speech pathology, including dyslexic and poor reading children and adults, language disordered and articulation disordered children, and minimal brain damaged and Down's syndrome children. Some of these studies will be briefly discussed.

Dichotic investigations of individuals with reading disability were comprehensively reviewed by Satz (1976) who showed that results have been equivocal with some studies demonstrating an REA and others failing to produce significant ear advantages. The issues are discussed by Beaumont and Rugg (1978) and Wilsher (1981). Witelson (1976, 1977) used dichotic digits and visual tactile tests to examine lateral advantage in dyslexic children. Her results indicated that such children demonstrate left-hemisphere advantage for verbal material, but right-hemisphere advantage for non-verbal material. This led her to suggest that dyslexia is due to a dysfunction of the right hemisphere, imposing extra non-verbal responsibilities on the left. The left becomes overloaded, responsible as it is for verbal and non-verbal processing, and its verbal efficiency is reduced. Support for Witelson's hypothesis has come from Newell and Rugel (1981). Using dichotic melodies and digits they found an REA for digits in normal and disabled readers, but disabled readers also produced an REA for music in contrast to the LEA found in the normal group.

The opposing view, that dyslexia represents a right-hemisphere specialization for language, has received some support from dichotic studies by Chasty (1981). Using four sets of digits, he obtained an LEA in dyslexic children, which he suggests reflects a less efficient neurological organization for language for such children. (As in other areas of dichotic research, comparisons between studies are precarious due to such factors as design differences, dichotic test differences and subject criteria.) In contrast, a three-pair dichotic digit study of illiterate adults (Tzavaras, Kaprinis and Gatzoyas, 1981) showed a highly superior REA with near extinction of the left ear, suggesting that reading and writing skills in *educated* adults involve considerable right-hemisphere involvement.

A series of studies conducted by Sommers and associates examined ear advantages in a range of speech and language disordered children. Most of these studies have used the simple single CVC rhyming word pair test described earlier. Sommers and Taylor (1972) examined the ear preferences of speech and language delayed children used a two- and three-pair digit test. These children produced significantly greater LEA scores in contrast to the control group's significantly better REA. Sommers *et al* (1972) compared the performance of normal, mild articulation disordered, severely articulation disordered and minimally brain damaged articulation disordered children on the single-pair word test. They found a relationship between severity and ear preference. The more severe the articulation problem, the greater the tendency towards an LEA for words; the severe group produced no ear preferences suggesting a lack of left-hemisphere specialization for language.

Sommers and Starkey (1977) investigated the ear preferences of Down's syndrome children in a high speech and language performance and a low speech and language performance group. Controls produced the expected REA but both groups of Down's syndrome subjects failed to produce any ear preference. Examinations of the phonetic effects of the test showed that the high performance group tended to produce similar phonetic preferences to the normal group, but the low performance group tended to produce different phonetic preferences. This is in contrast to the result produced by Hartley (1981), who found an LEA in 11 young Down's syndrome female subjects. Hartley used a single-syllable 38 word-pair test with oral report.

Prior and Bradshaw (1979) examined the performance of 19 autistic children on a 24 single-syllable word-pair test. They found considerable variability in results, with five subjects showing an REA, seven an LEA and the remaining seven no ear preference. There were correlations also between ear preferences and the presence or absence of speech before the age of 5 years as well as a relation with IQ level. The authors suggest that the LEA group may have developed right-hemisphere dominance for language.

Clinical applications

Dichotic listening is an experimental paradigm about which there is still considerable uncertainty concerning stimulus material, test length, response methods and the power of dichotic listening to tap and measure hemispheric advantage for auditory perception. Already there are clinics which use dichotic listening as a simple non-invasive method for investigating hemispheric advantage on a routine basis, although it is clear that there are a number of questions concerning general reliability that remain to be answered. Bearing this in mind, the state of the art is such that dichotic listening is a useful non-invasive, relatively simple and cheap technique, the results of which, especially with the brain damaged, need to be supplemented by other forms of investigation. With current knowledge it is safer to suggest that the technique can have only a contributory role.

We have seen that there are indications that dichotic listening may have a contribution to make in the future as a non-invasive method for localizing lesions. In the management of aphasia, the planning of treatment methods that are designed to utilize the undamaged hemisphere (Buffery and Burton, 1982; Burton *et al*, 1987; Code, 1989, 1994) can be aided by dichotic assessment. More information can be obtained if non-verbal as well as verbal dichotic processing is assessed and tachistoscopic hemifield viewing might be utilized to supplement dichotic results. At present, however, dichotic listening is predominantly an experimental technique, and its general clinical application remains to be determined more fully.

Therapeutic applications

There are, as yet, few reports of the application of dichotic listening in the treatment of communication disorders. However, it would appear that there is much scope for the development of such treatment methods. The experiment described by Code (1989) employed specially made dichotic tapes to direct material to the undamaged right hemisphere of an aphasic patient in an attempt specifically to improve his auditory-verbal comprehension. One to three pairs of digits were employed to increase auditory-verbal memory span and dichotically contrasting CV syllables were used to improve phonemic discrimination. Dichotic and hemifield viewing methods were also combined in a cross-model programme. The patient improved dramatically on digit retention and other specific areas, but made only modest improvement in general communicative ability as determined by aphasia battery assessment. The results were considered promising, however, and indicated that the method should be examined further.

Burton, Kemp and Burton (1987) used a tighter experimental design in a single-case study that used a modified dichotic task to examine the effects of semantic priming of the right hemisphere on picture-naming performance in a 55-year-old aphasic man of 2 years post-CVA. The study ran for six treatment sessions and entailed treating (priming) and testing on four sets of pictures in a pre-test and post-test and a priming condition. The patient had to use a 'Yes' or 'No' response to indicate whether the picture he was shown matched the word he heard. In two sessions the material was presented in dichotic competition and the patient had to attend to his left ear; in two other sessions material was presented for attention of the right ear and in the final two sessions the presentation was binaural and the patient had to attend to the left and then the right ear. No support was found for priming the right hemisphere and there was no difference between right and left dichotic presentation and binaural presentation, and there was no evidence of improved naming. Semantic priming of the right hemisphere failed to improve naming, at least in the short term and in this patient (see Code, 1987 and 1994, for further discussion of the role of the right hemisphere in treatment of aphasia).

It is clear that relationships have been inferred between neuropsychological dysfunction or abnormality and a range of communication disorders. It would seem logical, therefore, for those concerned with the treatment of such disorders to consider the possibilities of employing techniques such as dichotic listening, possibly in combination with hemifield viewing. For specific disorders, which may be characterized by difficulties in deriving sound from print, for instance, a combined method could direct material to just one or to both hemispheres (auditory to one, visual to the other).

Dichotic listening: summary

We have examined in some detail the major studies that have been carried out with individuals exhibiting a variety of communication disorders. We have spent more time considering those studies in aphasia and stuttering as other areas are less well developed. A number of conclusions emerge. First, it is clear that many investigators feel that ear advantages which differ from those of normal control groups reflect a different neurocognitive organization in many groups. Different neurocognitive organization, whether right-hemisphere dominance, bilateral representation, disordered or inefficient interhemispheric transmission, has been proposed as a major contributory factor in many human communication disorders. Indeed, the disorder which does not have such neurocognitive abnormalities as part of its underlying aetiology would appear, on the basis of the interpretations made of dichotic results, to be very rare!

We have seen also that it is by no means certain that there is a cause and effect relationship between ear and hemispheric advantage, that the reliability of dichotic tests is low (at least with some tests) and that brain damage will cause ear advantages which may have more to do with the nature and site of the lesion than with the hemispheric advantage for particular kinds of material.

We have also seen that a number of response modes have been used in dichotic studies as well as a variety of materials. Furthermore, subject selection criteria have been different, as well as analysis of results. While researchers will continue to adopt the methods that appear most appropriate to them, the lack of consistency between studies with regard to these critical variables makes comparison of results difficult and replication with 'non-normal' groups disappointing.

Clearly, a great deal more research is required to establish the most appropriate forms of dichotic tests and the best methods of administration for clinical use that are reliable and valid measures of hemispheric preference for various aspects of language.

References

Adams SG, Lang AE. Can the Lombard effect be used to improve low voice intensity in Parkinson's disease? European Journal of Disorders of Communication 1992; 27: 121–27.

Beaumont GJ, Rugg MD. Neuropsychological laterality of function and dyslexia.

Dyslexia Review 1978; 1: 18–21.

Beaumont JT, Foss BM. Individual differences in reacting to delayed auditory feedback. British Journal of Psychology 1957; 48: 85–89.

Berlin CI, Cullen JK Jnr. Acoustic problems in dichotic listening tasks. In Segalowitz SJ, Gruber FG. (Eds), Language Development and Neurological Theory. New York: Academic Press, 1977.

Blumstein S, Goodglass H, Tartter V. The reliability of ear advantage in dichotic listening. Brain and Language 1975; 2: 226–36.

Boller F, Marcie P. Possible role of abnormal auditory feedback in conduction aphasia. Neuropsychologia 1978; 16: 521–24.

Boller F, Vrtunski PB, Kim Y, Mack JL. Delayed auditory feedback and aphasia. Cortex 1978; 14: 212–26.

Borden GJ. An interpretation of research on feedback interruption in speech. Brain and Language 1979; 7: 307–19.

Borden GJ, Dorman MF, Freeman FJ, Niimi S. Coordination of phonation and articulation during delayed auditory feedback. Paper presented at the American Speech and Hearing Association Convention, Houston, Texas, 1976.

Brady JP, Berson J. Stuttering, dichotic listening and cerebral dominance. Archives of General Psychiatry 1975; 32: 1449–52.

Broadbent D. The role of auditory localization in attention and memory. Journal of Experimental Psychology 1954; 47: 191–96.

Bryden MP, Allard F. Dichotic listening and the development of linguistic processes. In Kinsbourne M. (Ed.), Asymmetrical Function of the Brain. Cambridge: Cambridge University Press, 1978.

Bryden MP, Ley G, Sugarman JH. A left-ear advantage for identifying the emotional quality of tonal sequences. Neuropsychologia 1982; 20: 3–7.

Buffery AW, Burton A. Information processing and redevelopment: towards a science of neuropsychological rehabilitation. In Burton A. (Ed.), The Pathology and Psychology of Cognition. London: Methuen, 1982.

Burton A, Kemp R, Burton E. Hemispheric priming and picture naming in an aphasic patient. Aphasiology 1987; 1: 41–51.

Buxton LF. An investigation of sex and age differences in speech behaviour under delayed auditory feedback. PhD thesis, Ohio State University, 1969.

Castro-Caldas A, Botelho MAS. Dichotic listening in the recovery of aphasia after stroke. Brain and Language 1980; 10: 145–51.

Chapin C, Blumstein SE, Meisser B, Boller F. Speech production mechanisms in aphasia: a delayed auditory feedback study. Brain and Language 1981; 14: 106–13.

Chase RA, Sutton S, First D, Zubin J. A developmental study of changes in behavior under delayed auditory feedback. Journal of Genetic Psychology 1961; 99: 101–12.

Chasty H. Dichotic stimulation effects in dyslexics and normal children. Dyslexia Review 1981; 4: 8–9.

Cherry C, Sayer B. Experiments upon the total inhibition of stammering by external control and some clinical results. Journal of Psychosomatic Research 1956; 1: 233–46.

Code C. Genuine and artificial stammering: an EMG comparison. British Journal of Disorders of Communication 1979; 14: 5–16.

Code C. Delayed auditory feedback and auditory feedback masking with stammerers and normal speakers. Australian Journal of Human Communication Disorders 1980; 8: 40–48.

Code C. Dichotic listening with the communicatively impaired: Results from trials of a Short British-English Dichotic Word Test. Journal of Phonetics 1981; 9: 375–83.

Code C. The validity of dichotic listening as an indicator of hemispheric shift in aphasia: Dominance vs lesion effects in the performance of fluent and non-fluent subjects. Paper presented at Dysphasia Conference, Middlesex Hospital, London, 1983.

Code C. Language, Aphasia, and the Right Hemisphere. Chichester: Wiley, 1987.

Code C. Hemispheric specialization retraining in aphasia: possibilities and problems. In Code C, Muller DJ. (Eds), Aphasia Therapy. London: Whurr, 1989.

Code C. Role of the right hemisphere in the treatment of aphasia. In Chapey R. (Ed.), Language Intervention Strategies in Adult Aphasia, 3rd edn. Baltimore: Williams & Wilkins, 1994.

Code C. Models, theories and hearistics in apraxia of speech in neuropsychology. Clinical Linguistics and Phonetics. In press

Crosson R, Warren RL. Dichotic ear preferences for C-V-C words in Wernicke's and Broca's aphasia. Cortex 1981; 17: 249–58.

Curlee RF, Perkins WH. Conversational rate control therapy for stuttering. Journal of Speech and Hearing Disorders 1969; 34: 245–50.

Curry FKW, Gregory HH. The performance of stutterers on dichotic listening tasks thought to reflect cerebral dominance. Journal of Speech and Hearing Research 1969; 12: 73–82.

Damasio H, Damasio AR. 'Paradoxic' extinction in dichotic listening: possible anatomic significance. Neurology 1979; 29: 644–53.

Darley FL, Aronson AE, Brown JR. Motor Speech Disorders. Philadelphia: WB Saunders, 1975.

Darwin CJ. Ear differences in the recall of fricatives and vowels. Quarterly Journal of Experimental Psychology 1971; 23: 46–62.

Darwin CJ. Ear differences and hemispheric specialization. In Schmidt FO, Worden F. (Eds), The Neurosciences, vol. 3. Cambridge, MA: MIT Press, 1974.

Dewar A, Dewar AD, Anthony JFK. The effect of auditory feedback masking on concomitant movements of stammering. British Journal of Disorders of Communication 1976; 11: 95–102.

Dorman MF, Porter RJ. Hemispheric lateralization for speech perception in stutterers. Cortex 1975; 11:181–85.

Downie AW, Low JM, Lindsay DD. Speech disorder in Parkinsonism: usefulness of delayed auditory feedback in selected cases. British Journal of Disorders of Communication 1981; 16: 135–39.

Fairbanks G. A theory of the speech mechanism as a ServoSystem. Reproduced in Experimental Phonetics: Selected Articles by Grant Fairbanks (1966). Illinois: University of Illinois Press, 1954.

Fairbanks G. Selective vocal effects of delayed auditory feedback upon articulation. Reproduced in Experimental Phonetics: Selected Articles by Grant Fairbanks (1966). Illinois: University of Illinois Press,1955.

Goodglass H, Peck EA. Dichotic ear order effects in Korsakoff and normal subjects. Neuropsychologia 1972; 10: 211–17.

Goldiamond I. Stuttering and fluency as manipulatable operant response classes. In Krasner L, Ullman L. (Eds), Research in Behaviour Modification, New York: Holt, 1965.

Gordon MC. Some effects of stimulus presentation rate and complexity on perception and retention in brain damaged patients. Cortex 1970; 6: 723–86.

Gregory AH. Ear dominance for pitch. Neuropsychologia 1982; 20: 89–90.

Gruber L, Powell RL. Responses of stuttering and non-stuttering children to a dichotic listening task. Perceptual and Motor Skills 1974; 38: 263–64.

Haggard MP. Encoding and the REA for speech signals. Quarterly Journal of Experimental Psychology 1971; 23: 3445.

Haggard MP, Parkinson AM. Stimulus and task factors as determinants of ear advantages. Quarterly Journal of Experimental Psychology 1971; 23: 168–77.

Hall JL, Goldstein MH. Representation of binaural stimuli by single units in primary auditory cortex of unanesthetized cats. Journal of the Acoustical Society of America 1968; 43: 456–61.

Harrington J. Stuttering, delayed auditory feedback and linguistic rhythm. Journal of Speech and Hearing Research 1988; 31: 36–37

Hartley XY. Lateralisation of speech stimuli in young Down's syndrome children. Cortex 1981; 17: 241–48.

Hugdahl K. (Ed.), Handbook of Dichotic Listening: Theory, Methods and Reserarch. Chichester: Wiley, 1988.

Hugdahl K, Wester K. Auditory neglect and the ear extinction effect in dichotic listening: a reply to Beaton and McCarthy (1993). Brain and Language 1994; 46: 166–73.

Hugdahl K, Wester K, Asbjornsen A. Auditory neglect after right frontal and right pulvinar thalamic lesions. Brain and Language 1991; 41: 465–73.

Huggins AWF. Accurate delays for auditory feedback experiments. Quarterly Journal of Experimental Psychology 1967; 19: 78–80.

Johns DF, LaPointe LL. Neurogenic disorders of output processing: apraxia of speech. In Whitaker H, Whitaker HA. (Eds), Studies in Neurolinguistics, vol. 1. New York: Academic Press, 1976.

Johnson JP, Sommers RK, Weidner WE. Dichotic ear preference in aphasia. Journal of Speech and Hearing Research 1977; 20: 116–29.

Kalinowski J, Armson J, Stuart A, Mieszkowski M, Gracco V. Effects of alterations in auditory feedback and speech rate on stuttering frequency. Language and Speech 1993; 36: 1–16.

Kimura D. Cerebral dominance and the perception of verbal stimuli. Canadian Journal of Psychology 1961; 15: 166–71.

Kimura D. Left-right differences in the perception of melodies. Quarterly Journal of Experimental Psychology 1964; 16: 355–58.

Kimura D. Functional asymmetry of the brain in dichotic listening. Cortex 1967; 3: 163–78.

Kinsbourne M. The ontogeny of cerebral dominance. In Aaronson O, Reiber RW. (Eds), Developmental Psycholinguistics and Communication Disorders, vol. 263. New York: New York Academy of Sciences, 1975.

Knox C, Kimura D. Cerebral processing of nonverbal sounds in boys and girls. Neuropsychologia 1970; 8: 227–37.

Lee BS. Effects of delayed speech feedback. Journal of the Acoustical Society of America 1950; 22: 824–26.

Lenneberg EH. Biological Foundations of Language. New York: Wiley, 1967.

Liberman AM, Cooper FS, Shankweiler D, Studdert-Kennedy M. Perception of the speech code. Psychological Review 1967; 74: 431–61.

Lombard E. Le signe de l'elevation de la voix. Ann. Mal. Oreil. Larynx. 1911; 37: 101–119.

Low JM, Lindsay DD. A body-worn delayed auditory feedback fluency aid for stammerers. Journal of Biomechanical Engineering 1979; 1: 235–39.

Lozano RA, Dreyer DE. Some effects of delayed auditory feedback on dyspraxia of speech. Journal of Communication Disorders 1978; 11: 407–15.

Mackay D. Metamorphosis of a critical interval: age-linked changes in the delay of auditory feedback that produces maximum disruption of speech. Journal of the Acoustical Society of America 1968; 43: 1–21.

Milner B, Taylor L, Sperry R. Lateralized suppression of dichotically presented digits after commissural section in man. Science 1968; 161: 184–86.

Moore WH Jr, Weidner WE. 'Dichotic word-perception of aphasic and normal subjects. Perceptual and Motor Skills 1975; 40: 379–86.

Muellerleile S. Portable delayed auditory feedback device: a preliminary report. Journal of Fluency Disorders 1981; 6: 361–63.

Neelly JN. A study of the speech behaviour of stutterers and non-stutterers under normal and delayed auditory feedback. Journal of Speech and Hearing Disorders 1961; Suppl 7: 63–82.

Newell D, Rugel RP. Hemispheric specialization in normal and disabled readers. Journal of Learning Disabilities 1981; 14: 296–97.

Niccum N, Rubens AB, Speaks C. Effects of stimulus material on the dichotic listening performance of aphasic patients. Journal of Speech and Hearing Research 1981; 24: 526–34.

Orton ST. A physiological theory of reading disability and stuttering in children. New England Journal of Medicine 1928; 199: 1045–52.

Pettit JM, Noll JD. Cerebral dominance in aphasia recovery. Brain and Language 1979; 7: 191–200.

Prior MR, Bradshaw JL. Hemisphere functioning in autistic children. Cortex 1979; 15: 73–81.

Rosenfield DB, Goodglass H. Dichotic testing of cerebral dominance in stutterers. Brain and Language 1980; 11: 170–80.

Ryan BP. Operant procedures applied to stuttering therapy for children. Journal of Speech and Hearing Disorders 1971; 36: 264–80.

Ryan BP, Van Kirk B. Re-establishment, transfer and maintenance of fluent speech in 50 stutterers using delayed auditory feedback and operant procedures. Journal of Speech and Hearing Disorders 1974; 39: 3–10.

Sark S, Kalinowski J, Armson J, Stuart A. Stuttering amelioration at various auditory feedback delays and speech rates. Paper presented at the Annual Convention of the American Speech-Language-Hearing Association, Anaheim, California, 1993.

Satz P. Cerebral dominance and reading disability: an old problem revisited. In Knights RM, Baker DJ. (Eds), The Neuropsychology of Learning Disorders. Baltimore: University Park Press, 1976.

Satz P, Aschenbach K, Pattishall E, Fennell E. Order of report, ear, asymmetry, and handedness in dichotic listening. Cortex 1965; 1: 377–96.

Schulhoff C, Goodglass H. Dichotic listening, side of brain injury and cerebral dominance. Neuropsychologia 1969; 7:149–60.

Shanks J, Ryan W. A comparison of aphasic and non-brain-injured adults on a dichotic CV-syllable listening task. Cortex 1976; 12: 100–12.

Shankweiler D, Studdert-Kennedy M. Identification of consonants and vowels presented to left and right ears. Quarterly Journal of Experimental Psychology 1967; 19: 59–63.

Siegel GM, Fehst CA, Garber SR, Pick HL. Delayed auditory feedback with children. Journal of Speech and Hearing Research 1980; 23: 802–13.

Singh S, Schlanger B. Effects of delayed sidetone on the speech of aphasic, dysarthric, and mentally retarded subjects. Language and Speech 1969; 12:167–74.

Soderberg G. Delayed auditory feedback and the speech of stutterers. Journal of Speech and Hearing Disorders 1969; 33: 20–29.

Sommers RK, Taylor ML. Cerebral speech dominance in language-disordered and normal children. Cortex 1972; 8: 224–32.

Sommers RK, Starkey KL. Dichotic verbal processing in Down's syndrome children having qualitatively different speech and language skills. American Journal of Mental Deficiency 1977; 82: 44–53.

Sommers RK, Moore WH Jr, Brady WA, Jackson P. Performance of articulatory defective, minimal brain dysfunctioning, and normal children on dichotic ear preference, laterality and fine-motor tasks. Journal of Special Education 1972; 10: 5–14.

Sommers RK, Brady WA, Moore WH Jr. Dichotic ear preferences of stuttering children and adults. Perceptual and Motor Skills 1975; 41: 931–38.

Sparks R, Goodglass H, Nickel B. Ipsilateral versus contralateral extinction in dichotic listening resulting from hemispheric lesions. Cortex 1970; 6: 249–60.

Speaks C, Carney E, Niccum N, Johnson C. Stimulus dominance in dichotic listening. Journal of Speech and Hearing Research 1981; 24: 430–37.

Stanton JB. The effects of DAF on the speech of aphasic patients. Scottish Medical Journal 1958; 3: 378–84.

Starkey K. The dichotic testing of young children: a new test for the speech and hearing impaired. Masters thesis, Kent State University, Ohio, 1974.

Studdert-Kennedy M, Shankweiler D. Hemispheric specialization for speech perception. Journal of the Acoustical Society of America 1970; 48: 579–94.

Sussman HM, MacNeilage PF. Hemispheric specialization for speech production and perception in stutterers. Neuropsychologia 1975; 13: 19–27.

Tiffany W, Hanley C, Sutherland L. A simple mechanical adaptor for variable sidetone delay. Journal of Speech and Hearing Disorders 1954; 19: 504–6.

Timmons B, Boudreau J. Auditory feedback as a major factor in stuttering. Journal of Speech and Hearing Disorders 1972; 37: 476–84.

Travis LE. Speech Pathology. New York: Appleton-Century, 1931.

Tzavaras A, Kaprinis G, Gatzoyas A. Literacy and hemispheric specialization for language: digit dichotic listening in illiterates. Neuropsychologia 1981; 19: 565–70.

Van Riper C. Speech Correction. Principles and Methods. Englewood Cliffs, NJ: Prentice-Hall, 1954.

Van Riper C. The use of DAF in stuttering therapy. British Journal of Disorders of Communication 1970; 5: 40–45.

Van Riper C. The Nature of Stuttering. Englewood Cliffs, NJ: Prentice-Hall, 1971.

Van Riper C. The Treatment of Stuttering. Englewood Cliffs, NJ: Prentice-Hall, 1973.

Venkatagiri HS. The relevance of DAF-induced speech disruption to the understanding of stuttering. Journal of Fluency Disorders 1980; 5: 87–98.

Vincent T, Bradshaw J. A simple device for the preparation of exactly aligned dichotic tapes. Behavior Research Methods and Instrumentation 1975; 7: 534–38.

Vrtunski PB, Mack JL, Boller F, Kim YC. Response to delayed auditory feedback in patients with hemispheric lesions. Cortex 1976; 12: 395–404.

Wilsher CR. Right hemisphere dominant or left hemisphere dysfunction. Dyslexia Review 1981; 4: 5–7.

Witelson S. Sex and the single hemisphere: specialization of the right hemisphere for spatial processing. Science 1976; 193: 426–27.

Witelson S. Developmental dyslexia: two right hemispheres and none left. Science 1977; 195: 309–11.

Yates A. Delayed auditory feedback. Psychological Bulletin 1963; 60: 213–32.

Yeni-Komshian GH, Gordon JF. The effects of memory load on the right ear advantage in dichotic listening. Brain and Language 1974; 1: 375–81.

Chapter 9
Microcomputer-Based Experimentation, Assessment and Treatment

WOLFRAM ZIEGLER, MATHIAS VOGEL, JÜRGEN TEIWES AND
THOMAS AHRNDT

Introduction

With the continuous advance in microcomputer technology computers
have become a common tool in clinical phonetics. They are widely used
to collect and handle the large amounts of data that are produced by the
different speech measurement devices reviewed in this volume, and clinicians become more and more acquainted with computerized versions
of analogue instrumentations such as the sound spectrograph, the
Nasometer or the Visipitch. It goes without saying that all areas of instrumental clinical phonetics have profited considerably from the versatility
and the economy of microcomputer applications. Yet, in many instances,
the use of a computer in itself makes no particularly novel methodological contribution and therefore deserves no separate consideration
within the present volume.

Beyond the subsidiary functions in the acquisition and analysis of
analogue signals, however, microcomputer applications bear a number
of novel options that are highly relevant in speech science and in the
clinical management of speech disordered patients. Among these, a
microcomputer's capacities to organize extensive stimulus-databases
and to control complex stimulus-response-chains are considered most
important, for these capacities provide the basis for constructing clinically and experimentally appropriate speaking and listening tasks.
Endowed with a sufficiently flexible architecture, a computer-based
system may allow researchers and clinicians to realize a great variety of
experimental paradigms. In the light of the increasing importance of a
'cognitive neurolinguistic approach' towards an understanding of
speech and language disorders it seems particularly attractive to dispose
of an 'experimental toolbox' that permits flexible examination of differ-

ent language processing modules by appropriately tailored experiments. Moreover, the recording of speech-related potentials and modern techniques of functional brain mapping such as PET-scanning or functional magnetic resonance imaging (FMRI) require a high flexibility in stimulating experimental subjects.

Finally, clinical work may profit considerably from the availability of facilities to construct diversified production and comprehension tasks: in neurophonetics, for instance, patient management can benefit from an 'experimental' approach to remediation, in that it allows therapists to link the construction of efficient training methods with the discovery of a patient's residual speech capacities. The design of computerized motor-learning tasks based on artificial feedback can be of particular relevance in this field.

Several microcomputer-based systems for clinical speech examinations are already commercially available, such as the Computerized Speech Lab (CSL; Kay Elemetrics Corp), the Speech Viewer (IBM), CSpeech (Paul Milenkovic, Madison, WI) or SoundScope (GW Instruments, Inc) (see Read *et al*, 1990, 1992; Ryalls and Baum, 1990; Thomas-Stonell, 1989). Most of these systems have a strong focus on speech signal-processing routines, providing facilities for waveform acquisition and display, editor operations, time- and frequency-domain signal analysis, and even speech synthesis. Barlow, Suing, Grossman, Bodmer and Colbert (1989) have devised a more physiologically oriented software system for the acquisition, display and analysis of electrophysiological, dynamic, kinematic and aerodynamic data, including also some stimulus control functions. As regards the assessment of perceptual processes, a highly specialized system for use in auditory physiology has been developed by Fuzessery, Gumtow and Lane (1991), comprising a variety of hardware filters and a precise clock to generate complex waveforms with a particularly high temporal and frequency resolution. These systems, and many others that have not been mentioned here, supply clinicians with a rich stock of analysis tools.

However, most of the software systems currently available are less powerful as far as the control of task variables in speech and listening experiments is concerned. Therefore, this chapter outlines the field of microcomputer applications in clinical phonetics under the particular aspect of a flexible management of complex stimulus materials and a flexible control of stimulus-response settings. The whole chapter is divided into applications where the experimental subject is a *speaker* and others where he or she is a *listener*. Thus, the chapter covers PC-based approaches towards disorders of phonetic processes in both the production and the comprehension of spoken language, with a particular focus on neurogenic dysfunctions. Most of the paradigms mentioned below have been known long before the age of microcomputers. What is new, however, is that modern technologies allow us to integrate these paradigms into a comprehensive and flexible unit and thereby make them more easily available for clinical purposes.

A General Framework for Neurophonetic Experimentation

Figure 9.1 presents the architecture of a universal system for the design of speech and listening tasks in neurophonetics. The system consists of two structurally similar components, one for speech production tasks ('SPEAKING') and one for auditory perceptual tasks ('LISTENING'). The SPEAKING component includes a chain of processing steps from the generation of stimuli to be spoken to the recording and analysis of the patient's spoken responses. Likewise, the LISTENING component includes consecutive steps from the generation of acoustic stimuli to be perceived to the acquisition and analysis of a listener's responses to these stimuli. The two chains are connected such that the verbal responses of a patient recorded within the SPEAKING component can be fed into a LISTENING experiment for auditory evaluation.

Within the SPEAKING component, verbal responses can be stimulated in different modalities, i.e. by pictured (*naming*), written (*reading*) or spoken stimuli (*repetition*). Vocal responses can further be controlled by visual targets, such as in tracking tasks, or by acoustic signals, such as in synchronization or reaction time tasks. The system's stimulus generator (GEN) allows for the generation and modification of such materials, and for the storage of stimuli in a database (STO). During an experimental or training session, the stored stimuli are selected (SEL)

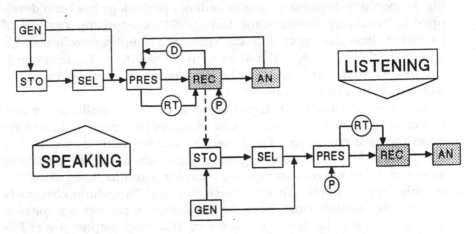

Figure 9.1. A universal architecture of a microcomputer-based system for experimentation, assessment and treatment in neurophonetics.
GEN: Stimulus generation, STO: Stimulus store, SEL: Stimulus selection,
PRES: Stimulus presentation, REC: Response recording, AN: Response analysis,
RT: Reaction time measurement, D: Feedback delay, P: Perturbation

and, following a given experimental protocol, presented to a patient (PRES). The patient's vocal response is recorded by a microphone or, in principle, by any other 'front-end' device (REC). The response delay (reaction time) can be measured (RT) and the response or any parameter derived from it can be fed back to the speaker, with or without a specified delay (D). Further, perturbations such as, for instance, a masking noise can be added during a patient's response (P). Speech recordings can finally be stored and analysed by signal processing methods (AN).

The LISTENING component has a very similar structure: its input consists of acoustic signals, which may either be generated within the system or fed into the system from an external medium (GEN). Again, these stimuli are stored (STO) and, during listening sessions, selected appropriately (SEL) and presented to a listener (PRES). The dashed arrow in Figure 9.1 indicates that the system is particularly designed to make the speech samples resulting from a SPEAKING task available in the LISTENING component, where they can be analysed by auditory methods. The listener's response can be acquired in different ways (REC), e.g. as a manual keypress, a transcript, a rating score, or a vocal utterance, and analysed appropriately (AN). Again, reaction times can be measured. In the case of a spoken response, the circle is closed because the listener acts as a speaker and his or her response can be treated again by the facilities of the SPEAKING component.

This architecture contains a sufficient number of degrees of freedom to realize most of the paradigms that are currently used in clinical and experimental phonetics and in neurolinguistics. The present authors have developed computerized systems that are based on the described architecture. In particular, the PHONX (Phonetic experimentation) system implements a comprehensive sample of experimental paradigms which, taken together, exhaust the components of the model of Figure 9.1. Owing to the history of this research, two further subsystems have been developed, each of them with a focus on a subset of particularly relevant clinical applications:

1.   The TheDiaS (Therapy and Diagnostics of Speech) system is confined to the SPEAKING branch of Figure 9.1 and is particularly specialized for the management of tracking tasks based on microphone, aerometer and pneumograph signals.
2.   The TUS (Testing Unit for Speech Disorders) implements facilities to record and replay speech, with a focus on standard clinical applications such as intelligibility testing, auditory rating scales and syllable repetition tasks.

These systems are implemented on an IBM-compatible PC 486 with a digital signal processor and an AD/DA converter, allowing for a 200 kHz 12-bit sampling on a total of four analogue input channels (for details see Ahrndt and Ziegler, 1993; Ahrndt *et al*, 1993; Finsterwald, 1990; Teiwes *et al*, 1993; Ziegler *et al*, 1994).

The following describes a selection of PHONX, TUS and TheDiaS-applications in the field of neurogenic disorders of the production and perception of spoken language. This overview, although necessarily incomplete, should be considered as an outline of the scope of a micro-computer-based speech assessment and treatment unit.

The SPEAKING component

The SPEAKING component of the system sketched in Figure 9.1 provides users with a number of facilities for the management of stimulus materials and for the control of complex stimulus-response settings. A systematic overview of the task variables that can be handled by this 'toolbox' is given in Table 9.1.

Management of complex stimulus materials

In reading, naming or repetition tasks, materials of a more or less complex variable structure must be presented to the patient, most often in a random order, while in the evaluation the patient's responses have to be re-ordered according to the underlying linguistic or phonetic factors (see columns 1 and 2 of Table 9.1). These requirements typically impose a number of technical problems in paper-and-pencil applications, with the consequence that clinicians often dispense with the most appropriate methods and resort to less adequate substitutes.

The scope of the problem and a possible solution can be illustrated by the computer implementation of the Munich Intelligibility Profile (Ahrndt *et al*, 1993; Ziegler *et al*, 1992). In order to assess a dysarthric patient's intelligibility reliably and in some therapeutically relevant detail, word identification methods based on the rhyme-test principle are generally considered most appropriate. The patient is asked to pronounce words from a phonetically balanced list, and the recorded utterances are later presented to one or more listeners in order to be identified among ensembles of 'similar sounding' alternatives. The target words and the multiple choice alternatives are chosen such that the profile of a listener's misidentifications may serve as a profile of the patient's articulation disorder (Kent *et al*, 1989; Weismer and Martin, 1992; Ziegler *et al*, 1988).

This methodological approach presupposes the use of highly stan-dardized materials, which is at odds with the requirement that the verbal message conveyed by the speaker must be unknown to the listener: if a fixed standard word list were used over and over again in clinical diag-nostics, clinicians would soon run short of listeners who are unfamiliar with the materials. Thus, efforts must be taken to pair the requirement of

Table 9.1. Task variables of the SPEAKING component of a microcomputer-based speech assessment and treatment.

Stimulus type	Structure of materials	Stimulus-response-timing	Feedback condition
— pictures	— linear word-/sentence— lists	*Sequential S-R-order*	*Extrinsic feedback*
— written language	— lists of minimal pairs, triples etc.	**No time requirements**	— knowledge of result
— spoken language	— rhyme test format	— naming, reading, repetition	— real-time biofeedback
— non-verbal acoustic stimuli	— continuous text	— imitation (pitch, rhythm)	*Modified auditory feedback*
— visual targets		**Reaction time (RT) condition**	— noise masking
		— simple RT, choice RT	— delayed auditory feedback
		— pronunciation	
		— implicit priming	
		— rhyme-/verb-generation	
		Continuous stimulation	
		— visuomotor tracking	
		— synchronization	
		— shadowing	

highly structured, standardized linguistic materials with the goal of keeping listeners maximally uncertain about the utterances to be identified.

The Munich Intelligibility Profile is based on word lists where each word is part of an ensemble of 12 'similar-sounding' words, i.e. words that differ from each other in one syllabic position. The phoneme that occupies this position within the target word is the *target phoneme*. The rationale of the test is that the patient has to articulate the target phoneme with sufficient accuracy in order to make the target word identifiable among the 12 alternatives. The target words of the test are grouped according to the phonetic features of the target phonemes, yielding a profile of the most relevant factors contributing to a patient's intelligibility problem (Ziegler *et al*, 1992). Figure 9.2, for instance, contains five contrastive profiles representing the relative contributions of labial, apical and dorsal consonants (left diagram), and of oral versus nasal consonants (right diagram) to these patients' intelligibility deficits. The five individual contours are related to the average MVP-scores of a sample of 120 dysarthric subjects. Subject A demonstrated a marked increase in error scores from front to back with above-average impairments in all places of articulation. In contrast, patient B scored above average only on apical consonants, whereas patient C had most problems with labials and dorsals. A similarly marked dissociation was found between patients D and E as regards the contribution of errors on nasal and oral consonants.

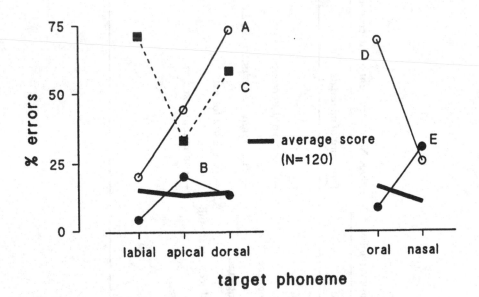

Figure 9.2. Dissociating intelligibility profiles in five dysarthric patients (A–E). Left: Differential affliction of labial, apical and dorsal consonants; Right: different intelligibility profiles due to hypernasal (D) and hyponasal (E) articulation. The bold lines represent average error scores of a group of 120 dysarthric patients.

An analysis of such detail can be achieved only when systematically balanced test lists are used. What can be done to make the test materials sufficiently variable despite the high demands on the structural make-up of the test? The PC-implementation of the Munich Intelligibility Profile contains a large and systematically structured store of stimuli (component STO in Figure 9.1) and various randomization procedures in stimulus selection (component SEL in Figure 9.1), in order to prevent listeners from predicting the target words of the test on the basis of their knowledge of the materials (see Table 9.2). The manipulations of the test materials, which can hardly be realized in a tape-recorder and paper-and-pencil method, increase the sensitivity of the test and prevent listeners from becoming familiar with the materials. They make the test suitable for repeated administration to the same listener and thus applicable as a standard assessment procedure in a clincial setting.

Similar, although less complex problems of handling stimulus lists are also encountered in other kinds of reading tasks, or repetition tasks, especially when paired stimuli, e.g. minimal pairs, are included. As a rule, it is advantageous in such tasks to have a patient produce the speech samples pertaining to different test variables in a randomized order, i.e. to avoid, for instance, the immediate succession of the two cognates of a minimal pair, or to have fillers between the target stimuli of a test. For an evaluation of the recorded utterances, the recordings have

Table 9.2. Randomization procedures in the SPEAKING component of the Munich Intelligibility Profile.

---

1. Parallel Lists
Each test item is represented by four parallel ensembles, which agree in most of the relevant test variables, such as target phoneme, target phoneme position or number of syllables. For each item, the selection among the four parallels is at random. Most of the target words may, in another item, occur as a foil.

2. Dummies
On each administration, 12 'dummies' are selected at random, meaning that each of the foils (from a pool of more than 2700 words) can in principle occur as a target.

3. Permutation
A permutation of the selected target words is performed on each administration, resulting in a randomized word list to be spoken by the patient.

4. Random embedding
Half of the target words are embedded into carrier sentences, with a transition probability of practically 0. To this end, the system stores a set of more than 2000 neutral carriers of differing lengths (between two and seven syllables) and differing positions of the embedding slot (initial, medial, terminal). The embedding respects the variable structure of the test and is balanced with regard to sentence length and embedding position.

---

to be de-randomized in order to obtain a structured view of the results. An interface to perceptual analysis procedures is necessary if the patient's utterances are to be entered into a structured evaluation by auditory rating scales (see the section on Scales) or by word identification procedures (see the section on Identification and discrimination tasks). Relational databases, such as the POET database used in the PHONX system, and object-oriented programming provide an efficient tool to handle complex linguistic materials and to relate a patient's stored responses and their acoustic or perceptual measures to the variable structure of these materials. Thus, any examination protocol, once configurated appropriately by an expert user of PHONX, can easily be administered and evaluated 'out of the box'.

Control of complex stimulus-response formats

While the preceding section was concerned with the structure of stimulus materials to be presented in speech tasks, a still more important aspect of neurophonetic examination is the presentation of stimuli. Microcomputer-based systems allow for a control of stimulus presentation, response acquisition and a precise synchronization of the events that may be relevant in a complex stimulus-response setting (see columns 3 and 4 in Table 9.1). This opens the field for a wide range of experimental and clinical applications.

Reaction time tasks

The general design of tasks that typically use vocal reaction times as one of their dependent variables is illustrated in Figure 9.3. Following this design, an experimental trial may include the presentation of a stimulus, which may or may not be preceded by a facilitating or inhibiting prime. The subject's response can be triggered by the stimulus itself or by a prespecified 'go' signal. At the beginning of each trial, a warning signal can be presented to alert the patient. Each of the events within this chain can be presented either visually (on the computer screen) or acoustically (over headphones), and the patient's response is recorded by a microphone. A subject's performance can be characterized both by the observed reaction time and the acoustic or perceptual quality of the response.

A number of well-known experimental paradigms can be cast into this general form. The most straightforward application is the *simple reaction* paradigm, where a stimulus, i.e. a vocalization, a syllable, a word, or even a sequence of words, is prespecified and must be produced as fast as possible upon presentation of a 'go' signal. In speech research, the simple reaction paradigm has been used extensively in investigations of the mechanism of retrieving a prepared motor program

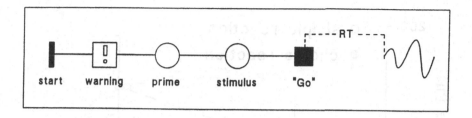

Figure 9.3. General format of a vocal reaction task.

from a hypothesized 'articulatory buffer' (for an overview see Levelt, 1989). A more complex paradigm is *choice reaction*, where two different responses are prespecified, each one being related to a specific 'go' signal. Experimental subjects are required to respond to each of the two 'go' signals by producing the corresponding utterance. Whereas in the simple reaction task the motor response can be programmed in advance, choice reaction times reflect the whole process of programming an utterance and of retrieving and unpacking the motor programs stored in the buffer. The choice reaction paradigm has, for instance, been used by Meyer and Gordon (1985) to study the implementation of phonetic features in the articulation process. Most obviously, it provides an attractive approach to the study of motor programming deficits in anterior aphasics, although it must be conceded that the choice between two reactions involves, beyond motor programming, other processes such as stimulus identification and stimulus-response translation (see Proctor *et al*, 1992), both of which may act as an additional source of response-delay in neurologic patients.

Figure 9.4 presents an application to a patient with apraxia of speech. A simple reaction experiment was designed, which required the subject to produce, in a blocked design, one of the syllables /ba/, /da/ and /ta/ as fast as possible upon presentation of a light square in the centre of the computer screen. Further, two choice reaction experiments were made using the syllable pairs /da, ba/ and /da, ta/, with the requirement that /da/ was to be produced when the square appeared in the upper part of the screen and /ba/ (or /ta/, respectively) was to be pronounced upon appearance of a square in the lower half. The two alternative positions were marked by orthographic labels.

The open circles in Figure 9.4 represent mean values of a total of 48 simple reaction times for each of /da/ and /ba/ (left) and for each of /da/ and /ta/ (right). The filled circles, on the other hand, represent mean values of 48 choice reaction times in the /da, ba/ (left) and the /da, ta/ (right) conditions. The substantially increased RT values in the choice reaction tasks reflect the additional processes that are required in the selection among two alternative articulations as compared with the

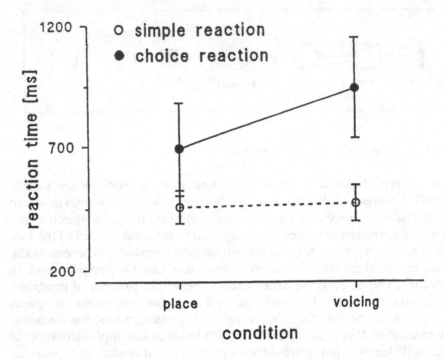

Figure 9.4. Simple (open circles) and choice reaction times (filled circles) for /da/ vs. /ba/ (left) and /da/ vs. /ta/ (right).

recall of a single, prespecified syllable. A comparison with normal subjects shows that this difference by far outweighs the difference one would normally expect, which points to some kind of 'programming' deficit in the examined subject. What is more revealing, however, is that the patient needed significantly more time to select between two voicing cognates than between two place cognates, which might be interpreted to reflect a specific problem of specifying the movement parameters that are relevant in voiced–voiceless distinctions.

Further tasks that fit into the format of Figure 9.3 are, for instance, the 'pronunciation task', where a stimulus is presented orthographically on each trial and the subject is required to pronounce it immediately or with a certain delay (e.g. Savage *et al*, 1990), or 'implicit priming tasks', where a subject responds to a given prompt by producing a learned associate (e.g. Meyer, 1990). Verb- or rhyme-generation tasks, where subjects are required to produce, to a given prompt, an associated verb or a rhyming word, have an equivalent format. Finally, any reading or repetition task may be understood as a special case of the task design depicted in Figure 9.3, although reaction times need not always be an important variable in these cases. In all instances, the input can be non-verbal as well, e.g. in tasks requiring the imitation of pitch using a musical scale or the imitation of the rhythmic pattern of a sequence of tones, and the patient can be required to produce his or her output with a fixed delay, like in the delayed response tasks often used in representational memory research (e.g. Goldman-Rakic, 1987).

The PHONX system disposes of the facilities that are necessary to configurate experiments of this format, to generate visual or acoustic warning signals, and to import and store lists of written or spoken primes and stimuli. RT measurements are supported by the system's speech editor on the basis of sound pressure level computations with adjustable thresholds, which is particularly relevant as traditional 'voice key' measurements of vocal reaction times are strongly influenced by a speaker's loudness, microphone distance or utterance type (e.g. Pechmann *et al*, 1989). The system disposes of an option to store the responses for off-line acoustic or perceptual analyses of their quality.

Continuous stimulation

In the paradigms described so far, speech tasks included stimulus-response cycles with a clear temporal separation of stimulus presentations and the subject's responses. There are a number of applications, however, where stimulation and response overlap in time. Some of these are of particular clinical relevance, as they derive from motor learning paradigms and, therefore, may be used in therapeutic exercises.

Synchronization

A paradigm that has obtained considerable importance in motor theory involves synchronization of a periodic signal by rhythmic movements, usually finger tapping. Part of the theoretical relevance of synchronization tasks lies in the fact that they are based on an interaction of an internal action timer with a perceived external rhythm (e.g. Aschersleben and Prinz, 1992). A further relevant aspect is that pacing signals can be used to examine the rhythmicity of a repetitive movement in close detail (Ivry and Keele, 1989).

In speech, repetitive articulation has frequently been examined by 'syllable repetition tasks', often with an instruction to perform maximally fast. Rhythmic auditory stimulation has been introduced, for instance, to study alternating articulatory movements in Parkinson's disease (e.g. Logigian *et al*, 1991). Although synchronization with the pace of a metronome may have some relevance in therapeutic approaches, there is only scarce scientific underpinning of this method.

Figure 9.5 illustrates the implementation of a synchronization task for clinical and experimental use in the Testing Unit for Speech Disorders (TUS). The system generates tones of adjustable length, loudness, pitch, and harmonic make-up, and with adjustable inter-stimulus intervals. Thus, tonal and rhythmic patterns of variable complexity can be presented to the speaker who is required to synchronize or imitate the signal by a given target syllable, e.g. /da/. As an example, the filled arrows in Figure 9.5 represent a rhythmic synchronization pulse (1500 Hz, 20 ms duration) at regular intervals of 444 ms and 888 ms, used to stimulate a short–long pattern of repetitive /da/-articulations in a patient with cerebellar dysarthria. The patient's response was transformed into a smoothed sound pressure level contour which reflects the rhythmicity of her vocal signal and its phase relation to the synchronization pulse. An adjustable threshold was used to determine syllable onsets from SPL-contours (vertical bars in Figure 9.5) and the relevant synchronization parameters. As the example shows, the patient was considerably variable in this task and appeared unable to anticipate the synchronization pulse at a regular pace, even at this slow rate. The overall period duration of the bisyllabic cycle was shorter than required and the duration of the short syllable relative to the total period was increased.

This program has a broad range of experimental and diagnostic applications and may furthermore be used as a therapeutic tool, providing patients with a rhythmic cue for the realization of multisyllabic utterances. It goes without saying that this unit can also be used to determine maximum syllable repetition rates, an examination which is part of almost all standard assessment protocols for dysarthric speakers.

Visuomotor tracking

Visuomotor tracking tasks are based on the principle that some physical measure reflecting movement performance is fed back visually in real

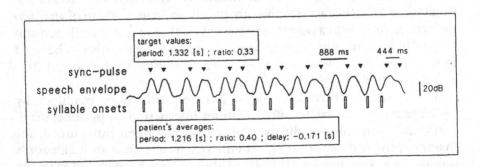

Figure 9.5. Performance of a patient with chronic cerebellar degeneration in a 1.5 Hz synchronization task. The filled triangles represent a 20 ms synchronization pulse, the solid line trace represents the smoothed and rectified speech envelope of the patient's vocal synchronization on /da/. Syllable onsets are marked by vertical bars.

time while a subject tries to match the signal with a static or moving visual target. It has been suggested that visuomotor tracking skills are based on an interplay between feedback processes integrating visual and intrinsic movement information and open-loop feedforward processes for the prediction of future positions of the moving target (Miall *et al*, 1993). As tracking tasks contain, as an essential component, a biofeedback condition, and as biofeedback is supposed to enhance the learning of novel motor skills (Mulder and Hulstijn, 1985), visuomotor tracking has become an important paradigm in motor learning research. As a consequence, tracking tasks have also been used in neurological rehabilitation to train motor functions of the extremities, e.g. the hand (Kriz *et al*, 1995). In speech therapy, too, a number of attempts have been made to utilize the visuomotor tracking paradigm, e.g. for the remediation of dysarthric patients (Barlow and Burton, 1990; McClean *et al*, 1987; Moon *et al*, 1993).

A special case of visuomotor tracking is *aiming*. In this task type, which has been used in studies of arm movements, the stimulus consists of a static visual target that is present during a number of successive trials and has to be hit by single goal-directed movements, e.g. of the arm. In speech, acoustic, aerodynamic, or even articulatory targets can be visualized on a computer screen, requiring a subject to hit the target by producing an appropriate sound, air pressure or articulatory configuration.

Therapeutic applications of tracking and aiming tasks are implemented in several commercial systems, such as the 'match-the-example' tasks of the IBM Speech Viewer or, in a certain sense, the 'feedback mode' operation of the EPG2 electropalatograph (Hardcastle *et al*, 1991), where a 'target' lingual contact pattern is modelled by the therapist and has to be imitated by the patient (see Goldstein *et al*, 1994). An overview of microcomputer-based systems providing biofeedback of speech parameters is contained in Volin (1991).

The TheDiaS system (Finsterwald, 1990) includes visuomotor tracking and aiming tasks based on respitrace, aerometer and acoustic measures, for use in the treatment of dysarthric patients. It offers several tracking functions such as constant or sine wave tracking and different feedback formats and allows therapists to compose tailored training programmes for individual patients. In a recent application of TheDiaS, a motor learning paradigm based on aerometer tracking tasks was used to study tracking skill acquisition in cerebellar patients and in traumatic dysarthrics (Deger, 1994; Deger *et al*, 1994). A therapeutic application of the system focused on respiratory functions is illustrated in Figure 9.6. The figure presents respitrace contours of thoracal and abdominal wall movements in a counting task. The two examples were obtained from a 66-year-old man who had suffered a bilateral brainstem infarction and had, among many other neurological symptoms, a severe dysarthria.

Before treatment

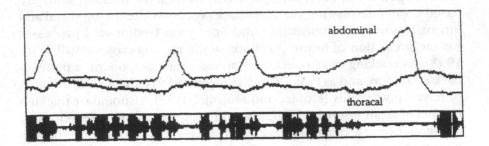

After treatment

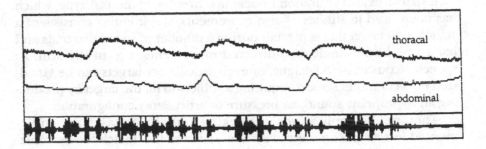

Figure 9.6. Display of abdominal and thoracal wall movements recorded by a strain gauge belt pneumograph during a counting task (10 s section) in a dysarthric patient with a speech breathing impairment. Top: Before feedback therapy. Bottom: After feedback therapy.

The traces in the upper half of the figure were recorded one year after the infarction, showing a marked disco-ordination between thoracal and abdominal movements, with only little thoracal activity and rapid and strong contractions of the abdominal system. Due to his poor respiratory control, the patient was entered into a therapeutic programme based on abdominal movement feedback. As a part of this programme, the patient was required to keep the feedback signal within a predetermined target region during speaking, in order to regain voluntary control over his respiratory system. The task requirements were progressively adapted to the patient's capacities by altering the specifications of the target field. The bottom panel of Figure 9.6 demonstrates the patient's speech breathing pattern after several periods of intensive therapy, showing a considerably improved co-ordination of the thoracal and abdominal wall movements, which was accompanied by a functionally significant increase in communicative skills.

When using a visuomotor tracking approach in the treatment of dysarthric talkers one should keep in mind that skilled motor acts like speaking are only to a minimal extent guided by external feedback and that automatized motor functions may even deteriorate with the utilization of feedback (see Koga, 1989). Moreover, the visual feedback modality is rather artificial in the context of speech motor control. A treatment approach based on visual feedback should therefore be confined to patients who, for their particular problem of gaining volitional access to one or several of the motor components required for speaking, can benefit transitorily from a provision of extrinsic feedback. Further, the treatment protocol should include a gradual fading-out of the feedback condition.

Modification of auditory feedback

In the tracking and aiming tasks described above, visual feedback is used to relate the subject's actual vocal performance to the goal of the task and thereby allow him or her to gain control over relevant vocal functions. Beyond the provision of artificial feedback, manipulations of the natural auditory afferent channel, too, can be clinically useful. There are two familiar methods of modulating a speaker's auditory feedback, i.e. *noise masking* and *delayed auditory feedback (DAF)*. Both of these are represented as separate modules within the SPEAKING branch of Figure 9.1.

Noise masking

Masking a speaker's auditory feedback by a sufficiently loud noise can be used to interrupt one of the afferent channels used during speaking. Auditory masking by a broad-band noise of between 80 and 100 dB causes speakers to involuntarily increase their voice volume ('Lombard effect'). The amount of loudness increase depends on the loudness of the masking noise (Howell, 1990). Further consequences of noise masking may be an increase in vocal pitch and duration and an alteration of the spectral quality of speech (Van Summers *et al*, 1988). Interestingly, these effects are largely uninfluenced by instructions to the speaker, meaning that they can be attributed to a relatively autonomous level of processing (Pick *et al*, 1989). On the other hand, normal speakers can utilize visual feedback to gain control over their vocal volume despite the application of a masking noise (Pick *et al*, 1989). One might speculate that a combination of noise masking and visual feedback can be useful in training patients with neurogenic voice disorder to regain control of their laryngeal musculature, although there is no experience of this kind reported in the literature.

Although auditory feedback is probably not essential in the on-line control of segmental aspects of speech production, speakers seem to monitor their own speech output constantly at various hierarchically ordered levels (Levelt, 1989). By the application of masking noise, a partial interruption of the monitoring of overt speech can be achieved. This may lead to a decrease in the rate to which speech errors are detected and repaired (Lackner and Tuller, 1979). The modification of a speech disordered person's constant awareness of his or her speech output may contain some therapeutic potential. It has for instance been demonstrated that the dysfluencies and self-repairs of stutterers can be influenced positively by noise masking (Postma *et al*, 1991). A similar mechanism can perhaps be expected for anterior as opposed to posterior aphasics, who are supposed to differ in their monitoring behaviour.

The generation of pink or white noise of a selectable sound pressure level during recording is among the facilities of several computer-based systems, such as the CSL. The PHONX system contains an option to use noise masking in any speech task implemented on the system, and a time pattern of alternating silence and noise can easily be programmed. Clinical applications can be imagined in both the assessment of the role of auditory afferent processes and the treatment of vocal control and monitoring deficits in speech disordered patients. PHONX also allows for a feedback modification, which in some sense is opposed to the masking effect, i.e. an amplification (and, as a matter of course, a reduction) of the speaker's own loudness level. A positive loudness gain in auditory feedback is known to lead to an involuntary loudness reduction ('sidetone amplification effect'; Garber *et al*, 1981) which, paired with visual feedback, can again be utilized in the treatment of voice volume control.

Delayed auditory feedback (DAF)

A speaker's auditory afference can also be influenced by feeding back his utterances with a certain delay. Delay intervals between 100 and 500 ms, preferably about 200 ms, result in characteristic alterations of the speech output, such as increased pitch and loudness, decreased rate, dysfluencies and speech errors ('Lee effect'; see Howell and Archer, 1984). Not all speakers are equally susceptible to this effect, and there is an interaction between a speaker's age and sex and the delay time producing maximum interference. Further, subjects differ in their ability to adapt to the DAF condition (for an overview and an explanatory model see MacKay, 1987).

There is considerable theoretical interest in the Lee effect in speech disordered patients of various aetiologies, in particular in stutterers (e.g. Jäncke, 1991). Like noise masking, DAF might also be useful in examining the influence of aphasic patients' awareness of their overt speech on their fluency and error rate. Therapeutic applications of DAF have primarily been suggested for the treatment of stuttering (see Harrington, 1988 for an overview and a discussion), yet there are also reports of a reduction of acceleration and hesitation phenomena in Parkinson's dysarthria by DAF (Downie *et al*, 1981). Pocket-sized, body-worn DAF instruments have been developed to be used as a permanent speech aid by these patient groups (Low and Lindsay, 1979).

PHONX contains an option to use speech delays between 0 and 1000 ms in any of the SPEAKING tasks offered by the system. In order to enhance the Lee effect, the subject's own speech can, in addition to being delayed, also be amplified. The utterances produced under delayed auditory feedback can be recorded, stored and analysed off-line by acoustic or perceptual methods.

LISTENING component

The second branch in the system architecture of Figure 9.1, the LISTEN-ING component, provides facilities for designing auditory-perceptual tasks. In the context of clinical phonetics, this component has two major fields of application, i.e. (1) the assessment of auditory perceptual dysfunctions and (2) the auditory evaluation of disordered speech. Within the former, investigations into aphasic disturbances of the comprehension of spoken language (e.g. Tyler, 1992), studies of phono-logical processing mechanisms (e.g. Praamstra *et al*, 1994), or the assess-ment of peripheral and central disorders of acoustic processing (e.g. Eustache *et al*, 1990) are most relevant. The speech evaluation aspects of the LISTENING component, on the other hand, include auditory assess-ment techniques ranging from simple scaling or transcription methods to more sophisticated experimental approaches.

Identification and discrimination tasks

A standard perceptual task requires subjects to label a stimulus by one of a given set of categories. Most typically, the stimulus is to be identified among two opposing categories like *voiced/unvoiced*, *word/non-word*, *animated/unanimated*, etc. A related, although more basic, task is to decide whether or not two stimuli pertain to the same category ('discrimination'). Both of these paradigms play a fundamental role in experimental perceptual phonetics and in psycholinguistics. In particu-lar, the classical phonetic theory of categorical perception is built on identification and discrimination experiments (see Repp, 1984) and much of the research in auditory word recognition uses these paradigms (e.g. Frauenfelder and Tyler, 1987).

A most straightforward application in clinical phonetics is presented in Figure 9.7. These data illustrate the phonetic and acoustic processing capacities of a patient with apraxia of speech relative to a group of 12 normal listeners. There were two non-phonetic acoustic tasks (left diagram), one requiring subjects to label tones as being higher or lower than a reference tone ('pitch'), the other one requiring subjects to label tone intervals as being longer or shorter than a reference interval ('time'). In each of the two conditions the probes to be matched with the reference stimuli formed a 10-step continuum. Two phonetic tasks (right diagram) required subjects to label stimuli from a /da/ - /ba/ ('place') and a /ba/ - /pa/ continuum ('voicing'), respectively.

The apraxic patient presented a differential pattern of identification errors: in the two non-phonetic tasks he was fairly within normal limits, whereas in consonant identification he was definitely impaired, with a clear preponderance of misidentifications within the voicing dimension. This would support the hypothesis of a specifically phonetic processing disorder with a focus, in this particular case, on the processing of the voicing feature.

The data of Figure 9.7 were obtained using the PHONX system. Whereas the two tonal continua were generated within the system's 'signal-generator' component, the two phonetic continua were imported from an external medium (see Figure 9.1). Experimental details like the duration of inter-stimulus intervals and the number of presentations per stimulus were specified in the 'configuration' compo-

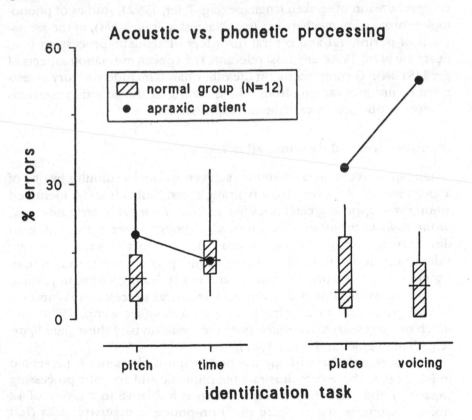

Figure 9.7. Acoustic and phonetic processing skills in a patient with apraxia of speech: identification tasks.

nent of the system. The system also provided the relevant statistics and graphs for the analysis of response errors and reaction times.

The format of this experiment can, with only slight modifications, be used in another important psycholinguistic paradigm, i.e. auditory lexical decision, where listeners are required to decide if a spoken utterance is a word or a non-word. A specific form of this paradigm, which exploits the structure outlined in the model of Figure 9.3, for instance, was used by Praamstra *et al* (1994) in a combined ERP and reaction time study of phonological processing. These authors used rhyming and alliterating prime-target pairs and a comparison between immediate response and delayed response conditions to investigate the extent to which phonological information is used in lexical decision. A similarly sophisticated modification of the lexical decision paradigm was introduced by Zwitserlood (1989), who used a cross-modal priming condition to tap into the temporal course of auditory processing mechanisms. A comprehensive collection of examples illustrating the application of discrimination and identification tasks in aphasic patients is contained in Tyler (1992).

Whereas the examples mentioned so far were focused on auditory processing of normal speech and the disturbances of these mechanisms, identification tasks may also find an application in the assessment of disordered speech by normal listeners. In an earlier experiment, for instance, we used a combination of the gating paradigm with an auditory identification task to measure the extent to which, in apraxic speech, coarticulatory information on an upcoming vowel is already contained in the segments preceding it (Ziegler and von Cramon, 1985). As a further example, we designed a reaction-time identification task to analyse the contrast between tense and lax vowels in the speech of dysarthric and aphasic patients (Ziegler and Hoole, 1989). Following the principles of these studies, identification tasks based on minimal pairs may be considered an appropriate method to assess specific articulatory impairments in various patient groups.

Monitoring tasks

Monitoring tasks differ from identification and discrimination tasks in that subjects are required to respond if, and only if, a prespecified stimulus, e.g. a particular phoneme ('phoneme detection') or word ('word detection'), occurs. The relevant stimuli are usually embedded in larger stretches of speech, like sentences or a piece of text. If the items to be decided on are separate linguistic units (words, sentences) instead of a continuous text, the term 'GO-NOGO' is used to express that a keypress is required only if the critical stimulus is present in a single item. The rate of hits/misses and of false alarms, respectively, and the delay of responses to the target stimuli are used to measure a subject's performance in monitoring or GO-NOGO tasks.

The technical realization of monitoring experiments within the framework of the system sketched in Figure 9.1 is straightforward: What is needed is a facility to replay a stored speech sample and, at the same time, record the subject's manual keypresses. Response delays can be calculated from the response-onset times and the stimulus-related time information, which must be pre-specified for a particular speech sample within the signal editor.

Although the PHONX system provides all these facilities, experiments with neurologic patients have not been performed so far. Potential applications in neurophonetics and neurolinguistics may include the assessment of phonological processing deficits on the basis of phoneme or syllable detection tasks (Tyler, 1992) or error monitoring tasks (e.g. Postma and Kolk, 1992), the examination of auditory comprehension in aphasics by tasks requiring the detection of words of a given semantic category (e.g. Metz-Lutz *et al*, 1992), or the examination of a subject's capacity to utilize prosodic cues for the detection of phonemes in stressed and unstressed syllables (e.g. Cutler 1976). Monitoring tasks are known to be sensitive to sustained attention or vigilance deficits, which makes them a useful component of attention batteries (for an overview, see Zimmermann *et al*, 1993). In neurophonetic and neurolinguistic applications it should be kept in mind, therefore, that a patient's performance may reflect attentional deficits as well as language processing deficits.

Applications in speech technology (Nix *et al*, 1993) suggest that monitoring tasks may also play a role in assessing the quality of disordered speech. Nix *et al* (1993) stressed that listening to synthetic speech may, even in the case of complete intelligibility, place great capacity demands on a listener's processing resources. This difficulty finds an expression in prolonged phoneme detection times when listeners are required to monitor synthetic speech for a given phoneme. There is a very obvious parallel to the processing of dysarthric speech, since listening to a dysarthric talker, even when he or she is completely intelligible, may be a hard task as well. Phoneme monitoring tasks may provide, therefore, a valid measure of the ease of phonetic processing of dysarthric or any other kind of disordered speech.

Scales

In the perceptual tasks described so far, listeners' responses are confined to simple keypresses (monitoring) or two-choice manual responses (identification/discrimination). This response format can easily be extended by allowing for 'scales' of more than two response categories or even for graded responses on a continuous scale-bar. Applications of this type of listening task are manifold. First, a listener may be required to relate a speech sample to one of several categories of a nominal scale, e.g. the consonant of a spoken CV syllable to one of several consonants, the meaning of a spoken word to one of several semantic categories, or the prosody of a spoken sentence to one of several emotions. Not least, the perceptual task of identifying a spoken word among several rhyming alternatives, which is part of the Munich Intelligibility Profile described in the section on Management of complex stimulus materials (pp. 266–270), turns out as a special case of a nominal-scale rating task. Second, a listener's task may also be to rate, on ordinal or interval scales, the extent to which a given feature is present in some speech sample, e.g. the syntactic regularity of a sentence, personality traits of a speaker, or a speaker's age. Most evidently, these facilities can be used for both the examination of patients with perceptual disorders and the auditory evaluation of samples of disturbed speech.

Users of the PHONX system have access to this category of listening tasks. Individual scales and a rating protocol determining the sequential order of the stimuli to be rated and/or the scales to be used can be specified freely by the examiner.

An application, which is part of a standard clinical assessment procedure, is the Munich Dysarthria Scales (MDS). This assessment protocol uses three-point rating scales to obtain auditory-based scores for a number of features of disturbed articulation, voice, and prosody. A list of the variables is presented in Table 9.3. For each variable to be rated, the computer presents between 10 and 20 items spoken by the patient, meaning that the total score obtained for a variable results from a sufficiently large number of elementary judgements. The test items are part of the Munich Intelligibility Profile (see pp. 266–270), which contains sufficiently systematic verbal materials.

The computer implementation of the MDS bears a number of specific advantages:

1. The system selects, for each variable to be rated, only those utterances that are particularly suited for a perceptual judgement of the feature in question. For the judgment of the feature *Place and manner: labial consonants* (see Table 9.3), for instance, only utterances with labial target consonants are presented, which allows listeners to focus their attention on labial articulation.
2. Each utterance to be rated or any part of it can be played back deliberately on command. Thus, listeners can repeatedly make sure of their decision without being obliged to rewind their tape each time.
3. During the rating procedure, listeners have access to any information that may be relevant for them: the utterance is presented orthographically on the screen, the phonemes to be judged (if any) are marked in red, the oscillogram of the patient's utterance

Table 9.3. Variables of the Munich Dysarthria Scales (MDS). Each variable is represented by at least 10 items. Scores: 0 = normal/absent, 1 = mild to moderate, 2 = severe.

Voice	Articulation	Prosody
Voice quality	**Consonant articulation: place and manner**	**Speech rate, rhythm and fluency**
— rough	— labial consonants	— slow rate — increased rate
— breathy	— apical consonants	— pauses
— tense	— dorsal consonants	— scanning speech
Pitch and loudness		— iterations
— high pitch — low pitch	**Consonant articulation: voicing**	**Sentence intonation**
— soft voice — loud voice	— voiced consonants	— monotone pitch/loudness
Vocal stability	— voiceless consonants	
— excessive pitch or loudness variation		
— intermittent devoicing	**Oral-nasal distinction**	
— voice tremor	— hypernasal — hyponasal	

is displayed on the screen, and an extra window contains a description of the scale points to be used. Finally, 'anchor stimuli' illustrating the feature in question by a particularly expressive acoustic reference can be played back on command.

Compared with traditional tape-recorder-based evaluations of disordered speech, computer-supported methods are more economical and probably also more reliable. The fact that anchor stimuli can easily be provided and that listeners may, in the future, have access to voice or articulation databases, adds a new quality to the use of rating scales in clinical diagnostics. Finally, computer-based auditory profiles can easily be supplemented by acoustic measures of syllabic rate, absolute pitch, pitch variation, and so on.

Transcription tasks

In a transcription task, listeners produce written protocols of a speaker's utterances. Again, this task can be used in two different ways: a patient's transcription of normal speech ('writing to dictation') can be used to examine his or her perceptual, comprehension, or writing proficiency, and a normal listener's transcription of a sample of disordered speech can be used to characterize the nature and degree of the speaker's output disorder. In the latter case, expert listeners may use the International Phonetic Alphabet (IPA) or extensions of this alphabet (e.g. extIPA, VoQS; see Duckworth *et al*, 1990; Ball *et al*, 1994) to describe the features of a speech impairment in closer detail.

'Writing to dictation' belongs to the standards of aphasia examinations: The patient is presented a sample of spoken language and is asked to write down what he or she has understood. If orthographically regular and irregular words and non-words are used in a systematic manner, a patient's capacity to use a semantic route or phoneme-to-grapheme conversion rules, respectively, can be examined by this paradigm. This may help to localize a patient's linguistic deficit within a hypothesized language processing model.

Orthographic transcriptions of disordered speech have predominantly been applied in intelligibility assessment. The correct transcription of a disordered patient's utterances selectively presupposes that the listener understands his speech; therefore, the proportion of correctly transcribed words of a standard text is considered a valid (and a reliable) measure of intelligibility (Samar and Metz, 1991). Phonetic transcriptions, on the other hand, play an important role in the analysis of aphasic or apraxic speech (e.g. Kohn, 1993) and of phonological or dyspraxic disorders in children (e.g. Thoonen *et al*, 1994).

The advantage of computer-supported transcription methods is self-evident: the microcomputer has 'direct access' to a stored utterance, allowing transcribers to replay a target utterance or any portion of it several times by a single keypress and thereby to make sure of the adequacy of their transcript. In contrast, the 'sequential access' principle of tape recorders makes repetitive playbacks of taped speech probes considerably harder. Microcomputers can further provide transcription aids, e.g. by acoustic examples illustrating the use of symbols or diacritical markings. Finally, transcripts stored in a computer can easily be evaluated along many dimensions (Long, 1991).

The International Phonetic Association (1989) has agreed on a coding system for IPA symbols, which is intended to serve as a computer-independent basis for creating computer-code translation tables. IPA symbols have already been implemented in PC-based speech analysis systems, such as the CSL, and extensions by extIPA and VoQS alphabets are projected (J. Esling, personal communication). Further, particular PC-based tools such as CLEAR (Baker-Van den Goorbergh, 1990), SALT (Miller and Chapman, 1990), or LIPP (1991) have been developed to support clinicians in structuring the transcription data and help them in analysing errors, creating tables and graphs, and drawing inferences from the numerical results (for a review see Long, 1991).

Conclusions

When considering the use of microcomputers in a clinical environment one should not be too enthusiastic about the potential effect of computerized therapies. In cognitive rehabilitation programmes for brain-injured patients, for instance, there is no clear evidence of a superiority of computer-assisted approaches over more traditional educational training methods (Middleton *et al*, 1991). Thus, for the time being, and as far as neuropsychological rehabilitation in general is concerned it seems more honest to justify the clinical use of microcomputers on practical or on motivational grounds rather than on their therapeutic efficacy.

Nevertheless, in some specialized disciplines a more differentiated view of the situation is in order (see Stachowiak, 1993 for a review). As far as clinical phonetics is concerned there is still an enormous potential in the introduction of microcomputer applications. On the one hand, the growing popularity of instrumental measurement systems makes the microcomputer an indispensable tool in the recording and the analysis of the incoming data. On the other hand, and this was the focus of the present chapter, the use of microcomputers permits clinicians to construct, with little expenditure and within a short time, a great variety of useful tasks and experimental conditions. The fact that microcomputers can be used to record and play back sound at high sampling rates opens to clinicians and clinical researchers a wide field of experimental methods, most of which have thus far been reserved to experimental laboratories. In particular, investigations into the production of spoken language can exploit the capacities of a computer to store complex stimulus databases and to control even most sophisticated stimulus-response chains. The computer integrates a number of specific functionalities into one unit, such as a presentation screen, a recorder, a voice key, a speech delayer, a noise generator, a sound spectrograph, etc, and the processor works as a 'central executive' to bring these different functions into play under a precise time schedule. In listening tasks, traditional tape-recorder applications are severely constrained by the problem that taped stimuli require sequential access. Acoustic stimuli stored on a computer, on the contrary, can be accessed directly, which makes them available for all kinds of controlled presentation. This offers clinicians a great variety of experimental applications, both in the assessment of auditory processing deficits and in the perceptual evaluation of disordered speech, and makes techniques such as monitoring, auditory identification, or 'anchoring' of auditory judgements available for clinical use.

References

Ahrndt T, Ziegler W. Control of vocal intensity: a computer-based system for the assessment and treatment of neurogenic voice disorders. IEEE Engineering in Medicine and Biology Society, 15th Annual International Conference, Proceedings, pp. 1365–66, San Diego, 1993.

Ahrndt T, Ziegler W,Teiwes J. Computer-based auditory analysis of neurogenic speech disorders. IEEE Engineering in Medicine and Biology Society, 15th Annual International Conference, Proceedings, pp. 1363–64, San Diego, 1993.

Aschersleben G, Prinz W. What gets synchronized with what in sensorimotor synchronization? Paper read at the 33rd Annual Convention of the Psychonomic Society, St Louis, MO, November 1992. Working Papers, vol. 13, pp. 1–9. München: Max-Planck-Institute for Psychological Research, 1992.

Baker-Van den Goorbergh L. CLEAR: computerized language-error analysis report. Clinical Linguistics and Phonetics 1990; 4: 285–93.

Ball MJ, Code C, Rahilly J, Hazlett D. Non-segmental aspects of disordered speech: developments in transcription. Clinical Linguistics and Phonetics 1994; 8: 67–83.

Barlow SM, Burton MK. Ramp-and-hold force control in the upper and lower lips: developing new neuromotor assessment applications in traumatically brain injured adults. Journal of Speech and Hearing Research 1990; 33: 660–75.

Barlow SM, Suing G, Grossman A, Bodmer P, Colbert R. A high-speed data acquisition and protocol control system for vocal tract physiology. Journal of Voice 1989; 3: 283–93.

Cutler A. Phoneme-monitoring reaction time as a function of preceding intonation contour. Perception and Psychophysics 1976; 20: 55–60.

Deger K. Sprechmotorisches Lernen mit Feedback. Pfaffenweiler: Centaurus, 1994.

Deger K, Ziegler W, Marquardt C. Airflow tracking in dysarthria. In Aulanko R, Korpijaakko-Huuhka AM. (Eds), Proceedings of the Third Congress of the International Clinical Phonetics and Linguistics Association, vol. 39, pp. 19–26. Helsinki: University of Helsinki, 1994.

Downie AW, Low JM, Lindsay DD. Speech disorder in Parkinsonism; use of delayed

Instrumental Clinical Phonetics

auditory feedback in selected cases. Journal of Neurology, Neurosurgery, and Psychiatry 1981; 44: 852–53.

Duckworth M, Allen G, Hardcastle W, Ball M. Extensions to the International Phonetic Alphabet for the transcription of atypical speech. Clinical Linguistics and Phonetics 1990; 4: 273–80.

Eustache F, Lechevalier B, Viader F, Lambert J. Identification and discrimination disorders in auditory perception: a report on two cases. Neuropsychologia 1990; 28: 257–70.

Finsterwald M. Methoden zur Diagnose und biofeedbackgesteuerten Therapie sprechmotorischer Störungen (Dissertation). München: Universität der Bundeswehr, 1990.

Frauenfelder UH, Tyler LK. The process of spoken word recognition: an introduction. Cognition 1987; 25: 1–20.

Fuzessery ZM, Gumtow RG, Lane R. A microcomputer-controlled system for use in auditory physiology. Journal of Neuroscience Methods 1991; 36: 45–52.

Garber SR, Siegel GM, Pick HL. Regulation of vocal intensity in the presence of feedback filtering and amplification. Journal of Speech and Hearing Research 1981; 24: 104–8.

Goldman-Rakic PS. Development of cortical circuitry and cognitive function. Child Development 1987; 58: 601–22.

Goldstein P, Ziegler W, Vogel M, Hoole P. Combined palatal-lift and EPG-feedback therapy in dysarthria: a case study. Clinical Linguistics and Phonetics 1994; 8: 201–18.

Hardcastle WJ, Gibbon FE, Jones W. Visual display of tongue-palate contact: electropalatography in the assessment and remediation of speech disorders. British Journal of Disorders of Communication 1991; 26: 41–74.

Harrington J. Stuttering, delayed auditory feedback, and linguistic rhythm. Journal of Speech and Hearing Research 1988; 31: 36–47.

Howell P, Changes in voice level caused by several forms of altered feedback in fluent speakers and stutterers. Language and Speech 1990; 33: 325–38.

Howell P. Archer A. Susceptibility to the effects of delayed auditory feedback. Perception and Psychophysics 1984; 36: 296–302.

International Phonetic Association. The IPA 1989 Kiel Convention Workgroup 9 report: Computer coding of IPA symbols and computer representation of individual languages. Journal of the International Phonetic Association 1989; 19: 81–82.

Ivry RB, Keele SW. Timing functions of the cerebellum. Journal of Cognitive Neuroscience 1989; 1: 136–52.

Jäncke L. The 'audio-phonatoric coupling' in stuttering and nonstuttering adults: experimental contributions. In Peters HFM, Hulstijn W, Starkweather CW. (Eds), Speech Motor Control and Stuttering, pp. 171–80. Amsterdam: Elsevier, 1991.

Kent RD, Weismer G, Kent JF, Rosenbek JC. Towards phonetic intelligibility testing in dysarthria. Journal of Speech and Hearing Disorders 1989; 54: 482–99.

Koga S. Acquisition of self-control of a novel muscular activity with EMG and video feedback. Perceptual and Motor Skills 1989; 69: 19–26.

Kohn SE. Segmental disorders in aphasia. In Blanken G, Dittmann J, Grimm H, Marshall JC, Wallesch CW. (Eds), Linguistic Disorders and Pathologie, pp. 197–208. Berlin, New York: W. de Gruyter, 1993.

Kriz G, Hermsdörfer J, Marquardt C, Mai N. Feedback based training of grip force control in patients with brain damage. Archives of Physical Medicine and Rehabilitation 1995; 76: 653–59.

Lackner JR, Tuller BH. Role of efference monitoring in the detection of self-produced speech errors. In Cooper WE, Walker ECT. (Eds), Sentence Processing: Psycholinguistic Studies Presented to Merrill Garrett. Hillsdale, NJ: Lawrence Erlbaum, 1979.

Levelt WJM. Speaking. From Intention to Articulation. Cambridge: MIT Press, 1989.

LIPP. Logical International Phonetics Program. Version 1.40. Miami, FL: Intelligent Hearing Systems, 1991.

Logigian E, Hefter H, Reiners K, Freund HJ. Does tremor pace repetitive voluntary motor behaviour in Parkinson's disease? Annals of Neurology 1991; 30: 172–79.

Long SH. Integrating microcomputer applications into speech and language assessment. Topics in Language Disorders 1991; 11: 1–17.

Low JM, Lindsay DD. A body worn delayed auditory feedback fluency aid for stammerers. Journal of Biomedical Engineering 1979; 1: 235–39.

MacKay DG. The Organization of Perception and Action. A Theory for Language and Other Cognitive Skills. New York: Springer-Verlag, 1987.

McClean MD, Beukelman DR, Yorkston KM. Speech muscle visuomotor tracking in dysarthric and nonimpaired speakers. Journal of Speech and Hearing Research 1987; 30: 276–82.

Metz-Lutz MN, Wioland F, Brock G. A real-time approach to spoken language processing in aphasia. Brain and Language 1992; 43: 565–82.

Meyer AS. The time course of phonological encoding in language production: the encoding of successive syllables of a word. Journal of Memory and Language 1990; 29: 524–45.

Meyer DE, Gordon PC. Speech production: motor programming of phonetic features. Journal of Memory and Language 1985; 24: 3–26.

Miall RC, Weir DJ, Stein JF. Intermittency in human manual tracking. Journal of Motor Behaviour 1993; 25: 53–63.

Middleton DK, Lambert MJ, Seggar LB. Neuropsychological rehabilitation: microcomputer-assisted treatment of brain-injured adults. Perceptual and Motor Skills 1991; 72: 527–30.

Miller JF, Chapman RS. Systematic Analysis of Language Transcripts (SALT) Version 1.3 (MS-DOS) [Computer Program]. Madison, WI: Waisman Center, 1990.

Moon JB, Zebrowski P, Robin DA, Folkins JW. Visuomotor tracking ability in young adult speakers. Journal of Speech and Hearing Research 1993; 36: 672–82.

Mulder T, Hulstijn W. Sensory feedback in the learning of a novel motor task. Journal of Motor Behaviour 1985; 17: 110–28.

Nix AJ, Mehta G, Dye J, Cutler A. Phoneme detection as a tool for comparing perception of natural and synthetic speech. Computer Speech and Language 1993; 7: 211–28.

Pechmann T, Reetz H, Zerbst D. Kritik einer Meßmethode: zur Ungenauigkeit von voice-key Messungen. Sprache und Kognition 1989; 8: 65–71.

Pick HL, Siegel GM, Fox PW, Garber SR, Kearney J. Inhibiting the Lombard effect. Journal of the Acoustical Society of America 1989; 85: 894–900.

Postma A, Kolk H. Error monitoring in people who stutter: evidence against auditory feedback defect theories. Journal of Speech and Hearing Research 1992; 35: 1024–32.

Postma A, Kolk H, Povel DJ. Disfluencies as resulting from covert self-repairs applied to internal speech errors. In Peters HFM, Hulstijn W, Starkweather CW. (Eds), Speech Motor Control and Stuttering, pp. 141–47. Amsterdam: Elsevier, 1991.

Praamstra P, Meyer AS, Levelt WJM. Neurophysiological manifestations of phonological processing — latency variation of a negative ERP component timelocked to phonological mismatch. Journal of Cognitive Neuroscience 1994; 6: 204–19.

Proctor RW, Reeve TG, Van Zandt T. Salient-feature coding in response selection. In Stelmach GE, Requin J. (Eds), Tutorials in Motor Behaviour, vol. II, pp. 727–41. Amsterdam: Elsevier, 1992.

Read C, Buder EH, Kent RD. Speech analysis systems: a survey. Journal of Speech and Hearing Research 1990; 33: 363–74.

Read C, Buder EH, Kent RD. Speech analysis systems: an evaluation. Journal of Speech and Hearing Research 1992; 35: 314–32.

Repp BH. Categorical perception: issues, methods, findings. In Lass NJ. (Ed.), Speech and Language: Advances in Basic Research and Practice, vol. 10. New York: Academic Press, 1984.

Ryalls J, Baum S. Review of three software systems for speech analysis: CSpeech, Bliss, and CSRE. Journal of Speech-Language Pathology and Audiology 1990; 14: 49–52.

Samar VJ, Metz DE. Scaling and transcription measures of intelligibility for populations with disordered speech: where's the beef? Journal of Speech and Hearing Research 1991; 34: 699–702.

Savage GR, Bradley DC, Forster KI. Word frequency and the pronunciation task: the contribution of articulatory fluency. Language and Cognitive Processes 1990; 5: 203–36.

Stachowiak FJ. Micro-computers in the assessment and rehabilitation of brain-damaged patients. Technology and Health Care 1993; 1: 19–43.

Teiwes J, Ziegler W, Ahrndt T. PhonX — a flexible system for experimentation, assessment, and therapy in neurophonetics. IEEE Engineering in Medicine and Biology Society, 15th Annual International Conference, Proceedings, pp. 1367–68. San Diego, 1993.

Thomas-Stonell N. Speechviewer review. Journal of Speech-Language Pathology and Audiology 1989; 13: 59–60.

Thoonen G, Maassen B, Gabreels F, Schreuder R. Feature analysis of singleton consonant errors in developmental verbal dyspraxia (DVD). Journal of Speech and Hearing Research, 1994; 37, 1424–1440.

Tyler LK. Spoken Language Comprehension. An Experimental Approach to Disordered and Normal Processing. Cambridge, MA: MIT Press, 1992.

Van Summers W, Pisoni DB, Bernacki RH, Pedlow RI, Stokes MA. Effects of noise on speech production: acoustic and perceptual analyses. Journal of the Acoustical Society of America 1988; 84: 917–28.

Volin RA. Microcomputer-based systems providing biofeedback of voice and speech production. Topics in Language Disorders 1991; 11: 65–79.

Weismer G, Martin RE. Acoustic and perceptual approaches to the study of intelligibility. In Kent RD. (Ed.), Intelligibility in Speech Disorders, pp. 67–118. Amsterdam: Benjamins, 1992.

Ziegler W, Cramon D. von. Anticipatory coarticulation in a patient with apraxia of speech. Brain and Language 1985; 26: 117–30.

Ziegler W, Hoole P. A combined acoustic and perceptual analysis of the tense-lax opposition in aphasic vowel production. Aphasiology 1989; 3: 449–63.

Ziegler W, Hartmann E. Das Münchner Verständlichkeits-Profil (MVP): Untersuchungen zur Reliabilität und Validität. Der Nervenarzt 1993; 64: 653–58.

Ziegler W, Hartmann E, Cramon D. von. Word identification testing in the diagnostic evaluation of dysarthric speech. Clinical Linguistics and Phonetics 1988; 2: 291–308.

Ziegler W, Hartmann E, Wiesner I. Dysarthriediagnostik mit dem 'Münchner Verständlichkeits-Profil' (MVP) — Konstruktion des Verfahrens und Anwendungen. Der Nervenarzt 1992; 63: 602–8.

Ziegler W, Ahrndt T, Teiwes J. PC-based experimentation, assessment, and treatment in neurophonetics. In Aulanko R, Korpijaakko-Huuhka AM. (Eds), Proceedings of the Third Congress of the International Clinical Linguistics and Phonetics Association, pp. 207–13. Helsinki: University of Helsinki, 1994.

Zimmermann P, North P, Fimm B. Diagnosis of attentional deficits: theoretical considerations and presentation of a test battery. In Stachowiak FJ. (Ed.), Developments in the Assessment and Rehabilitation of Brain-Damaged Patients, pp. 3–15. Tübingen: Narr, 1993.

Zwitserlood P. The locus of the effects of sentential-semantic context in spoken-word processing. Cognition 1989; 32: 25–64.

Index